An Impossible Inheritance

An Impossible Inheritance

POSTCOLONIAL PSYCHIATRY AND
THE WORK OF MEMORY IN
A WEST AFRICAN CLINIC

Katie Kilroy-Marac

UNIVERSITY OF CALIFORNIA PRESS

University of California Press, one of the most distinguished university presses in the United States, enriches lives around the world by advancing scholarship in the humanities, social sciences, and natural sciences. Its activities are supported by the UC Press Foundation and by philanthropic contributions from individuals and institutions. For more information, visit www.ucpress.edu.

University of California Press
Oakland, California

Library of Congress Cataloging-in-Publication Data

Names: Kilroy-Marac, Katie, 1974- author.
Title: An impossible inheritance : postcolonial psychiatry and the work of memory in a West African clinic / Katie Kilroy-Marac.
Description: Oakland, California : University of California Press, [2019] | Includes bibliographical references and index. |
Identifiers: LCCN 2018048200 (print) | LCCN 2018055288 (ebook) | ISBN 9780520971691 (Epub) | ISBN 9780520300187 (cloth : alk. paper) | ISBN 9780520300200 (pbk. : alk. paper)
Subjects: LCSH: Centre psychiatrique du C.H.U.F. de Dakar. | Psychiatric clinics—Senegal—Dakar. | Psychiatry—Senegal—Dakar—History.
Classification: LCC RC451.S62 (ebook) | LCC RC451.S62 K55 2019 (print) | DDC 362.2/109663—dc23
LC record available at https://lccn.loc.gov/2018048200

28   27   26   25   24   23   22   21   20   19
10   9   8   7   6   5   4   3   2   1

To my mom, Kitty Marac
In loving memory of my dad, Walt Marac

CONTENTS

ILLUSTRATIONS

ACKNOWLEDGMENTS

The Wolof word *teranga* signals a special kind of hospitality that overflows with generosity and weaves people together in powerful and enduring ways. I wish first to express gratitude to my dear friends in Senegal and across the diaspora who have, over these past twenty years, invited me into their homes and lives, who have shared with me their laughter and tears, and who have come to call me daughter, sister, tata, and friend. A heartfelt thanks to ñoom Liberté 4 and Usine (now also ñoom Connecticut and New Jersey), to the Hanne and Ly families, and especially to Yaay, Yaayu yaay, Maxu, Emma, Isseu, El Hadj, Mansour, Djibril, Seynabou, Abou, and their wonderful partners and children. Thanks also to Chico, Sylvie, Sidi, Modou, Gnagna, Eric, Jean, Joe Badji, and so many others for your friendship along the way, for patiently explaining to me all of the jokes that I was never quite able to get, and for all of the music and dancing of our younger years.

This project could not have been undertaken without the support of both the former and current director of the Fann Psychiatric Clinic (Service de Psychiatrie—Clinique Moussa Diop), the larger Centre Hospitalier National Universitaire (CHNU) de Fann in which it is located, and the UCAD (l'Université Cheikh Anta Diop de Dakar) Faculté de Medecine (FMPOS) and Faculté des Lettres et Sciences Humaines (FLSH). I owe a deep debt of gratitude to all of the doctors, nurses, medical students, social workers, interns, administrators, and support staff who have so graciously taken the time to talk with me over the years, who have let me tag along to meetings and consultations, and who have patiently answered so many of my questions. I am beyond grateful to the patients and *accompagnants* at Fann who have entrusted me to hold their stories and experiences, hopes and dreams. A special thanks also to the brilliant René Collignon, whose intellectual generosity and kindness helped me find my way. I would like to acknowledge Fann's document center, under the direction of Octavie Ndiaye, for providing a constructive research and writing environment while I was in Dakar, as well as the library at WARA (West African Research Association) and the Archives Nationales du Sénégal (ANS).

Lesley Sharp took me under her wing when I began graduate school at Columbia University, so many years ago. I am incredibly grateful for the unfailing support and encouragement she has offered me over the years. She remains an important intellectual role model to me today, and I am also lucky to call her a friend. Mick Taussig's curiosity for the world—his way of turning things upside down, his playfulness and incisiveness, all at once— likewise made a profound and lasting impression on me during graduate school. I thank him for his brilliant seminars, his living room gatherings, and his High Falls retreats. Brinkley Messick, John Pemberton, Marcia Wright, Lee Baker, Val Daniel, Sherry Ortner, Mahmood Mamdani, Brian Larkin, Paige West, Rosalind Morris, and Ann McClintock also inspired and guided me with their excellent teaching and writing during my time at Columbia. As dissertation committee members, Mamadou Diouf, Marilyn Ivy, and Stefan Andriopoulos were generous readers and interlocutors, offering valuable insights and critical commentary.

Many fantastic colleagues, dear friends, and excellent students—from Colombia University, Sarah Lawrence College, the University of Toronto, and elsewhere—have inspired me and pushed my thinking about this project over the years. Many others have offered their support, advice, and encouragement along the way. A special thanks to Kristen Drybread, Jenny Sime, Richard Kernaghan, Narges Erami, Bob Desjarlais, Mary Porter, Alejandro Paz, Krista Maxwell, Sarah Hillewaert, Michael Lambek, Sandra Bamford, Farzi Hemmasi, Janice Boddy, Jessica Blatt, Knut Graw, Bianca Schreiber, and Dima Saad, all of whom have offered feedback on parts of this book at various stages, or have intervened in other critical (and sometimes magical!) ways. An enormous thanks to Donna Young and Anne Meneley for generously reading an early version of the full book manuscript, and to Amira Mittermaier, who was subjected to multiple manuscript drafts—I am so grateful for our enduring friendship and our ongoing exchange of writing and ideas. I would like also to thank the book's reviewers, Matthew Heaton, Jonathan Sadowsky, and Caroline Melly, for their careful reading and astute feedback, and my editor at University of California Press, Kate Marshall, for her vision and support of this project.

Research for this book was made possible by a number of generous grantors and institutions, including a Scheps Summer Research Travel Grant, a FLAS (Foreign Language / Area Studies) Summer Research Fellowship Award, a Fulbright-Hays DDRA Fellowship Award, a Columbia University Travel Grant, a Zeising Travel Grant from Sarah Lawrence University, and two SSHRC Institutional Grants at the University of Toronto. The finishing touches of the book were completed during a Core Program residency at the Camargo Foundation in Cassis, France; I thank all of these institutions for their support. Parts of the Introduction and "Rupture: Chasing a Ghost" first appeared in "Speaking with Revenants: Haunting and the Ethnographic Enterprise," *Ethnography* 15, no. 2 (2014): 255–76. I thank Sage Publications Ltd. for allowing the modification and reuse of this piece. I am likewise grateful to the Taylor and Francis Group for allowing me to revise "Nostalgic for Modernity: Reflecting on the Early Years of the Fann Psychiatric Clinic in Dakar, Senegal," *African Identities* 11, no. 3 (2013): 367–80, into what would become chapter 3. Finally, parts of my article "Of Shifting Economies and Making Ends Meet: The Changing Role of the *Accompagnant* at the Fann Psychiatric Clinic in Dakar, Senegal," *Culture, Medicine and Psychiatry* 38, no. 3 (2014): 427–47, have made it into chapters 2 and 5; I thank Springer Nature for allowing their revision and reproduction.

My deepest gratitude goes to my mother, Kathleen (Kitty) Kilroy Marac and my late father, Walter Marac, for their unfailing support, encouragement, and love. The story of my adoption and my becoming-family, which they told me from the time I was little and which quickly became family lore, was one of my very first lessons against biological determinism, and in favor of an understanding of family that extends far beyond the confines of biological kinship. This might have been what drove me to study anthropology in the first place. Finally: to Tod, Odin, and Fiona Levi. How lucky I am to share this life with you, to laugh and learn and play and see the world with you! You are my home. Thank you for seeing me through the writing of this book, and thank you for the inspiration, love, and kindness that you bring to each and every day.

A note on names: As is the convention in anthropological writing, I have used pseudonyms for my interlocutors throughout the book to protect their privacy. An exception to this is Demba, whose true name I have chosen to give posthumously, both to properly credit his writing and artwork and to honor his memory. Admittedly, there exists an awkward tension in the book; many of the Fann doctors I refer to pseudonymously have also authored articles cited in this text. While this book owes everything to the people who contributed to its production, I alone am responsible for any errors of fact or omissions.

———

Entanglements

The individual can be said to be "tangled up in stories" which
happen to him before any story is recounted.

—PAUL RICOEUR,
"Life in Quest of Narrative"

DEMBA VIVIDLY REMEMBERS THE FIRST TIME he was brought to the
Fann Psychiatric Clinic, in the early 1970s. Over the course of many months
he told me different parts of the story, mostly in French but peppered in
Wolof, which I eventually put together and read back to him, hoping to get
it all right.

*Heavy traffic, scorching sun. An old green car—old, even then—lurches
toward the city. Inside of it sit two men. They are brothers, same mother and same
father. Elder brother is driving. The window next to him is rolled down even
though black exhaust and deafening noise are pouring into the car; it is much too
hot to keep the window up. His head buzzes. He is frustrated by the traffic. He can
feel his heart beating hard in his chest. He wishes he could drive faster, but he
cannot.*

*Younger brother is laid out on his stomach in the back seat. He is positioned
awkwardly, uncomfortably. His legs are bound, his knees are bent, and his arms
are tied behind his back. The right side of his face is pressed into the worn plush
of the seat. Younger brother cannot move. He howls.*

*Elder brother ignores younger brother and his howling for as long as he can,
and then finally turns back to scream at him. Elder brother curses and hits him
hard. Younger brother continues to howl. All the way into the city, their noise fills
the car and pours out the windows, mingling with the sounds of the busy road.*

*Finally, they reach their destination. Elder brother pulls up to the front steps
of the whitewashed building. He quickly parks the car, gets out, and runs
panting inside. A few seconds later he returns with doctors, nurses, and a social
worker in tow.*

*"Dafa dof, bilâhi! He is crazy, I swear on god's name. I cannot do anything
for him. He cannot stay with us any longer." Elder brother is saying this as the*

group scrambles down the steps to remove the howling man from his agony. Perhaps elder brother is already feeling a wave of relief that this terrible burden will now belong to someone else.

"Untie him NOW!" booms a man's voice. All move to untie younger brother, and they somehow manage to pull him out of the back of the car. He is still folded upon himself and howling. He is hot and sick. The doctor leans down and speaks firmly in French. He grabs the man by the arms and pulls him up. "Stand up! Quiet. Be quiet. Calm yourself. Stand up."

Younger brother stands up and looks at the man. That was the first time he, Demba, saw Dr. Henri Collomb.

But it is not as though Demba has been at Fann ever since. Fann is not a long-term hospital. It is not an asylum or a prison. There are no cells, no bars on the windows, no locks on the doors. Patients feeling well enough are free to walk around clinic grounds; many come and go as they wish. The boundary between inside and outside is monitored but never patrolled. Through the building's multiple exits there is a fairly constant in-and-out flow of people, cats, and birds.

According to one psychiatrist at Fann, the clinic's main priority is to restore patients to what he referred to as "baseline mental health"; in other words, to restore their ability to function normally. For most patients, he says, this seems to take about a month, or maybe a bit longer. The nurses agree that this is all many need. Often, when the nurses are asked what is wrong with one of the patients, they say, "Oh, she's not sick, she's just tired. She will be better in no time, *inchallah* (God willing)." Most patients are admitted, stay a spell, leave, and never return.

Some patients, though, are admitted over and over again, at regular or irregular intervals. There are also patients who come back on their own. Sometimes they return for treatment or medication; sometimes simply to visit, check in with doctors or nurses, watch TV, or to look for odd jobs they might do around the clinic to make a little money. Some even stay a while, temporarily claiming unused rooms as their own and going about their business. *Les anciens* (the elders, the old-timers), as people call them, know and understand the place, although doctors and nurses sometimes complain that they are meddlesome and cause trouble.

Demba is one of these folks, one of *les anciens*. This man I have come to call Demba, whose real name is Magatte Ndiaye, has been a regular at Fann, coming and going, longer than any of the other patients, longer even than the doctors currently working at the clinic. When he comes around, he stays in room number 4 *rez-de-chaussée droite* (first floor, right corridor) and refers to it as his own. He even has his own key.

. . .

The Fann Psychiatric Clinic (*Service de Psychiatrie—Clinique Moussa Diop*) in Dakar, Senegal, is one of a number of specialized medical facilities that make up the *Centre Hospitalier National Universitaire (CHNU) de Fann*, a large teaching hospital that provides clinical instruction to medical students affiliated with the adjacent Cheikh Anta Diop University. The neighborhoods adjacent to Fann, now officially joined together as the *commune d'arrondissement* de Fann / Point E / Amitié, have historically been among the wealthier residential areas of Dakar. Since the 1950s and 1960s, they have been considered *scolarisés* (educated) neighborhoods, quiet and calm compared to the nearby "popular" neighborhoods of Medina, Yoff, and Grand Dakar. Back then, the area was also home to many *tubaabs* (white foreigners, especially French expatriates) and NGOs, although in recent years, as the urban landscape in Dakar has shifted away from the downtown area and toward a nearby coastal area called *Les Almadies*, the prestige of this area has also waned. Alongside the psychiatric clinic, the CHNU compound is also home to a drop-in consultation center, a dental clinic, an HIV / AIDS clinic, a center for infectious diseases, a tuberculosis service, a neurology clinic, and several other services. Together with *l'Hôpital Aristide Le Dantec* and *l'Hôpital Principal* in Dakar, the CHNU complex is among the most important medical facilities in the country, offering medical services to tens of thousands of people each year.

The psychiatric clinic itself is a building shaped like a fat letter H, located near the northwest wall of the compound and not far from *Ker Xaleyi* (the "Children's House," a children's psychology center), a new (as of 2015) addictions clinic, and the morgue. Years ago, during my first research stays at Fann, the psychiatric clinic's weathered façade was cracked and crumbling, discolored to a dirty beige, and a handful of trees and small shrubs grew hesitantly in the sandy earth around the building. At that time, the most remarkable features of the building's exterior were two small murals that had been painted by Demba. Visible to all who approached the clinic, they pictured horses, calabashes, a distant desert oasis, and veiled women with minarets

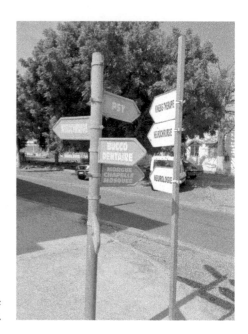

FIGURE 1. Signage inside the
CHNU compound (2013).

and towers rising up out of a mythical city. Since then, however, Fann's exterior has been resurfaced; the building is now much brighter than it was before, and all signs of Demba's mural have been erased.

A plaque above the clinic's main entrance, which is located at the bottom center of the H's crossbar, reads *Clinique Moussa Diop,* thus bearing the name of a promising young psychiatrist who was to become the first Senegalese director of the unit, but who passed away before this could take place. His untimely (and according to some, mysterious) death in 1967 sent shockwaves through the clinic. Many people who were affiliated with Fann back then remember the event in terms of the impact it had on the clinic's future, a story that I shall tell later in the book.

The clinic's main entrance leads into a small foyer, then to a hallway that runs left to right. To the left is a triage and consultation room where nurses convene, then an archive center and a doctor's office. Across the hallway is the social workers' office, next to which is located the director's office, his secretary's antechamber, and the waiting room. The hallway to the right of the entrance is lined with offices occupied by doctors, a therapist, a clinical psychologist, and his secretary. The left leg of the H is the *Division Sud*; it

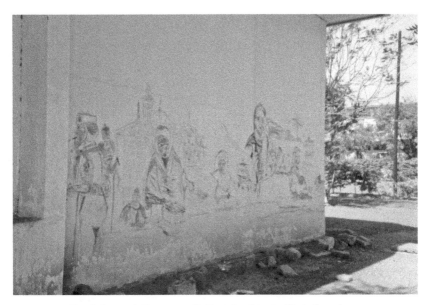

FIGURE 2. Demba's mural. Exterior wall, Fann Psychiatric Clinic (2003).

used to be called the *Pavillon des Dames*. The right leg, which is the only part of the building that is two stories high, is separated into four divisions: the *Rez-de-Chaussée Gauche* and *Droite* (first floor left and right) and *l'Étage Gauche* and *Droit* (second floor left and right). *L'Étage Droit*, which had been closed since the 1990s due to budgetary constraints, disintegrating conditions, and a shortage of personnel, was reopened in 2014. Two small external buildings were also added a few years before that. Each division is monitored by its own team of nurses and headed by a psychiatrist, who also teaches at the university and oversees a cohort of medical students. Fann currently has the capacity to take in 50–60 inpatients at a time, although many more are seen on an outpatient basis. In 2012, for instance, Fann records showed that between 300 and 400 outpatient consultations were performed at the clinic each month.

At first glance, it might be difficult to guess that the institution's rich and remarkable history made it the subject of both local intrigue and international renown during the 1960s and 1970s. The clinic was established in 1956, just four years before Senegalese independence, and a French military doctor by the name of Henri Collomb was named director in 1959. Over the next

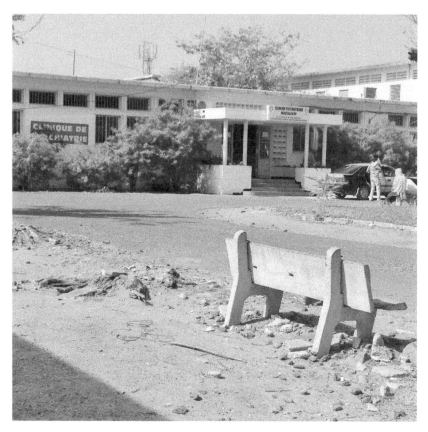

FIGURE 3. Entrance, Fann Psychiatric Clinic (2015).

two decades, Collomb and his (mostly European) colleagues at Fann channeled their energy and resources into anthropological research, clinical practice, and theoretical inquiry. They also trained the first generation of
Senegalese psychiatrists. *L'Ecole de Fann*, or the Fann School, as the group
came to be called, not only positioned itself as a departure from colonial
psychiatry, it also challenged conventional Western psychiatric and psychoanalytic models by attempting to establish a truly transcultural psychodynamic psychiatry that would, among other things, bring local ideas about
madness and therapy into conversation with Western approaches.

Taking the concept of culture—and "African culture" in particular—as
their point of departure, Collomb and the Fann School studied traditional
(mostly Wolof and Lebu, but also Serer[1]) healing customs as well as daily life
in Senegal with the goal of creating a more effective psychiatric practice at

Fann. Importantly, the group's focus on African culture privileged some forms and traditions over others—Negritude ideas and values, for example, were emphasized over the centuries-old impact of Islam on West African life.[2] The group's ethnographic and ethnological research, which still stands as a significant contribution to the fields of anthropology and transcultural psychiatry, inspired a reassessment of both the physical space of the clinic and the model of patient care offered at Fann. For all of this, Fann was touted as an exemplary institution of the nascent Senegalese state by Léopold Sedar Senghor, who served as Senegal's first president from 1960–80.

As the first generation of Senegalese psychiatrists replaced Collomb and his European colleagues during the late 1970s, however, things began to change at Fann. The new generation of Fann doctors distanced themselves not only from the brand of transcultural psychiatry that had been established as its trademark, but also from the question of "culture" more generally. As members of this group relayed to me in interviews conducted in the early 2000s, Collomb's departure and the *sénégalisation* of the clinic was quite a long time coming. Many experienced Collomb's extended presence as stifling, a few even framed their relationship with him in Oedipal terms. Others were more ambivalent about his departure. Across the board, however, this new generation began to put distance between Collomb's culture project and their own orientation. In contradistinction, the young doctors took as their point of departure the universality of the human psyche as well as the universal applicability of psychiatric medicine. Collomb's heirs were as wary of his collaboration with local healers and healing traditions as they were reluctant to engage with the cross-cultural research that had been produced by the Fann School.

With its focus on Collomb's distinctive project in transcultural psychiatry and the eventual disavowal of such project, this book tells a story of postcolonial transformation, both within the realm of psychiatry and in the Senegalese state more broadly. As I investigate the shifting place of "culture" within Senegalese psychiatry, I also seek out the afterlives of Fann's contested past that linger in the present-day clinic. Here I take haunting—and the work of memory more broadly—as a key analytic device. At another level, I consider the institution as a powerful lens through which the late colonial and postcolonial Senegalese state has been reflected and refracted over the last six decades. By paying special attention to how stories about the past and present-day clinic are made to speak to larger narratives of postcolonial and neoliberal transformation and vice versa, this book examines the complex relationship between memory, history, and power—both within the institution and beyond.

Since its very beginnings, the Fann Psychiatric Clinic has existed as a border zone of sorts. It has been, and continues to be, a space of constant and ongoing contact, friction, mediation, and entanglement—between the colonial and the postcolonial, between local exegeses of mental distress and Western psychiatry, between madness and its other, and between the multiple affective, cosmological, therapeutic, and temporal orientations of those who inhabit it. It is also a place in which "culture," and cultural difference in particular, has been alternately acknowledged, misrecognized, and refused. On the one hand, I endeavor to write a history of this extraordinary place that might also stand as a history of postcolonial Senegalese psychiatry and its relation to the Senegalese state. On the other, I resolutely insist upon the unsettledness and uncontainability of Fann's past, which itself stands as a central thematic of the book. In some ways, then, the objectives I have set for this book are irreconcilable in their contradiction. These dual motivations work against each other throughout the following chapters; they constitute a tension that I have chosen, in the end, to accentuate rather than resolve. In the pages that follow, I gather up "multiple [and oftentimes unassimilable] strands of remembrance" (Bissell 2005: 16) and imagination in order to produce a coherent historical narrative of Fann that I also, at the same time, will work to unsettle and disrupt. My efforts to tell (while also untelling) such a story and to grapple with ghosts find their form within ethnography, which, poised as it is "between powerful systems of meaning" (Clifford 1986: 2), has its own special affinity for border zones and in-between places.

ETHNOGRAPHY AND / AS HISTORY

I build this book upon historical research and my own ethnographic engagement with the Fann Psychiatric Clinic that has spanned nearly twenty years and multiple visits (though with some substantial gaps as well, as I note below). What this means is not only that this work brings together perspectives that are at once historical and ethnographic, but that much of my own early ethnographic material that I draw on here has, in its own way, become history.[3] The social, economic, and infrastructural transformations that have taken place in Dakar over the past two decades have made the city a very different place than it was at that time. Fann has changed a great deal, and the clinic's past has been continually reconfigured in response. Over the years, several of my key interlocutors—the Senegalese doctors, nurses, translators, healers, and past patients who worked at or frequented Fann during the 1960s and 1970s and with whom I held numerous interviews between 2001 and 2003—have passed away. I have also changed, of course, as have my friends and surrogate families in Dakar, many of whom I have known since the very first year I spent in Senegal, as a university exchange student, during the mid-1990s. In his preface to *Behold the Black Caiman: A Chronicle of Ayoreo Life*, Lucas Bessire (2014: xii) notes that he and his ethnographic project "have grown up together." In a very real sense, I feel the same way about my own project and this book.

During my first extended stay in Senegal as an exchange student from 1995–96, I split my time between my host family in Dakar and the northern Senegalese city of St-Louis, where I attended the Université Gaston Berger St-Louis. I became interested in local conceptions of health, illness, and healing, and I spent part of that year volunteering in the maternity ward in *l'Hôpital de St-Louis* and working as a surveyor for the INSERM (*Institut national de la santé et de la recherche médicale*) study of maternal morbidity and mortality in West Africa. I also conducted ethnographic research related to cooperative indigenous and biomedical health care efforts at ENDA Santé tiers-monde in Dakar and at the Malango Center (officially named the *Centre Expérimental de Médecine Traditionnelle*, or CEMETRA) in Fatick.[4] This project fueled my desire to embark upon PhD work that would allow me to further investigate the relationship between local or "traditional" forms of healing and Western medical practices in Senegal, especially psychiatric medicine. How, I wondered, did these different healing systems (and the vastly different metaphysical orientations from which they arise) coexist in the present?

Historically, how and when did the French colonial regime begin to include psychiatry as part of its larger colonizing project, and how have biomedical models attempted to suppress, supplant, or co-opt local forms of healing? How do contemporary Senegalese psychiatrists view these "traditional" forms of healing, and how do doctors as well as patients negotiate multiple—and oftentimes competing—therapeutic possibilities? It was with these questions in mind that I entered Columbia University's PhD anthropology program in the late 1990s.

My ethnographic engagement with Fann began during the summer of 1999. I spent much of my time that summer in the *Pavillon des Dames,* or women's wing, of the clinic, which supported eight or nine women at a time.

Since 1972, inpatients at Fann have been required to have a family member or close friend—an *accompagnant*—stay with them for the duration of their hospitalization, so their *accompagnants* were also present. I attended weekly *pénc* sessions, or town hall–type meetings that function as group therapy sessions, in which clinic staff, patients, family members, and guests were encouraged to participate. I was also allowed into Fann's small but rich document center and given access to patient files.

That summer, against a backdrop of rolling blackouts, water shortages, and the widespread rumors of government corruption that marked the end of Abdou Diouf's nearly twenty-year presidency (1981–2000), many Fann doctors I spoke with fantasized about leaving Senegal to work elsewhere, and nurses peddled purses and other goods within the clinic to supplement their paltry incomes. The heavy-handed structural adjustment policies put into place in Senegal during the 1980s and 1990s had a profound effect on the clinic. Doctors and staff alike complained that they were overworked, undercompensated, and demoralized. The institution's infrastructure was crumbling and resources were difficult to come by. In terms of therapeutic strategies, the clinic leaned heavily on pharmaceutical treatment regimes, despite oftentimes prohibitive medication costs and chronic shortages.

During my next extended fieldwork stay at Fann, which stretched from December 2001 until March 2003, I continued to observe the daily routines of the clinic and participate in the activities that took place there. I conducted many informal interviews and a total of sixty-three formal interviews with doctors, nurses, social workers, and other support staff currently working at Fann, as well as retired doctors, staff members, and past patients. Doctors and staff continued to be consumed with the difficulties and demands of their day-to-day occupations at the clinic, where they had to deal with shortages and constraints at every turn. They were also still concerned with what the future would bring, both in terms of the clinic and in their own lives, although many saw a glimmer of hope in the fact that the former opposition leader, President Abdoulaye Wade, had been elected as Senegal's third president in 2000 under the battle cry of "*Sopi!*" (Wolof: change).[5] The clinic, too, was under its third directorship by this time, a transition that had inspired optimism in a portion of its doctors and staff. In the meantime, still lacking the resources necessary for them to do their jobs, those working at Fann had to make do with what they had, thereby exhibiting the same degree of creative bricolage in their practice that so many other Dakarois exhibited in their daily lives. Their approach to the past was equally creative and strategic during this period, a point to which I shall return later in the book.

The city of Dakar changed dramatically during Abdoulaye Wade's two terms as president (2000–12) and continues to transform under Macky Sall, who became Senegal's fourth president in 2012 after wide-scale popular protest against Wade's reelection bid. Wade's government prioritized infrastructural development over social service provision in its march toward modernization, and in an effort to attract more foreign investment. This was most visible in the massive road and port construction projects undertaken during his presidency. Many residents of Dakar saw evidence of the rising prosperity of a select few when they looked to the new shopping and entertainment facilities constructed along the Corniche around 2010, but for most Dakarois, these were distinctly out of reach. Indeed, one of the most startling changes I noted when I was finally able to return to Dakar in 2013 were the ways in which new wealth, prosperity, and status were put on display, as a matter of distinction. Often in very close proximity to the increasingly desperate living conditions of others, the wealth of the few who had prospered (either at home, or much more likely, abroad) during Senegal's neoliberal turn was upheld by the state as sign of the nation's progress—as a possibility available to all citizens. For those struggling to make ends meet, however, such displays did little more than affirm the disjuncture between the prosperity of others and the precarity of their own lives. Although many continue to count on Macky Sall to ensure a more equitable future for the people of Senegal, others insist that his pedigree—as well as his pro-capitalist, neoliberal stance—can only mean more of the same. During my research stay in Senegal in March 2017, I observed public favor turn against him when Dakar's popular mayor, Khalifa Sall (no relation to the president), and his entourage were imprisoned for embezzlement. Amidst widespread protests and sit-ins, many Dakarois insisted that the action was ordered by Macky Sall, and that it was politically motivated. The president, people told me, was troubled by the mayor's rising popularity and bold style, and feared that he might enter the presidential race in 2019.

The long gap between my earlier fieldwork stays at Fann and my subsequent returns presented a dramatic picture of how things had changed within the clinic. As with greater Dakar, new distinctions of wealth and status had cropped up within the Fann Psychiatric Clinic during the same period. In the mid-2000s, Fann had begun to offer a new "VIP" level of patient accommodation. This move generated much-needed revenue for the clinic, but it also institutionalized new distinctions of status and hierarchy.

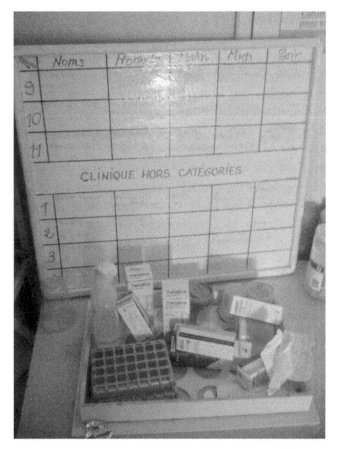

FIGURE 4. Medication timetable and patient medications. Nurses' station, Fann Psychiatric Clinic (2013).

During the three research visits I made to Fann between 2013 and 2017, I saw how the informal economy operating at Fann became even more visible—and indeed, enterprising—than it had been during my first fieldwork stays. For many people searching for work in and around Dakar, the gaps created by personnel shortages and material insufficiencies at Fann provided an opening—informal and unstable, but the possibility of work nevertheless—within the clinic. It is not an exaggeration to say that doctors, nurses, and social workers depend on this informal support staff in order to do their jobs; their presence at Fann fills a critical gap.

When asked about Collomb or the Fann School, most current Fann doctors and staff offer vague praise for the group's innovative approach to psychiatry while also making clear that the group's insistence upon culture is simply less relevant today than it was back then. Current doctors and staff are quick to name the practices that have endured at Fann since Collomb's time—*pénc* (group therapy) meetings still take place and patients still have *accompagnants* stay with them for the duration of their hospitalization, although both practices have changed over the years. Art therapy was also resurrected several years ago. However, as they continue to stress the universal basis to mental illness, downplay psychodynamic approaches, and lean heavily on pharmaceutical strategies for treatment, culture is seen to be important only insofar as it supplies the patient with a language of affliction and provides clues about the "really real" condition that exists underneath or behind it; here, "culture" must be translated into the universal language of psychiatry before it can be properly treated and cured.[6]

· · ·

Here is what Demba remembers of his first day at Fann:

Food to eat. Injection to sleep. The morning after Demba's arrival, a young nurse escorts him to Collomb's office. Collomb is still making his rounds, so Demba is told to sit down in a small, empty waiting room. Even though all of the chairs are identical, he selects his seat carefully and sits on its edge. He folds his hands in his lap and looks at the wall of green metallic filing drawers in front of him. He does not try to make out what is written on their labels. He hums softly under his breath.

Enter Collomb. Demba jumps up and wipes the palms of his hands on his pants. Collomb smiles at him and shakes his hand, tells Demba he hopes he has slept in peace. He motions for Demba to come with him, and Demba follows him from the waiting room into his office. Collomb shuts the door behind him and motions for Demba to take a seat. They sit facing each other, Collomb's desk between them.

Collomb leans forward and says, "Demba, I think you should stay here with us for a while. You will be comfortable here, and I think we will be able to help you."

Demba gets angry. His hands are squeezed into fists and his face is tense. "You see me and you think I am crazy, but I am not. If you think you can cure me, you are wrong. You do not know what my problem is. You are just as crazy as I am." He stands up again.

Collomb is not the slightest bit fazed. He remains entirely composed. He stays seated. "Why do you say that? What do you mean?" His voice is gentle, but it fills the office just the same; it seizes Demba.

Demba pauses and looks around, says nothing.

"What did you say then, Demba?" I ask him. I am impatient to hear the rest of this story. This much has already taken me months to piece together. I am well aware that he could be done talking to me for the day, or that he might prefer to talk to me all afternoon, but about something else. I am equally aware that the next time I ask him to tell me this part of the story, it could be completely different, or he will tell me that I got it all wrong and become angry with me for wasting his time.

We are sitting on a broken concrete bench in the courtyard behind Fann. It is morning, and there is a brownish tint to the hazy sky. The air is gritty, almost palpable. I look over at Demba again, who is sitting cross-legged on the bench, holding on to a pile of notebooks and folders in his lap. His eyesight has deteriorated these last couple of years, he says; his vision is foggy. I wonder what he sees. His old glasses don't work at all, so he doesn't bother using them anymore. He wears a black and white knit hat on his head, "to keep the wind out of his ears," as he says, and he is clothed in his standard fashion: a dark green army jacket over an old T-shirt, black *bubu* pants rolled to the knee, and blue flip-flops on his feet.

I try him again. "Then what happened, Demba? Then what did you say to Collomb?"

Demba blinks. He looks back at me and crinkles his face into a grin. His few remaining teeth are brown, decaying, jagged.

"I said, give me a cigarette! Then I will smoke and we will talk." He glances down at the pack of Marlboro Reds in my bag. He knows to look for them there; he has already smoked several since we sat down together.

I hand Demba the pack. Chuckling, he reaches for them. He takes two, sticks one behind his ear, and bites the filter off of the other. With a loud *thwwwp*, he spits it out onto the ground in front of us, lights the cigarette, inhales, and starts back in on his story:

Demba says nothing as he lights the cigarette that is handed to him by Collomb. He sits down again.

"My brothers are jealous of me—they have always been jealous." Demba starts, his voice quivering and resonating in Collomb's office. "We are like lions with each other. In primary school one of the teachers told me I was very smart and encouraged me to continue with my studies. They hated me for that. I went away with the priests for secondary school. That was the first reason. Later, my father took me aside and told me that I was his heir—that I was the eldest in his eyes even though I was actually his fourth-born son. I was his chosen one. He

confided in me his secrets, the family secrets. This caused a terrible conflict between my brothers and me. They made my life hell. After my father's death it got even worse. We used to fight with our fists after that. I left the house then to be on my own. I was working with wood. But I got in some trouble; I got a few women pregnant. A little funny business, you know. That brought me big problems. Someone put a spell on me [m'a marabouté], tried to attack me. I don't know who it was. Maybe one of the women's sisters, maybe an aunt. I got really sick after that. I had to quit my job and go back to the house, to where my brothers are. I have children, you know. Everyone calls me impotent, but I am not impotent! I have children! I am not married but I have children. When I went back to the house, well that is when things got really bad. They didn't try to help me. Instead, they said that I was crazy and locked me up. My oldest brother hates me the most. He tied me to the tree and hit me with a stick. And then he was talking to my brothers—I heard him talking to them in the courtyard. 'We are going to take him to Fann,' he said. 'He is too crazy to stay here with us, and he is too crazy to be out wandering around.'"

Demba talks and talks to Collomb. He talks about spirits [tuur, rab, djinné] and witches [dëmm] and invisible worlds. He talks about philosophy, about Senegal, about life in general. After many hours of attentive listening, Collomb leans forward to close the distance between them, and says, "You, Demba—you are my friend. You are going to stay here with me for a while. You are sick, but you are not crazy. You have many ideas. Because you have worked with wood and say you are good with your hands, I am going to give you some paper and some watercolors and you are going to see what you can do with them. You are a philosopher, Demba. Put your thoughts and ideas on paper. Everything that is in your head—draw it, write it, paint it."

Demba looks down at the notebooks and papers he had been holding in his lap. Tears collect in the corners of his eyes. "That was when I started to paint, to write, to be an artist. It was all because of Collomb. His family did not know him at all, you know. He was here in Senegal all alone. His family was far away. He was not here with his wife. He had a daughter, but even his daughter did not know him. He rarely saw her. He did not have a son of his own. I was like a son to Collomb, ask anyone! I could walk into his office at any time. I was the first to see Collomb in the morning and the last to see him when he left the clinic each night. He was always here. As he was leaving, he would say, 'Now guard the place for me, Demba.' And I would walk him to his car, and he would give me a few *sous* for coffee the next morning."

Demba pauses and looks back up at me. He sits up straight, puffs his chest out a little. "I know everything about Collomb, everything! Now what is it you want to know?"

· · ·

Beyond simply constructing a history of the Fann Psychiatric Clinic up to the present day, this book pays close attention to forms of historical consciousness (or better yet, historicity[7]) that may disrupt, exceed, or offer alternate imaginings to conventional historical narrative and the linear, progressive model of time upon which it is hinged. As it pauses before the images, material objects, practices, and people who index—but also always complicate—the pastness of the past, it gets caught up in the multiple temporal inflections and indices of the stories it tells, ultimately revealing an entanglement of time itself. The chapters of this book linger on ghosts and follow rumors of witchcraft as they pay special attention to the complex forms of memory work that are undertaken by Fann's current and retired doctors, nurses, staff, and a few longtime patients. By way of the stories recounted throughout the book, I show memory work to be both an act of the imagination and a moral practice (Lambek 1996) with oftentimes unexpected temporal, affective, and political dimensions. But let me turn back to Demba for a moment before embarking upon a more theoretical discussion.

As an (ex)patient who had been returning to the clinic for more than three decades, Demba had experienced Fann as a patient, a visitor, a critic, and a witness. In some ways, he knew Fann better than anyone. To be sure, many of the stories Demba told me about his life and his experiences in the clinic bordered on the fantastical; many resembled iterations of desire, hope, hopelessness, and regret rather than objective, chronologically ordered facts. Here I am reminded of Tuhami's stories as recounted by Vincent Crapanzano, many of which, writes the latter, could be said to "stand midway between history and fairytale" (Crapanzano 1980: 6). And yet, as Crapanzano explains, even those stories that could not be fit into Tuhami's life history as "real" (as in, verifiable as having really happened, like the tale of the pasha's son, for instance) bore upon its very truth. This, too, I came to understand, not just in relation to the many stories Demba told me, but about remembrance more generally. Above all, Demba's stories led me to question my own assumptions about the equivalence of the real and the true (i.e., the assumption that truth can only spring for that which is empirically sound, and conversely, that whatever cannot be observed, measured, cross-checked, or chronologically accorded cannot possibly be true), which Crapanzano (1980: 5) has called a distinctly "Western presumption" (see also Comaroff and Comaroff 1987; White 2000).

All of this is not to say that I have chosen to do away with the "real" in this book; there is, of course, much about Fann's past that is discernable as "fact." But I am reminded here of Michel-Rolph Trouillot's (1995: 25) brilliant intimation that "between the mechanically 'realist' and naively 'constructivist' extremes, there is the more serious task of determining not what history is—a hopeless goal if phrased in essentialist terms—but how history works." Somewhat surprisingly, though, it has been precisely in grappling with "how history works" and has worked at Fann that I have been led, by way of memory, to the imaginative practices that constitute it. Trouillot is cautious: "not any fiction can pass as history" (29). But I do not equate imagination with fiction, nor do I understand all fiction to be untrue. Rather, I insist that any attempt to apprehend and make sense of "what really happened" in the past is necessarily an imaginative endeavor; it must grapple with ghosts and, in turn, allow itself to be haunted. It must also account for the conditions of its own production, and the deeply uneven fields of power out of which it emerges and within which it circulates. Following my interlocutors' lead, this book moves between and holds together the "real" and the "true," the factual and the fictitious, and the ghostly, the routines and the performances, the present and its others (absence, the past). It is not just Demba's life history or his memories of Fann's early years that "stand midway between history and fairytale" or contain both at once, but all of my interlocutors' invocations and elaborations about the past, and indeed, the very narrative I have constructed here.

MEMORY / HISTORY, TRACES,
AND THE IMAGINATION

Much has been written about the relationship between memory and history in recent years, and often the two have been plotted against each other in antagonistic terms. Olick and Robbins (1998) remind us that the ascendancy of social memory as a field of inquiry in the social sciences and humanities was paired from the start with a critique of history and historicism.[8] But the relationship between memory and history has been described in less oppositional terms as well.⁹ In *Remembering War*, historian Jay Winter (2006: 6) notes that "the space between history and memory has been reconfigured" during the past century. Within this space has emerged "a varied set of cultural practices that may be described as forms of historical remembrance" (9), which he describes as "a way of interpreting the past which draws on both history and memory, on documented narratives about the past and on the statements of those who lived through them" (9). This shift to talking about memory as *remembrance*, as a process and a practice, is a crucial point that I shall take up in greater detail in the next section. Here, however, I want to note Winter's insistence on the fact that memory and history complement—even *need*—each other; that they may, in fact, serve to enrich each other and keep each other in check. History may be challenged or contested by memory and vice versa, he writes. At the same time, "those who try to reconstruct their 'memory' of past events need historians to establish the boundary conditions of possibility" (10). Ricoeur (2006) likewise argues that one of the primary tasks of the historian—and the goal of what he refers to as the "historiographical operation" more generally—is to enter into dialogue with collective memory, and ultimately, to affirm or challenge its claims. To him, memory's "truth-claim" is of ultimate ethical importance, for "there [can] be no *good* use of memory if there [is] no aspect of truth" (Ricoeur 1999b: 14–15; see also Ricoeur 1999a).

"What happened leaves traces," Trouillot (1995: 29) reminds us, "some of which are quite concrete—buildings, dead bodies, censuses, monuments, diaries, political boundaries—that limit the range and significance of any historical narrative." While Trouillot would seem to agree with Winter's intimation about the "boundary conditions of possibility" that historical facts place upon what can be said about the past, he also insists that historical inquiry must begin and not end with these traces. "The production of traces is always also the creation of silences. Some occurrences are noted from the start; others are not. Some are engraved in individual or collective bodies; others are not. Some leave physical markers; others do not." There are other kinds of traces, too, other ways that the past might be found in the present that are less concrete but no less significant: personal and collective memories; affective orientations; manners of speaking and not speaking; institutional habits and routines, incorporated bodily practices. Diana Taylor (2003) refers to the concrete and enduring remnants of the past as the *archive* and to these latter, more ephemeral performances as the *repertoire*. Of the relationship between the two, Taylor writes that the archive "constitutes

materials that seem to endure" and thus "exceeds the 'live,'" while the repertoire, "because it is 'live,' exceeds the archive's ability to capture it" (19–20).
Both are crucial to history, she says, because "both exceed . . . the limitations
of the other" (21). To apprehend the conditions of the production of historical narratives is to pay attention to traces of all sorts, as well as to their
absences and erasures, and to the silences, too.

But calling something a trace is already setting it into a particular kind of
relationship with the event that is presumed to have brought it into being. It
assumes correspondence and connection, but it also always stands apart from
its referent; there is always a gap. A trace always marks the absence of a presence, but it is also always an object in itself (Derrida 1976, 1978). According
to Ricoeur (2006: 13), the trace has "continued to overwhelm not only the
theory of memory, but also the theory of history" since Plato's *Theaetetus*,
which first described memory as an imprint upon a wax slab in the soul.
From the start, the central problem with imagining memory this way has had
to do with the relationship between the original event (which was assumed
to be the source of the impression) and the memory (the impression or the
trace itself), and especially with the correspondence or (lack thereof) between
the two. Plato interrogated memory for its capacity to stand as a source of
true knowledge, where the truth (or falsity) of a memory hinged primarily
upon "its identity with, or perfect correspondence to, something that is"
(Komaromy 2011: 63). For something to be true, it had to correspond to the
real. The troubling issue, for Plato, was that in absence of the original event
(and the original event was always absent), the memory-imprint's correspondence to it could not but be in doubt. A memory, like an image, might be
either *eikastic* (in correspondence with the original) or *phantastic* (a distortion or deviation from the original that issues from the imagination, and thus
for Plato, of a lower order and not a source of true knowledge). The distinction between the two forms emerges in the dialogue between *Theatetus* and
the Stranger in Plato's *Sophist*, revealing that the truth of memory can never
be certain. This is the *aporia*, or impasse, of memory.[10] And it is also why
Ricoeur (2006: 7) reminds us that "[t]he entanglement of memory and imagination is as old as Western philosophy" itself.

This entanglement of memory and imagination was troubling to Ricoeur,
who, in a similar vein to Plato, saw the effect of the imagination on memory
as a distortion, and thus a move away from the *real* of the past to which we
carry an ethical obligation, even a debt. Ricoeur (1999b: 15) recalls Sartre's
insistence, in *The Psychology of Imagination*, that "the imagination is about

the unreal and memory is about the (past) real ... there is an unrealising of history in imagination." Relating memory to perception and imagination to fiction, Ricoeur admits that the two do intersect at times. But then he adds, "sometimes fictions come closer to what really happened than do mere historical narratives, where fictions go directly to the *meaning* beyond or beneath the facts. It is puzzling." In the end, however, Ricoeur notes that it is what "really happened" in the past that matters most. In the end, he says, "we have to return to the body count. You have to accurately *count* the corpses in the death camps as well as offering vivid narrative *accounts* that people will remember" (15).

This book, then, emerges out of the space between the facts and the meaning "beyond or beneath" them. Instead of thinking about traces of Fann's past as indexical of a historical reality that can only be distorted or contaminated by imagination, this book takes memory to be a fundamentally imaginative endeavor from the start—a creative process or practice that is every bit as socially mediated and culturally shaped as it is individually experienced. In this I find more affinity with Spinoza, who understood memory—as a process of conjuring that which is not present—to fall within the domain of the imagination, than I do with Ricoeur.[11] In these chapters, then, I approach traces of Fann's past not so much as a detective apprehends evidence in order to pin down "what really happened," but as nodes of elaborative imagination—at once personal and social, moral and political—that often both illuminate and complicate (and sometimes, even defy) the "what really happened" of the past.

MEMORY WORK

Riffing on Nietzsche's assertion that that the nineteenth century was plagued by a hypertrophy of history, Andreas Huyssen (2003: 3) notes that our current age is marked by a "hypertrophy of memory." Indeed, a veritable "memory boom" (Winter 2006) has taken place in North America and Europe in recent years, both within and outside of academia—a combined effect, perhaps, of an overarching suspicion of grand historical narratives, a privileging of subjective experience, and the aggressive commodification of the past. Anthropology too has been occupied with memory; over the past three decades, studies concerning social and collective memory, cultural memory, the politics of memory, embodied memory, and trauma have abounded.[12]

Reacting to the pervasiveness of this trend, Johannes Fabian (1999, 2007), David Berliner (2005), and others have expressed deep concern about the epistemological dangers of overextending the concept.[13] Berliner (2005: 198) argues that "memory" has become a catchall phrase in anthropology that, quite problematically, "tends to encompass many features of the notion of culture itself." Following Fabian, he urges us as anthropologists to be as careful and critical with the concept of " 'memory' . . . as we have learned to be of 'culture' and 'identity' " (206).

Many historians have likewise wearied of the overextension of memory, and collective memory in particular.[14] While the idea remains relevant that it is "in society that people normally acquire[,] . . . recall, recognize, and localize their memories" (Halbwachs 1992: 38), both the haziness of the concept of memory as "some vague cloud which exists without agency" (Winter 2006: 11) and the reification of "the social" supra-individual force have come into question. Winter and Sivan (1999) suggest moving away from the term "memory" altogether to focus rather on "remembrance" for its emphasis on process over product and action over object. "To speak of 'remembrance,' " Winter (2006: 3) writes, "is to insist on specifying agency, on answering the question of who remembers, when, where, and how?"; it is to be just as concerned with the person or people doing the remembering and their social location(s) as it is with the memories being produced. Remembrance marks the transience and dynamism of the performative act of remembering, stressing how the conscious and active invocation of the past happens *in* and *through* the present. Above all, the focus on "remembrance" draws attention to the very conditions and scenarios that allow (and inhibit) remembrance to take place.

This shift away from memory to remembrance, and not just as an agentive social process but as a moral practice, had already been proposed by Michael Lambek in "The Past Imperfect: Remembering as Moral Practice" (1996). Here he looks beyond a characterization of memory as that which is a possession of—and also constitutive of—the individual self to instead consider memory as active, relational, intersubjective, and dialogical, necessarily "situated in time" and acted out and through social contracts (239). Lambek's concern is with the acts of remembrance themselves, which are always much more than just "past in the present." "To remember," he writes, "is never solely to report on the past so much as it is to establish one's relationship toward it" (240). Rather than thinking of memory as a neutral representation of facts about the past, he insists, we might do better to think of it as a claim that always carries a moral valence. Such a claim is necessarily selective,

creative, and performative; it is carefully tailored and imaginatively elaborated and it positions the person doing the remembering in relation to both
the past and to his or her present-day audience (cf. Cole 2001).

It is precisely this taking up and reworking of the past, as both an imaginative endeavor and a moral practice, that I refer to throughout this book as
"memory work." Following Stoler and Strassler (2000: 9), my thinking about
"memory work" takes as its point of departure the idea that memory is not so
much a "privileged [means of] access[ing] . . . a real past" nor a mere construction in and of the present, but rather what they describe as an "interpretive
labor." This is not to say that the past is "out there" like a complete text waiting to be interpreted. Rather, what is being interpreted is itself already an
assemblage of traces, selected and lifted out of the debris of the past in order
to make a claim on the present. Its coherence is always the result of a certain
degree of bricolage, and the construction of the text is itself always also the
first act of interpretation.

Although the memory work I detail in these chapters always mediates the
personal and the social (as well as the institutional and the postcolonial), I
remain cautious of the way psychological and therapeutic discourses have
infiltrated these other realms in recent years, especially relating to the concept
of trauma.[15] I look to Freud's work, then, not so that I might offer a psychoanalytic reading of the clinic, but to take up his characterization of memory as a
kind of work that *transforms* (cf. Ricoeur 1974, 1999a). In his more clinical
than philosophical "Remembering, Repeating, and Working-Through" (1914),
for example, Freud describes the process of "working-through" as a labor that
transforms one kind of memory (unconscious repetition) into another (conscious, integrated remembrance), thereby bringing about a reordering and
reworking of time.[16] In "Mourning and Melancholia" (1917), Freud describes
mourning as a kind of labor that transforms and eventually severs affective
attachment; it reworks affect as it seeks to disentangle desire from reality and
past from present. This he contrasts with melancholia, which refuses to give
up or let go of what has been lost—it instead *lingers, fixates*, and *ruminates*.

Throughout this book, then, I take up memory work at Fann as a creative
practice of bricolage, a labor of interpretation, and a process with the capacity
to transform action, affect, and time. I also show memory work to be an ongoing process without resolution or end–not because it resembles something
more akin to melancholia than to mourning, but because it is always poly-
phonic and intersubjective, and because the sheer inexhaustibility of the past
means that the multiplicity of meanings that can be drawn from it change

over time. Memory work includes a range of practices and orientations toward the past that extends beyond simple remembering to include selection, omission, erasure, and disavowal, and as such, it brings to the fore a seemingly naïve but nonetheless important question: *Why remember, anyway?* The assumption that remembering (and remembering *accurately*) is always better than not remembering—and that it provides a pathway to liberation, to justice, to self-knowledge, and to a better future—is central to historiographical thinking and foundational to Freud's psychoanalysis. It also operates as a powerful truism, so obvious that it often goes unquestioned in everyday life.[17]

When I began this project, I carried with me a deep suspicion of *not remembering*. I operated under the assumption that to *not remember* was to be ignorant, or that it was tied up in coercion or deceit or a play of power, or that it was representative of some sort of pathology; I likewise assumed historical remembrance to be an ethical obligation and a condition for living in the present. Such assumptions guided my early research, but they also limited my ability to apprehend other points of view. Early on, for example, I felt great sympathy toward the views of the retired nurses, social workers, and translators who had worked alongside Collomb and his colleagues at Fann when they accused the current Fann institution of operating as though it had no memory of its past and no acknowledgment of its history. "The doctors currently working at Fann use the prestige of Collomb's name," a retired nurse named Seynabou told me, "but in reality the clinic is not like it used to be. They have forgotten the past. They don't want to remember." The irony of a psychiatric clinic with memory troubles was, of course, not lost on her. I was struck by what I saw to be a kind of double disavowal of memory—on the one hand, the current doctors did not want to remember the past, and on the other, the clinical orientation of Fann had itself shifted away from orientations that privileged memory. I took Seynabou's indictment seriously without interrogating my own expectations about remembrance, what it should do, and what it should look like.

But why remember, indeed? Certainly it can be argued that remembering the victims of violence and oppression and constructing counterhistories to challenge dominant narratives of the past is a precondition to achieving social justice in the present.[18] But what of other kinds of pasts, especially those belonging to the people and institutions that had power on their side? Are some memories, and some acts of remembering, more important or valid than others? What sort of political project would I be engaging in if I were to suggest that Senegalese psychiatrists who inherited Fann from Collomb and his mostly European colleagues should remember (and pay homage to, and even try to integrate into their own practices) the innovations of their (colonial) predecessors? Might it not be necessary to remember selectively and creatively, or even to forget sometimes, if indeed as Nietzsche (1874) has suggested, "[f]orgetting belongs to all action" and the *unhistorical* is as crucial to the present as is the historical?[19] But here too, haunting has the capacity to complicate and disrupt forgetting as much as it does memory.

ENTANGLEMENTS

To focus on memory work and haunting at Fann is also necessarily to pay attention to the different temporal orientations and indices, layerings and inflections, trajectories and imaginings that continually disrupt the possibility (or expose the impossibility) of linear time and progressive historical narrative, both within the Fann clinic and in postcolonial Senegal more generally. These disruptions, I argue, are also openings for imagining other pasts, presents, and futures—and indeed, for reimagining temporal, social, therapeutic, and political orders writ large. In this book, then, I call upon and interrogate what Achille Mbembe has famously referred to as the "time of entanglement" that stands as a kind of temporal signature of postcolonial Africa. "The postcolony," Mbembe (2001: 14) writes, "encloses multiple *durées* made up of discontinuities, reversals, inertias and swings that overlay one another, interpenetrate one another, and envelop one another." To address memory work at Fann necessarily requires one to consider time not as a linear series of events but as "an interlocking of presents, pasts, and futures, that retain their depths of other presents, pasts, and futures, each age bearing, altering, and maintaining the previous ones" (16). Any consideration of memory work and haunting at Fann, or in postcolonial contexts more broadly, it seems to me, must not limit itself to a simple past-orientation, but must begin by thinking with the very notion of entanglement itself.[20]

If the concept of entanglement is a powerful metaphor for thinking about time and temporality at Fann, it is equally relevant for thinking about the people and generations that have occupied this post / colonial institution, and the different therapeutic and political orientations they have embraced. At the heart of these entanglements are questions about how sameness and difference—and especially that which is perceived as *cultural* difference—have been identified and negotiated within the clinic and by the state since the time of independence. That cultural difference should be acknowledged and even celebrated was the view of Senegal's first president, Léopold Sédar Senghor, whose vision for a distinctly Senegalese modernity hinged upon a political philosophy shaped by Negritude. To Senghor, cultural differences between Africa and Europe had an ontological basis—a claim much contested by Frantz Fanon, Aimé Césaire, and others for its essentialization and depoliticization of Black experience. As I describe in chapter 2, Senghor's efforts to put independent Senegal on the map—to secure the new nation's membership within the modern global community—were built upon the accentuation rather than the denial of difference. Likewise, the recognition of cultural difference was at the very center of the therapeutic orientation developed at Collomb's Fann during that same period. By the early 1980s, however, a new generation of politicians and psychiatrists was downplaying cultural difference—either by disavowing it or by reducing it to sameness—in order to stake its own claims in global membership. I argue throughout this book that these temporal, therapeutic, and political orientations remain entangled and are still perceptible in the present-day clinic, if only as traces, and that the place of culture within today's Fann is a far from settled affair.

Of course, it not just Fann or Senegal or "Africa" that might be described as entangled. Mbembe (2001: 8) emphatically reminds us: "all human societies participate in a *complex* order, rich in unexpected turns, meanders, and changes of course.... The torment of nonfulfillment and incompleteness, the labyrinthine entanglement, are in no way specifically African features." Any yet, there is something distinct about the postcolonial era in Africa, its unfolding, and its transformations. In a 2002 interview with Christian Höller, Mbembe describes the distinctiveness of the postcolony, calling it a "timespace characterized by proliferation and multiplicity. As a temporal formation, the postcolony is definitely an era of dispersed entanglements.... From a spatial point of view, it is an overlapping of different, intersected and entwined threads in tension with one another. Here, the task of the analyst is to tease out those threads, to locate those intersections, and entwinements." My historical and ethnographic engagement with Fann is an attempt to do precisely that.

· · ·

I had watched Demba for a long time before we exchanged more than passing greetings. I had watched him while pretending not to be watching. I had watched the way he moved his body; I had listened to his voice, to his words. There were days that his eyes looked yellow and dull, his gaze unfocused. On these days he would shuffle about, disoriented, quiet, not speaking but mumbling. Other days his eyes seemed glassy and his movements jerky. He would quickly become agitated on these days—his voice would rise and quiver, he would become frustrated, angry. He would complain about his general *malaise*, his old broken body. He would speak of injustice, of time taken from him, of money problems. He would talk desperately about how it was time for him to marry, time for him to build his house, time to have a family. He was already well into his sixties, after all.

And then there were the days when Demba's eyes were sharp, and his tongue and wit even sharper. On these days he would boss people around, get into everyone's business, give advice and roll his eyes arrogantly. He had a lot of energy on these days and would stand around with one hand on his hip. His paintings, drawings, and notebooks were never far away.

Our first real encounter had been of his making. As I sat reading through files in the clinic's document room one day, he walked in, greeted everyone, and sat down across from me. I swallowed hard and smiled, looking over at Madame Dieng (the secretary) and Monsieur Fall (the document room specialist) for some sort of support. Demba started talking and telling me he was writing a story, something he made up himself. All from his head, he said. He took a rolled-up notebook out of his pocket and opened it, showing me pages and pages of text that he had written, in French, with a red ballpoint pen. This, he told me, was the first of three parts. He had two other notebooks—both also full—in his room down the hall. He started to tell me the story, and then he stopped, pushed the notebook over in front of me, and said, "You read it yourself. Read it and tell me what you think." With that, he stood up and left as quickly as he had come in. I had not said a word.

One hour later, Demba came back looking for me with loads of paper and cardboard tucked under his arm. He sat down again and asked me if I had read his story yet. I told him, nervously, that I had looked at it, yes, but it would probably take me a few days to finish. "No problem," he said. "Here, look at my drawings and sketches. I'll sell them to you. They aren't expensive. Not for you, anyway," he winked and grinned, putting a stack of papers down on the table in front of me. "I did all these," he said. "They are part of my series of pen drawings." Most were done in red ballpoint pen, just like his story. And with that he got up and left, leaving the drawings in front of me.[21]

A few minutes later, Demba stormed back into the room. This time he was agitated—very obviously upset about something. He had wrapped his head up in a white cotton scarf, and he carried a small knapsack. He scooped up his drawings and tucked them under his arm. He was yelling in Wolof, translating and repeating himself in French (as he often did), and using Arabic exclamations for added emphasis. "I am leaving right now and going back to Rufisque! They cannot treat me this way! This doctor is young enough to be my grandson and he thinks he can tell me what to do! No respect! I have been coming to this clinic longer than he has been alive, *bilâhi* (I swear it)! I have been here longer than anyone! I was here when Henri Collomb was here, *bilâhi*! That is how long I have been here! I would not have been treated like this back then! Does anyone have money for a *car rapide*? I am leaving right now, and they can't stop me. I am free to go if I want to go. And I am going to Rufisque, right now."

Without looking up from his newspaper, and in a tone that told me this whole situation was nothing out of the ordinary, document specialist Fall told Demba to sit down for a second and calm himself. Demba cursed a response, and told him that nothing could make him stay. Then he turned to me and barked, "Give me your pen!" I quickly handed it to him, and watched him take the cap off with his rotted teeth. "Give me a piece of paper!" I tore out a piece of paper and gave it to him. On it, he scribbled: Artist-Écrivain, M. Magatte Ndiaye BP 1234 Rufisque. "Come see me after you read the story. I hope you will help me get it published. Come see me if you want to buy art—I will make you a deal. Hmph. I am never coming back here again!" Demba huffed and stormed out, slamming the door behind him.

Fall chuckled. He still had not looked up from his newspaper. Perhaps sensing my uneasiness, he told me that Demba sets off like this every so often, that he has been doing this for years. "Sometimes Demba disappears for a few days or weeks, but usually he doesn't get very far or go for very long," Fall explained. "He will be back in no time. Demba suffers from occasional *bouffées délirantes* [temporary delusional states]. He was treated for schizophrenia in the past, I think. But usually he is just fine." Madame Dieng sighed and shook her head. "*Sacré* Demba. What would Fann be without him? He is a fixture around here, *un des anciens*."

I remember sitting there for a moment, thinking about what I had just seen. Demba was clearly upset, but I could not determine whether his leaving meant he was well or not well. Nobody seemed too concerned, or acted as though any of this might be a problem. Fall had said that Demba is usually "just fine," but since he comes and goes at will, did that mean he stayed at the clinic when he was feeling well and normal, only to leave when he had an "episode"? As I sat scribbling this down in my own notebook, Fall motioned for me to look out the window. Sure enough, there was the army jacket–clad Demba walking back toward the clinic, holding his knapsack in one hand and his drawings in the other. I could not see his face, but the sight of him made me sad. I guess he could not make it home. Or maybe he had.

ORIENTATIONS

To both write a history and attempt to unsettle it, all at once—to do justice to stories that invoke hope and failure, nostalgia and haunting, crisis and erasure, endless waiting, witchcraft suspicions, dreams of the future, and events that may not have happened—calls for a different kind of writing. I have structured the book as a series of chapters, ruptures, and interludes, each of which takes up a different strand of memory or a different temporal lens. I begin with a ghost—that of Henri Collomb—not just because "haunting is historical" (Derrida 1994: 4), but because the repetition and return of ghosts has a way of unsetting linear time and "mak[ing] the present waver" (Jameson 1995: 83). Taking a cue from Avery Gordon, I approach the ghost as a social figure and take seriously the concept of haunting as I insist upon its relevance to anthropological inquiry.

In chapter 1, I turn to the archive as a repository of traces, gaps, and silences in order to imagine a genealogy of the Fann Psychiatric Clinic. Fann was in many ways a departure from the colonial psychiatric facilities and practices that had come before it in Senegal. What had come before it, however, was far from monolithic or consistent, nor was it the outcome of a coherent plan. Indeed, archival records reveal a remarkable amount of hesitation, frustration, and contestation among colonial officials at various levels regarding what should be done with the colony's "lunatics" (les aliénés), not to mention a wide array of proposed solutions. This chapter thus traces the history of French colonial psychiatry in Senegal from the construction of l'Hôpital Civil de St-Louis in 1853 until the establishment of the Fann Psychiatric Clinic in 1956, paying special attention to one of the more unfortunate colonial "solutions" to the problem: the forced transportation of lunatics from Senegal to the Metropole. Between 1897 and the beginning of the Great War, 144 West African men and women were shipped to France and institutionalized at l'Asile de St-Pierre in Marseille. The vast majority of these patients ended up dying in the French asylum and very few were ever repatriated.

Drawing on extensive archival and historical research that at times pauses to examine the logic of the archive, I show that debates about the colony's lunatics during this period expose tensions between colonial doctors and officials at various levels. Even more than simply indexing the Foucauldian transition (from madness to mental illness) in colonial psychiatry that was taking place in the years leading up to Senegalese independence, these debates were a key site in its transformation. In the end, I argue that the brutality of the early colonial treatment of madness itself haunted and became a kind of impossible inheritance to Collomb's Fann—one from which the group necessarily kept its distance, but one that would nevertheless remain present in this institution that bridged the colonial and postcolonial eras.

Between chapters 1 and 2 comes the first of three short interludes from Demba; here he tells of a colonial-era battle that set his life into motion, and that set the stage for many other battles he would face during his life. Chapter 2 likewise presents a story of origins, as it details the early independence era within the Fann clinic and beyond. Shortly after the death of Henri Collomb in 1979, President Senghor penned an obituary applauding Collomb for creating an institution that was as uniquely Senegalese as it was distinctively modern. In Senghor's view, the Fann Psychiatric Clinic was an exemplary institution of the newly independent nation, and Senghor saw no apparent contradiction in crediting a French military doctor with establishing such a place. In this chapter, I look carefully at the unique project in cross-cultural psychiatry that was initiated by Collomb and his colleagues during the 1960s, framing it within Senghor's vision for independence-era Senegal. Senghor, I argue, whose ideas about Negritude not only informed his political philosophy as president but also provided a national aesthetic for the new nation, viewed Collomb's project as one that articulated and accentuated elements of "traditional" Africa in the most modern of ways. In Collomb's work at Fann, then, Senghor saw the springing to life of a new kind of Senegalese modernity that actualized his vision of a "Civilization of the Universal."

A rupture appears between chapters 2 and 3 that takes up an unanswered letter that was sent by Frantz Fanon to Senghor, and briefly imagines how history might have been otherwise. Chapters 3 and 4 then engage with two contrasting sets of stories that circulate about the early years of Fann. Demba reappears in and between these chapters as well, with a poem of his featured in the second interlude. Chapter 3 examines the nostalgic memories of Fann's past (and also Senghor's Senegal) recalled by the Senegalese women and men who worked alongside Collomb and his colleagues as nurses, social workers, and translators during the 1960s and 1970s. As the "middle figures" of Collomb's project, these women and men were also part of a rising, educated Dakarois middle class that was deeply invested in the emerging Senegalese modernity of the post-independence years. I consider the nostalgic remembrances of these now-retired middle figures as both an affective narrative mode and a salient social practice. As their stories underscore the vast disjuncture between then and now, their nostalgia for the glorious past serves as an indictment for the failures of the present and the sense of hopelessness they feel for the future, both within Fann and toward the neoliberal state more generally. The object of their nostalgia, rather than being a pre-modern, idyllic "time before time," is modernity itself—both the distinctly Senegalese style of modernity promoted by Senghor and the potential futures it promised, which have since been foreclosed.

Chapter 4 tells a different story about the same period. It begins with the untimely passing of Dr. Moussa Diop, the promising psychiatrist who was expected to take Collomb's place and become the first Senegalese director of Fann. Diop's 1967 death was a harsh blow to the clinic; to this day, many people still whisper that he fell victim to invisible (occult) forces, namely witchcraft. In the wake of Diop's death, Collomb stayed on as the director of Fann until 1978, and although the clinic continued to flourish during his tenure, he faced growing dissent from the first generation of Senegalese psychiatrists who were ready to take his place. As this generation came into its own and began to seek legitimation in its own right, it put increasing distance between Collomb's project and its own orientation, which assumed— as its point of departure—the universality of the human psyche as well as the universal applicability of psychiatric medicine. The new group was as wary of Collomb's collaboration with local healers as it was reluctant to engage with the cross-cultural research that had been produced by the Fann School.

As told by many at Fann today, the story of Moussa Diop's death has come to stand as a reminder of the limits of the clinic as a site of collaboration between Western medicine and local models of illness and therapy. The tragic event is made to recall the impossibility of Collomb's project of transcultural psychiatry, all the while affirming the validity of Fann's philosophy vis-à-vis treatment and therapy *since* the era of Collomb. I argue that this particular framing of Diop's death also recalls the failures and limitations of Senghor's ability to build a distinctly Senegalese modernity predicated upon both the politicization of Negritude and the notion of a "Civilization of the Universal." Diop's death, then, was the beginning of the end of the era of collaboration and cooperation in which Collomb's Fann and Senghor's vision for Senegal flourished. I also, in this chapter, examine key points of contrast between Collomb's work and that of Frantz Fanon.

The third of Demba's interludes appears between chapters 4 and 5; here he tells a bitter story about the changes he has seen at Fann over the years. Chapter 5 moves between the ordinariness of the everyday within what had become, by the late 1990s, a struggling, resource-poor clinic and the major international event that was initiated by Fann in 2002. Known as the First Pan-African Conference on Mental Health (*Premier Congrès Panafricain de Santé Mentale*), the event took months to organize and required Fann's already-overtaxed doctors and staff members to take on extra work. Nevertheless, it drew over a hundred participants from more than thirty countries and was touted by many as a great success. In this chapter, I examine the conference as an ambitious attempt to rebrand Fann as an innovative institution that was neither tethered to nor dependent upon its past. Here I show how the success of the conference (which, quite tellingly and despite its name, was far from the first of its kind) hinged upon numerous erasures, willful omissions, and exclusions that were nevertheless visible to a handful of its participants during the three-day event. The production of the conference, I argue, was indicative of the same kind of "strategic ambivalence" toward Collomb's project that was present within the clinic at that time.

Between chapters 5 and 6 comes a final rupture. Here I describe and reflect upon my own failure to be present at a critical moment during my fieldwork. In late September 2002, the ferry *Joola* capsized off the Senegambian coast, resulting in the deaths of 1,863 people, including many children and youths returning to school in Dakar. The tragedy deeply affected the lives of everyone around me, both within and outside the Fann clinic, but I remained distant from its unfolding. Nevertheless, the event has stayed with me. I reflect upon my inabilities to cope with it at the time, a reaction that has caused me to think more broadly about the limits of both ethnographic fieldwork and ethnographic writing. It is a story of ethnographic failure.

Building upon chapter 5, chapter 6 details the afterlives of arrangements that were first put into place at Fann during Collomb's era, and are still perceptible in the present-day clinic. It also examines changes that have taken place at Fann—changes in care and caretaking practices, changes in therapeutic regimes, and modifications that have been made to the physical space of the clinic—against the backdrop of former president Abdoulaye Wade's neoliberal agenda. The Wade years marked a period of uneven, mostly foreign-sourced investment around Dakar. The investments translated into an uneven distribution of resources and opportunities, new forms of exclusion, and new forms of social distinction. Through a close examination of how the clinic operates and gets talked about today, I describe the distinct temporal and affective sense of the present moment within the clinic. I conclude by coming back around to Demba, to haunting, to impossible inheritances, and to the making and unmaking of history.

Chasing a Ghost

IT IS A FUNNY THING TO ADMIT, I know, but I had returned to Fann in search of Collomb's ghost. That was not exactly what I told Demba, though, at least not right away. During my first visit to Fann, a young intern had said something that surprised and stayed with me. As I sat reading through patient files in a small room adjacent to the *Pavillon des Dames*, I saw that each patient had been asked whether or not she had a *tuur* in her family. *Tuur* is a Wolof word meaning "to pour," but it also refers to a kind of invisible being that allies itself with—and protects—a particular family. Familial *tuur* can often be traced back to the founding ancestors of one's lineage; the *tuur* is passed from one generation to the next, normally making itself present to one person of each generation. The person chosen by the *tuur* must acknowledge and reaffirm his or her (usually her) relationship with the spirit lest she fall ill or suffer misfortune. In addition to the *tuur*, each patient had also been asked if her family was in possession of a *xamb*, a domestic altar where the *tuur* were thought to visit or reside, and at which sacrifices could be made by members of the family.

When I next crossed paths with the intern, I asked him about these notations: Why were patients asked about *tuur* and *xamb*, and what did the doctors do with the information? He laughed, and explained that Henri Collomb and his colleagues had begun asking patients about *tuur* and *xamb* during the early 1960s and documenting the responses. The habit at the clinic was an old one, he said, but really, there was no reason that such questions should be asked anymore. "Collomb and his colleagues were interested in traditional therapies," the young doctor told me. "They wanted to collaborate with healers to learn more about their ways; they wanted to figure out how and why these therapies worked to cure people. Of course we don't do that anymore here. If people want to consult healers or have their *ndëpp* (spirit possession ceremony), they can do it outside of the clinic. We don't do that here, not now anyway. This is a hospital, after all! I think Collomb may have been as crazy as his patients." The young intern paused and looked at me. "He still roams the halls of this place, you know. People have told me they have seen him, in any case. And it wouldn't surprise me, not one bit."

I thought about this brief exchange for a long time after it took place. The young intern had described the notations—and Collomb himself—as useless traces of a bygone era that, despite having no proper place within the present-day Fann, still make themselves visible from time to time. Then, in the very next breath, he had gone on to say that it was not just the notations that lingered in the present, but Collomb himself, in ghostly form. In his statement, both Collomb and his project were disavowed in an effort to distinguish the present from this other past.

Another reason I was struck by the intern's offhanded comment about Collomb roaming the halls of the clinic: The spectral landscape in Senegal is crowded with beings and nonbeings alike. Here, wild *rab* and domesticated *tuur* spirits exist alongside *djinné*.[1] Witches (*dëmm*) travel at night attempting to devour the vital energy (*fit*) of their victims. There are winds that can enter your body and make you sick or crazy (*febaru ngelaw*), and strange entities that can catch you when you are walking alone at night (*jommi*). As a friend in Dakar once told me, there are more invisible beings wandering through the world than there are visible beings. Some trouble humans and want their attention, while others move about quite oblivious to them. There are those who live in forests or near the water, and then there are those who choose to live in large cities. "There are probably even some in this room with us right now," she had said to me, laughing.

Somehow, the idea of Collomb's ghost milling about the halls of Fann and joining this already diverse and cosmopolitan group of spectral characters captivated me. As a number of people explained to me during my years in Senegal, spirits of the recently (or for that matter, the not-so-recently) dead do not normally make themselves manifest and wander about on their own; if they do, it is usually a sign that something terrible has happened. Perhaps the person died tragically or wrongfully? Perhaps she was not given a proper burial? In these cases, the recently dead person may haunt the site of her death. But this is quite rare, or so I was told, and it is always a very bad thing. No, Collomb's ghost roaming the halls of Fann did not fit this description. Clearly his was a ghost of another kind, a foreign ghost who haunted according to a different set of rules. What is more, this was a ghost from the West, from France, from a country that had once colonized Senegal. What was it doing at Fann? Why would Collomb's ghost have returned in the first place? What unfinished business might he have? What did people in the clinic make of this ghost? These were but a few of the questions that inspired my own return to the Fann clinic and led to my meeting of Demba. Just like that, I too had become a *revenant*. Following a ghost means you sometimes have to act like one.

I became interested in even more than Collomb's ghost. More generally, I wondered, why do ghosts haunt at all? They must have some *raison d'être*; they must have some sort of job to do. A ghost may come to demand redress for past injustices or warn of the future ahead. It may be unhappy and unsettled, or vengeful and angry, and it may want to stir things up. Whether conjured up or appearing of its own volition, the haunting figure seems to call out to those who encounter it. It beckons them to stop for a moment, look around, and take note of how both past and future come to play in the present.

"The ghost," writes Gordon (1997: 63), "imparts a charged strangeness into the place or sphere it is haunting." Here something unusual happens to time itself. Indeed, Derrida (1994: 39) describes the spectral moment as one "that no longer belongs to time," insisting that spectrality causes us to doubt the "linear succession" of time and "the border between the present . . . and everything that could be opposed to it." In discussing what he calls the "spectrality effect" and considering the way spectrality may complicate the relationship between presence and absence, present and past, he playfully coins the term "hauntology" to reference the logic of the ghost. Haunting, he writes, contains both a "first time" and a repetition; as such, haunting is "[a]ltogether other. . . . This logic of haunting would not be merely larger and more powerful than an ontology or a thinking of being. . . . It would harbor within itself . . . eschatology and teleology themselves" (10).

From this perspective, to acknowledge, address, and chase after ghosts is to complicate ideas of linear, homogeneous time and approach history not as the cumulative effect of events, or in the spirit of "progress," or as a justification for the present, but from a more radical perspective. Gordon calls on Walter Benjamin and likens his idea of the monad to the sign of a specter's presence, or in other words, the presence of a haunting of some kind. Benjamin (1969: 292–93) describes the monad as follows:

Where thinking suddenly stops in a configuration pregnant with tensions, it gives that configuration a shock, by which it crystallizes into a monad.

A historical materialist approaches a historical subject only where he encounters it as a monad. In this structure he recognizes ... a revolutionary chance in the fight for the oppressed past.

Benjamin's notion of "*Jetztzeit*" is similarly useful in building a theory of ghosts and haunting. He describes *Jetztzeit*, or "the now-time," as a dialectical relationship between the past and the present that is brought into being through the "blast[ing of] a specific era out of the homogeneous course of history" and into what he refers to as "the time of the now" (1969: 263). *Jetztzeit*, he explains, does not mean "that what is past casts its light on what is present, or what is present [casts] its light on what is past" (1999: 462), for this would affirm time as linear and keep the past anchored in the continuum of history. Instead, *Jetztzeit* is the "past charged with the time of the now," which is exploded out of this continuum (1969: 261). This dialectical movement, he explains, offers a radical approach to history that is based not on the view that the past is a chain of events that progressively lead up to the present, but on the idea that there is revolutionary potential to be found when a "part of the past [is] touched by the present instant [with] no continuity between them" (1999: 470). According to Benjamin, we must work both to discover— and to create—this dialectical relationship between the past and the now. One must be sensitive to the images and effects produced by these relationships, for they are repositories of revolutionary potential. Ghosts, I suggest, are not just the byproducts or bystanders of these dialectical relationships; they may also act as their mediators or instigators.

Why else might one search for a ghost? "It is essential," Gordon (1997: 196) writes, "to see the things and people who are primarily unseen and banished to the periphery of our social graciousness." Ghosts may very well return because "the very essence of humanity is at stake" (Derrida 1994: 44). Every engagement with a specter—no matter where, when, or what kind—is thus a political engagement of sorts:

> It is necessary to speak *of the* ghost, indeed *to the* ghost and *with* it, from the moment that no ethics, no politics, whether revolutionary or not, seems possible and thinkable and *just* that does not recognize in its principle the respect for those others who are no longer or for those others who are not yet *there*, presently living, whether they are dead or not yet born.
>
> No justice ... seems possible or thinkable without the principle of some responsibility, beyond all living present, within that which disjoins the living present, before the ghosts of those who are not yet born or who are already

dead, be they victims of wars, political or other kinds of violence, nationalist, racist, colonialist, sexist, or other kinds of exterminations, totalitarianism (Derrida 1994: xx).

The ghosts to which Derrida refers are undoubtedly ghosts of the oppressed and the silenced; at hand is a question of justice for the past, present, and future. Likewise, Gordon (1997: 64) also links the search for ghosts to a concern with justice: "The ghost is alive, so to speak. We are in relation to it and it has designs on us such that we must reckon with it graciously, attempting to offer it a hospitable memory out of a concern for justice. Out of a concern for justice would be the only reason one would bother." Although perhaps it should also be said that haunting might just as likely overflow the boundaries of these concerns, that haunting might not be altogether containable by the logics and desires of liberation, justice, or revolution.

Both Gordon and Derrida write of the ghosts of those who have been victimized, silenced, or disavowed (see also Kwon 2008; Mueggler 2001). Collomb, however, was neither invisible nor disenfranchised during his lifetime; the privilege and authority of his position should not be denied. What sense, then, is there to make of his ghost? To be sure, it is tempting to read Collomb's ghost as a specter of colonialism who, by roaming the halls of Fann, continues to haunt and disrupt the postcolonial present—he was, after all, a French military doctor whose tenure at Fann bridged the colonial and independence eras. As I show in the following chapters, however, the story of Collomb and his time at Fann is more complex than such an explanation would allow. Collomb did provide shelter for many, as Demba's own story shows. Further, while he was alive, Collomb occupied and moved within a border zone at Fann; he willfully cast himself as a figure between worlds, just as his ghost does today. And, thus, as Gordon (1997: 139) reminds us, "the ghost is haunted, too."

Demba laughed at me, of course, when I finally told him that I had come back to Fann to look for Collomb's ghost. He did not believe a word of the young doctor's story; he thought the doctor was pulling my leg. Demba would roll his eyes at me when I mentioned the ghost, and he barely put up with me when I asked questions about it. I tried to tell him that the ghost story was important to my project; it was the reason I even had a project in the first place. "Maybe," I suggested, "we could look at this poetically? I could explore the figure of the ghost as a way of approaching history? Look at it as a way that the past might come to inhabit the present?" Demba would just laugh. He could not believe I was awarded money for such a project, and he found this to be much more interesting (and amusing) than the possibility of Collomb's ghost milling about the halls of Fann. He often shook his head at me, grinning. "Shaaa-dut-dut-dut. They sure do have money to throw into the water over there, don't they?"

ONE

Archiving Madness

FROM COLONIAL PSYCHIATRY TO
THE ESTABLISHMENT OF FANN

LOOKING BACK, DR. JEAN RAINAUT REMEMBERS BEING horrified by the abject state of the hospital he had inherited. When the French military doctor became the director of *l'Ambulance du Cap Manuel* in Dakar in 1955, the place was no more than a miserable, prison-like, racially segregated dumping ground. Reflecting upon his experiences at *Cap Manuel* some twenty-five years later, Rainaut (1981: 431) still had not forgotten its awfulness; he carried with him the image of the "cage into which a number of nearly naked men and women were crowded, deprived of all outside contact," not to mention his memory of the suffering endured by the patients themselves.

In his recollections of *Cap Manuel* during the 1950s, Rainaut comes across as a sympathetic character. He paints a picture of himself as having been sensitive to issues of abuse and injustice as he highlights the strong objections he had to the dehumanizing conditions of the colonial hospital. Far from being an anticolonial radical, however, Rainaut might better be described as a colonial liberal, eager to implement reforms from the inside. And were it not for the fact that his 1981 testimony recalling the horrors of *Cap Manuel* quickly evolves into a heroic tale of overseeing its closure in 1956 and leading its patients to the newly built, state-of-the-art Fann Psychiatric Clinic, Rainaut's grim recollections of the place might have allowed him to cast himself as victim, in a role similar to that of what medical anthropologist Allan Young (2007: 156–57) describes as a "self-traumatized perpetrator," or in other words, one who "has been traumatized by the effects of his own violence" during a time when he himself was not a "morally autonomous agent" (158). Rainaut, as part of the colonial apparatus, might have scripted himself as having suffered the suffering of the caged patients under his care.

But that is not how Rainaut remembers *Cap Manuel*; it is not how his story goes. Rainaut's tale is one of liberation and enlightenment—one that, in scenes reminiscent of Philippe Pinel's liberation of *l'Hôpital Bicêtre*, moves from the dark horrors of confinement to the brightly lit spaces of modern psychiatric medicine; one that describes the dawning of a new era of psychiatry in late colonial Senegal. Rainaut writes that even he could not wait to escape the confinement of *Cap Manuel* and make the transition to Fann. And the patients! As Fann was being built, Rainaut recounts, patients would sometimes accompany staff from *Cap Manuel* to the construction site. Amazed at what they saw, they would return to *Cap Manuel* and tell the others about a "sumptuous palace" that was being built for them; Rainaut (1981: 433) jokes that "one could almost construct a new classificatory scheme based on how easily patients were able to project themselves into this wondrous future from the space of a sordid and real present." In his recollection:

> we were ecstatic about the fact that patients would have their own rooms; that these rooms would have windows and doors that would allow daylight in and be lighted by electric bulbs at night; that they would sleep in beds made with fresh linens; that they would take their meals at the table when their health allowed them to do so and if they so desired; and that they would also have forks, spoons, and knives. (432)

The "liberation" and progressive medicalization of madness, which Foucault (1965) has described as having taken place in France and England between the late eighteenth and early twentieth centuries, took place in Senegal on October 17, 1956, when the first convoy of patients was installed at the newly established Fann Psychiatric Clinic in Dakar. And while Megan Vaughan (1991: ix) reminds us that there had never been an "equivalent of what Foucault called the 'Great Confinement'" in colonial Africa—that is, the number of "lunatics" confined within institutions in the colonies had never reached the same dramatic proportions that it had in Paris from the mid-1600s onward—Fann nevertheless represented a departure from the carceral conditions of *Cap Manuel* and the other psychiatric facilities and practices that had come before it. At Fann, persons suffering from mental disorders would be treated as patients rather than prisoners; they would be referred to as *les malades mentaux* (the mentally ill) rather than *les aliénés* (lunatics / the insane; literally "the alienated"). And from the point of view of the late French colonial administration, addressing and treating madness as mental illness within this brand-new, ultramodern psychiatric clinic would serve the dual purpose of underscoring the civility and best intentions of the French colonial mission and itself serve as a civilizing force—one rooted not in the repressive power of the colonial state as was *Cap Manuel*, but rather in its productive function, through the creation of new habits, subjectivities, and orientations in the world (Bourdieu 1977, 1984; Foucault 1965, 1973). A rehabilitated patient at Fann, as Rainaut's recollection implied, would be restored to his or her self, life, family, and community. She also would be socialized to French manners and customs until these became second nature. Rather than eating around a communal bowl set upon a woven floor mat (as was, and still is, customary in most households in Dakar and throughout Senegal), patients would eat from a personal plate *à table* and learn the intricacies of silverware use.

But I am getting ahead of myself. The stories told in this chapter are not about the Fann clinic per se, but about the colonial psychiatric facilities, practices, and unheeded recommendations that came before it in Senegal. As an institution built during the late colonial era, a period in which French rule resembled something closer to welfare colonialism and "care" than brutal subjugation or coercive force, the legitimacy of the Fann Psychiatric Clinic was predicated on its rupture from this violent past. This chapter thus draws upon extensive historical and archival research to trace the vagaries of French colonial psychiatry in Senegal from the construction of *l'Hôpital Civil de St-Louis* in 1853 to the establishment of Fann in 1956, paying special attention to one of the more terrifying colonial "solutions" to the problem: the forced transportation of *les aliénés* from Senegal to the Metropole. Between 1897 and the beginning of the Great War, 144 Senegalese men and women were shipped to France and institutionalized at *l'Asile de St-Pierre* in Marseille. The vast majority of these patients would die in the French asylum; few would ever be repatriated. The violence of this and other early colonial psychiatric interventions stood as an "impossible inheritance" to the new Fann Psychiatric Clinic, which was imagined as a distinct departure from that which had come before it.

It would be a mistake to think that the early French colonial government's approach to managing madness in Senegal was monolithic or consistent, or that it was the outcome of a coherent scheme or plan. Rather, archival records reveal a remarkable amount of hesitation, frustration, and contestation among colonial officials at various levels regarding what should be done with the colony's "lunatics" (*les aliénés*), not to mention a wide array of proposed solutions. We are reminded here that "[c]ontrary to received conceptions of colonial encounters sui generis—and of medical encounters in particular—a mature system of knowledge was not simply exported to the edges of the empire, there ... to be bestowed or imposed upon indigenous peoples" (Comaroff and Comaroff 1993: 328). Psychiatry stands as a particularly apt example of this, for during the 1800s and even into the early twentieth century, there existed no coherent body of psychiatric knowledge or expertise to be exported to the colonies in the first place—the discipline itself was born during the very same period that European powers were expanding and consolidating their empires across the African continent. Indeed, the evolution of psychiatric science and the assertion of empire were more intertwined than one might imagine (Mahone and Vaughan 2007). For example, as Richard Keller (2007) has brilliantly argued in his examination of French psychiatry in Algeria, France's overseas territories allowed for a degree of experimentalism that was not possible in the Metropole, thus playing an important role in the advancement of psychiatry itself. What is more, theories of racial inferiority that hinged upon such concepts as the "Arab mind" and the "African mind" were elucidated within the space of the colonial psychiatric encounter and in turn served to reflect, affirm, and justify the French colonial mission. And yet, despite the fact that colonial medicine has often been described as a "tool of empire" (Headrick 1994), colonial regimes "overwhelmingly failed to establish hegemony" (Heaton 2013: 9) when it came to the management of madness in the vast majority of colonial Africa. Facilities and practices that could be called even remotely "psychiatric" touched only a tiny minority of the local populations; resources and manpower were lacking, as was the political will of most colonial governments. For most of the colonial period in Senegal, madness was perceived as a pressing concern to colonial authorities only when it constituted a threat to public order; in this vein Sarr, Seck, and Ba (1997: 214) remind us that most of the colony's *aliénés* "remained in the hands of traditional therapists," which should lead us to question the extent to which it is proper to say that madness was colonized in the first place.

Nevertheless, from the 1890s onwards, colonial doctors began pushing hard on both moral and medical grounds for the establishment of an asylum in Senegal that would usher in a new approach to treating madness in France's West African colonies.[1] In considering key debates and discussions surrounding *les aliénés* in colonial Senegal between 1896 and 1956, then, what becomes clear is not simply that ideas about the nature of colonial madness were evolving during the period, or that the French colonial administration's position vis-à-vis the management of madness finally or inevitably "caught up" to that of the Metropole. More than merely indexing a Foucauldian transition from incarceration to care in the practice of colonial psychiatry, this chapter illustrates the extent to which these debates and exchanges were a key site in which the moral legitimacy of French colonialism was questioned and even challenged from the inside—especially by many of the military doctors themselves. These debates were also key sites for the elaboration of changing ideas about the "African mind," and about the nature of culture and madness itself.

FRENCH COLONIAL ORDER AND
THE THREAT OF MADNESS

France's first permanent settlements in sub-Saharan Africa were established in the city of St. Louis (*Ndar*) and the island of Gorée in 1659 and 1677, respectively. More than anywhere else on the continent, France's early and sustained presence in these coastal enclaves transformed them into something of a testing ground for overseas administration and French colonial policy (Crowder [1968] 1976; Johnson 1971), not to mention a site in which (French) civilization came to be constructed against its "uncivilized" others (Conklin 1997). French policies in this region were marked by experimentalism, and they produced unique forms of exceptionalism throughout the colonial period: French Civil Code was applied in St. Louis and Gorée as early as 1830, and in 1872, the two enclaves were granted the status of French communes (as "*communes de plein exercice*") with representation in the French National Assembly (Clark and Phillips 1994; Collignon 1995; Diouf 1998; Johnson 1971). St. Louis and Gorée were later joined by Rufisque (in 1880) and Dakar (in 1887) to form what would come to be known as the Four Communes (*Quatres Communes*) of Senegal.[2]

The Four Communes were modeled after French municipalities, each with its own elected mayor and council. African and *métis* (persons of mixed European and African ancestry) inhabitants of the Four Communes were called *originaires*, and those who had "assimilated" to French culture were referred to as *les assimilés* or *les évolués*. In theory, *originaires* were permitted to apply for French citizenship, as were *les assimilés* or *les évolués* who could prove that they had been living within the Communes for at least five years. However, the administrative barriers to French citizenship were formidable. Unlike the residents of these four coastal cities who could in theory access the status of citizen (*citoyen*), those living in French-controlled territories outside of the Four Communes were strictly considered colonial subjects. There, the French colonial administration governed indirectly, and residents were subjected to the laws of *l'indigénat*—a body of colonial laws that enforced such things as taxation, labor drafts, and military conscription.[3]

During the early colonial era, the French experimented with a policy of assimilation in the Four Communes that aimed to socialize an elite stratum of indigenous inhabitants as French men and women (Crowder [1968] 1976). But local populations were, in fact, quite selective in what they variously incorporated and rejected. They often adopted French political sensibilities while asserting and maintaining values that were distinctly "non-French" and often distinctly Islamic (Lambert 1993: 243; see also Diouf 1998). Identifying with Islam may have even provided local populations with a tool for resisting the cultural force of France's *mission civilisatrice* (Johnson 1971).

French assimilation policy, which held that "Africans could and should be educated to assimilate to French culture" (Clark and Phillips 1994: 65), hinged first upon a belief in the superiority of French civilization, and second upon the notion that it was France's duty and responsibility—even a moral imperative—to bring its civilization to the rest of the world. The legitimacy of French colonial rule, both within the Four Communes and elsewhere, leaned heavily upon this notion of *mission civilisatrice*. But the notion was more than just a ruse to lend moral justification to the colonial project; by the period of the Third Republic, the civilizing mission was hailed as both "a duty and a right" of the French "to remake 'primitive' cultures along lines inspired by the cultural, political, and economic development of France" (Conklin 1997: 2).

By the early part of the twentieth century, although still operating under the banner of its *mission civilisatrice*, the French colonial administration began to restrict the rights of citizens in the Four Communes and replace the ideal of assimilation with a more "pragmatic" policy of association (Betts 1961). Contrary to the theory of assimilation, which had held that any given individual could be taught to embrace and inhabit French Republican values and dispositions, the theory of association was based on an assumption that peoples throughout the world occupied different rungs on the ladder of civilization, and that moving up this ladder was a long and arduous process that could take many generations. From this perspective, looser colonial "associations" were seen to be both more practical and more humane in that they encouraged colonized populations to move along the path of civilization in their own time. Growing approval for the new policy of association—and a growing distance from the policy of assimilation—was increasingly evident at the annual meetings of the French Colonial Congress during the early 1900s, and the policy of association was unanimously embraced by the Congress in 1907 (Betts 1961; Clark and Phillips 1994; Diouf 1998; Gellar 1982; Harrison et al. 1987; Idowu 1969; Lewis 1962; Vaughan 1985). A strong political conscience also began to develop in Senegal during this time and especially in the period following the Great War. Many Senegalese (both citizens and subjects) marked the hypocrisy of French policy and fought to obtain the rights and responsibilities to which they saw themselves entitled.

Despite France's assimilationist ideals and its early experimental application of French Civil Code within the Communes, its 1838 law regarding *les aliénés*, referred to by Goldstein (1990) as the French "lunacy law," was never applied in Senegal.[4] The 1838 law described *l'aliéné* in France as a person in need of public assistance; it was the first law to define mental disturbance or deficiency as a condition requiring medical intervention and state protection. In that the law cast *l'aliéné* as both a vulnerable person and a potential threat to others and to public health and safety more generally, the "state protection" it called for worked under the sign of a "conjoint philanthropy and police" (Goldstein 1990: 282). The law was as concerned with maintaining social order as it was with the welfare of those who were to be institutionalized. To that end, the 1838 law divided *les aliénés* into two groups—those who were considered dangerous and those who were not—and distinguished different ways of dealing with each. Persons deemed dangerous by the local prefect were to be subjected to what was known as *le placement d'office* (official placement) and incarcerated within regional institutions or asylums. Those not considered dangerous would be eligible for *le placement volontaire* (voluntary placement; committed by a family member) and would be institutionalized by the state if so requested by their families (de Bures 2006).[5] Finally, the 1838 law decreed that each French *département* should be responsible for the management and institutionalization of its mentally ill population. As such, the law served to "integrat[e] the new medical specialty [of psychiatry] into the apparatus of the [French] state" (Goldstein 1990: 276; Castel 1976).

If the 1838 lunacy law announced a new regime of monitoring and treating madness in France and signaled the exercise of new and "productive" (as opposed to repressive) state power (Foucault 1965, 1973), the fact that no attempt was ever made to apply the law within the Four Communes (despite the experimental application of the French Civil Code there) suggests not only that the colonial administration lacked the resources and infrastructure necessary to enforce it, but also that madness within the Communes was not identified as a site of medical intervention or state protection; rather, "mad natives" in the colonies appeared on the radar of the colonial administration only when they posed a threat to public order. Megan Vaughan (1991: 10) rightfully argues that the power exercised within colonial states was much more "repressive" than it was "productive"; there was, as noted earlier, no widespread institutionalization across sub-Saharan Africa, and the Four Communes of Senegal (and later, the federation of French West Africa) were no exception.

In the absence of lunacy laws or any systematic approach to madness within the Four Communes, then, it was the "repressive" function of the Royal Order (*Ordonnance organique*) of 1840 that would determine how madness was dealt with in the colony for many years to come (Reboul and Régis 1912: 212; Collignon 1995).[6] The Royal Order, which defined the roles and responsibilities of the French colonial administration in Senegal and outlined how the administration should go about dealing with "dangerous elements," did not even specifically address *les aliénés*, only colonial order. The Royal Order thus translated into "police action against potentially dangerous persons rather than one of medical action to care for ill patients" (Collignon 1995: 41). Researchers working within the ANS (*Archives Nationales du Sénégal*) came to realize this rather quickly; searching for traces of colonial madness in nineteenth-century Senegal means turning to the archive's F-series documents (Police and Prisons) more than the H-series documents (Health and Assistance). During the last half of the nineteenth century, persons judged to be mentally deranged and dangerous in Senegal were thus either locked up in jails or penal institutions, or held in a special section of *l'Hôpital Civil de St-Louis,* a large civilian hospital that was built in the city of St. Louis in 1853. Other colonial and military hospitals in the region, including *l'Hôpital de Gorée, l'Hôpital Colonial de Dakar,* and *l'Hôpital Militaire de St-Louis,* kept "lunatics" in specially designated sectors only until they could be relocated to *St-Louis* (Diouf and Mbodj 1997: 22–24).

The conditions faced by mental patients in these hospitals were grim, and overcrowding made them much worse. A detailed report written by medical officer Dr. Réné Morin to the director of health services for French West Africa, for example, described extremely degraded conditions at each of the colony's hospitals.[7] At *l'Hôpital Civil de St-Louis,* which was by far the best equipped to handle *les aliénés,* there were five small brick huts (2 × 2 × 2.5 m) with tiled roofs constructed behind the main building. At least one of the huts was even further subdivided, and in all of the huts it was common for several patients to be held together. The door of each hut was a heavy, bolted thing that locked from the outside with a small opening lined with wired mesh at the top. The insides of the huts were dark and stifling, and most contained small mats or nothing at all upon which to sleep. And yet this was luxury compared to the quarters offered to *les aliénés* at the other hospitals, which doubled as holding cells for prisoners and persons with infectious diseases.

By the mid-1890s, the situation had become so deplorable and overcrowded at *l'Hôpital Civil de St-Louis* that doctors had no choice but to "authorize the release of patients who were not cured, who still posed a danger to the public order, in order to make room for patients who were even more affected, more agitated, more dangerous" (Cheneveau 1938: 1; see also Reboul and Régis 1912: 81).[8] Although doctors working at *St-Louis* had been voicing their complaints about the conditions of the hospital for some time (Reboul and Régis 1912: 82), discourses surrounding the management of madness shifted during the 1890s from a concern with logistics, space, and containment to a language of pity and concern for the welfare of those prisoner-patients interned within the hospital. Even the director of the Interior of the Colony was compelled to speak out about the deplorable conditions he had witnessed while touring the hospital: "[The patients] are locked alone in narrow cells that can only be compared to airless lavatories. I saw a native breathlessly clinging to the sides of the wall, climbing like a monkey to breathe a bit of fresh air through the narrow bars of his prison."[9] In the director's eyes, the fact that patients at *St-Louis* were confined like animals accentuated their animality; his statement was a plea to recover their humanity. In response, the *Conseil Général du Sénégal* made a formal recommendation in 1896 that it hoped would ameliorate the problem. Unlike the British, however, who had long since established their first colonial asylums in the Cape Colony[10] and had more recently erected an asylum in the Gold Coast at Victoriaborg in 1888 (McCulloch 1995),[11] the French colonial government sought an altogether different solution. Instead of recommending a designated lunatic asylum be built within Senegal or elsewhere in the newly formed territory of French West Africa, General Councilor Faure made a case for the shared humanity of the suffering patients in the overcrowded *St-Louis* hospital (Borreil 1908) and recommended that at least a portion be evacuated to the Metropole, to be interned at *l'Asile de Saint-Pierre* in Marseille.

It is tempting to read Faure's formal recommendation—as well as the heightened concern for the welfare of the patients—as a turning point, or at the very least, a definitive step away from the repressive function of the Royal Order. There is clearly a discursive shift happening in the 1890s among the colonial administration on the ground in Senegal regarding how the "problem" is defined and how it should be remedied—from a language of management to a focus on the suffering patient as a site of intervention and state protection. Recommending that a number of the patients kept at *St-Louis* be shipped to Marseille might have been viewed as an act of "good faith" that would put late assimilation-era ideals into practice. This was an early claim to productive (bio)power over the lives and bodies of the interned mental patients "for their own good" (see Foucault 1978; Gagnon et al. 2010; Rabinow and Rose 2006). It is not hard to imagine, however, that the transportation of West African patients to Marseille was an abject failure on every count. For the unlucky souls forced to make the trip, it was little more than a death sentence.

THE PASSAGE TO MARSEILLE

In French colonial thought, the idea of transporting psychiatric patients from the overseas territories to receive treatment in the Metropole was not new. The *Saint-Pierre* asylum had, in fact, been receiving patients from abroad for many years. The transfer of mental patients from Algeria to France began in 1845, with the signing of a treaty between Algiers and *Saint-Pierre* (Bégué 1989, 1997; Collignon 2002).[12] In that many French colonial officers assigned to French West Africa had previously worked in Algeria, the earlier treaty almost certainly served as a model for the treaty with Senegal (Collignon 1999: 247). An important difference between the two treaties, however, was that the first aimed to evacuate French (specifically European-born or descendant) men and women living in Algeria rather than the country's indigenous inhabitants. Of the total number of patients transferred from Algiers to *Saint-Pierre* for care, only a small fraction were of North African descent (Planchon 2013: 141). In contrast, the treaty with Senegal was designed specifically with the transport of West African psychiatric patients in mind— not only those who officially held *citoyen* status as did the *originaires* of Senegal's Four Communes, but also colonial subjects from throughout the region who had ended up interned at *l'Hôpital de St-Louis*. The evacuation, then, was devised as a temporary solution to the overcrowded and untenable conditions at *St-Louis*. The hope was that it would cost the colony a great deal less than the price of building, maintaining, and staffing an asylum locally, while at the same time offering patients more humane and evolved forms of internment than could be found within the colony at that time.

The treaty outlining the terms of the transfer of patients was approved by the prefect of the *Bouches-du-Rhône* and the governor of Senegal in 1897, and the first group of patients was transported to Marseille on a Compagnie Fraissinet ship named *Taygète* that same year.[13] The treaty stated that the colony would be responsible for arranging and paying for the patients' transportation to Marseille. In terms of medical protocol, it stated that each patient should be accompanied by (1) an internment order (*ordre d'internement*) from the director of the interior, (2) a medical certificate written by a doctor in the colony, (3) a document providing as much information as possible regarding the civil status of the patient, and (4) an additional medical certificate stating that the patient was in good physical health at the time of embarkation and exhibited no sign of infectious disease. The treaty also noted that each patient would be supplied with clothing appropriate to Marseille's colder climate.

For each patient institutionalized at *l'Asile de Saint-Pierre*, the colony agreed to pay the sum of two francs per day to cover the cost of medical provisions, food, clothing, and care. This was a fair amount of money, not excessive, but it was expected to cover patient costs without too much trouble. In cases where a patient was cured and ready to be released, the treaty emphasized that he or she should under no circumstances be allowed to stay in Marseille. Instead, arrangements would be made for the released patient to be escorted to the port and given over to the captain of an authorized ship; the colonial administration would pay for their repatriation. Should the patient pass away while interned, the colonial administration would pay six francs to cover the cost of his or her burial, presumably in or near Marseille, as no mention was made of bodies being returned to Senegal.

Unfortunately, Senegalese psychiatric patients interned in Marseilles were much more likely to die in *l'Asile de Saint-Pierre* than be cured and released. In his 1908 medical thesis entitled *"Considérations sur l'internement des aliénés sénégalais en France,"* a young doctor named Paul Borreil wrote that a total of 72 patients had been shipped from *St-Louis* to Marseille and interned at *Saint-Pierre* between 1897 and 1907. Of these 72, a staggering 38 (52%) had passed away—26 (68% of the deaths) from tuberculosis. Thirty-one patients remained institutionalized, and only three had been repatriated. By the end of 1911, a total of 128 patients had been transferred to *Saint-Pierre*; 94 (74%) of them had already met their death.[14]

Borreil's medical thesis, which drew on his two years' work as an intern at *Saint-Pierre*, offered an illuminating look at the grim situation faced by Senegalese patients aboard the ships that transported them from the colony to the Metropole. He described the "convoys of negroes" (*"ces convois de negres"*) that he saw arrive at the asylum, "in shock from their 8- to 10-day voyage, numb no matter what the season, barely clothed, often even straight-jacketed, and bound like dangerous lunatics" (1908: 7). Patients were normally kept in the holding cell of the ship for the duration of the voyage and monitored by a nurse and police officers, Borreil explained. Two grim images come to mind when one imagines these passengers and the ships that carried them. The first is that of the *Narrenschiff*, or the Ship of Fools. Throughout early Renaissance Europe and especially in Germany, the *Narrenschiff* not only figured as a prominent motif in literary and artistic compositions; according to Foucault ([1964] 1988b), the practice of loading madmen onto ships was frequently embraced as a means of ridding cities of their madness. The Ship of Fools, a boatload of madmen drifting aimlessly downriver, was both a liminal space and prison, both journey and destination. "Confined on the ship, from which there is no escape, the madman is delivered to the river with its thousand arms, the sea with its thousand roads, to that great uncertainty external to everything," writes Foucault ([1964] 1988b: 11). He continues:

> He is a prisoner in the midst of what is the freest, the openest of routes: bound fast at the infinite crossroads. He is the Passenger par excellence: that is, the prisoner of the passage. And the land he will come to is unknown—as is, once he disembarks, the land from which he comes. He has his truth and his homeland only in that fruitless expanse between two countries that cannot belong to him.

The passage from *St-Louis* to the Metropole was likewise an extradition, a form of exile, though the eight- to ten-day journey was but a means to a final destination and not, as with the *Narrenschiff*, a destination unto itself.

The forced transportation of Senegalese psychiatric patients from *St-Louis* to the Metropole evokes another image as well, an image perhaps equally obvious to some readers—that of the transatlantic slave trade, which saw the forced transportation of as many as 20 million enslaved men and women from Africa to be sold in the "New World." It goes without saying that the scale of this forced migration was exponentially larger than the passage to Marseille; the seas were rougher, the journey longer, the conditions aboard the slave ships infinitely more brutal and horrific. For those enslaved men and women who managed to survive the Middle Passage, what awaited them at their destination was a gruesome fate of enslavement and forced plantation labor. For the Senegalese psychiatric patients en route to *Saint-Pierre*, what awaited them in Marseille was an imprisonment of a different kind—a death sentence or worse, a confinement to a purgatory between life and death.

If the forced passage was an unimaginable horror for the Senegalese patients, the situation awaiting them at *Saint-Pierre* was hardly better. Borreil's thesis offered frank testimony of the limitations—even the impossibility—of assisting the Senegalese patients at the asylum in a way that might affect a cure. What is more, his account describes what he saw to be the rapid deterioration of the patients' physical and mental health upon arriving at *Saint-Pierre*. "These unfortunate men and women," he writes, "whose language we do not speak and who do not speak our own, whose mannerisms and expressions elude us completely, arrive healthy but after little time, die exhausted" (1908: 7–8). The problem was not only that the barrier of language and culture rendered care inadequate and ineffective for these foreign patients, but that the transportation and internment of psychiatric patients in Marseille actually hastened their death. On average, Senegalese patients could expect to survive only 27 months at *Saint-Pierre* (31).

When a convoy of Senegalese patients first got to the asylum, they were placed in an area where they could be closely monitored. As Borreil insisted, however, doctors and nurses could do little more than observe; they had no way of knowing whether they were correctly interpreting the patients' behavior. To add to these difficulties, a patient's condition upon arrival did not always resemble the condition described in the medical documents that accompanied him or her. Take the patient Borreil (1908: 19) calls A., a 35-year-old woman of Joola ethnicity from Senegal's Casamance region. The medical certificate that traveled with her to Marseilles in November 1906 stated that she had been interned at *St-Louis* for dementia; it described her as suffering from "prolonged fits of melancholy" that caused her to be always lying about or lying down (*constamment couchée*). Once she arrived at *Saint-Pierre,* however, A.'s comportment bore no resemblance to this description. According to doctors' reports, A. never stayed still, not even at night. Constantly in motion, she wandered about the asylum, barely dressed and barefooted, speaking loudly and ceaselessly. She performed bizarre dances and spoke to people who were not there; she appeared to experience auditory and visual hallucinations. With virtually no way to communicate with A. (she spoke no French and little Wolof, only Joola, a language most commonly spoken in Senegal's southern Casamance region) and only her actions to observe, the doctors in *Saint-Pierre* were at a loss to interpret her behavior, which departed so dramatically from her medical certificate. It was not until A. died fourteen months later and an autopsy was performed on her body that she was found to have, among other physical ailments, an "enormous kidney stone" (*un enorme calcul de rein*) that doctors understood she had likely been in severe pain for a good deal of time (25).

If the treaty had devastating consequences for those patients who were transferred to the Metropole, it was a failure by a number of other measures as well. Conditions at *l'Hôpital Civil de St-Louis* were hardly ameliorated by the forced relocation of what amounted to only a small portion of its mental patients. In terms of the monetary cost to the colony, unforeseen expenses related to the patients' transportation, surveillance, treatment, and medication far exceeded the administration's expectations, making real costs much higher than had been anticipated (Morin 1910; Cheneveau 1938; Collignon 2006). Complicated contracts with naval companies likewise spurred many a logistical headache; over the years the treaty was in effect, the colony had contracts with four different shipping companies, three of which had distinct sets of regulations for the transport of mental patients (Reboul and Régis 1912). Within *Saint-Pierre*, the West African patients were themselves seen as a threat to the health and safety of the other patients (read French or European-born, and white) within the asylum (Borreil 1908). Already by the time Borreil published his thesis in 1908, it appeared that no party had benefitted from the implementation of this treaty.

Although Borreil was speaking from a medical, not an administrative or juridical, perspective and was not really in a position to make recommendations regarding colonial policy, he concluded his thesis by stating not only that the transportation of Senegalese patients to France should be terminated, but that suitable facilities should be built within the colony itself so that patients could be treated in place (1908: 52). Both the governor of Senegal and the director of *l'Hôpital Civil de St-Louis* shared his opinion. In Borreil's ongoing correspondence with the governor of Senegal, the latter wrote, "[i]n my personal opinion . . . I believe it would be preferable to treat them within the colony, but for the moment, we do not possess a suitable facility" (49). Likewise, the director of *l'Hôpital Civil de Saint-Louis* confided that "an asylum would be useful within the colony and . . . would certainly have clients (*une clientèle assurée*);" he further stressed that his opinion was shared by many other doctors in the colony and beyond (50). Such recommendations did not exactly fall on deaf ears. In 1909, for example, the *Conseil Général du Sénégal* made an appeal to the federal government of French West Africa that a central asylum be built in Dakar, and that the cost be defrayed by contributions from each of the colonies of the federation (Morin 1910). The recommendation was considered, but in the end it was denied. Over the next four decades, plans for a federal asylum would be floated again and again, in numerous forms and iterations, always to be struck down, or at best, to be stalled indefinitely.

For the occasion of the 22nd *Congrès des médecins aliénistes et neurologistes de France et des pays de langue française* in Tunis in 1912, doctors Henri Reboul and Emmanuel Régis built upon consultations with colonial doctors and data collected from all parts of the France's overseas dominion, including Borreil's thesis, to present a influential report in which they criticized the French government's reluctance to build asylums within its overseas territories and urged it to take definitive charge of madness within the colonies—the French, they announced, were lagging far behind the British and Dutch in this regard and must step up their efforts. Among their key recommendations, they put forth that: (1) more colonial psychiatrists be trained to work in France's overseas territories, (2) proper legislation be put into place regarding *les aliénés* in the colonies, and (3) special asylums, hospitals, or other facilities be established throughout France's colonial dominion (Reboul and Régis 1912: 188–201). Reboul and Régis likewise harshly condemned the forced transportation of patients from France's overseas territories as an example of disastrous policy and retrograde thinking. "It is not decent, it is not human, it is not worthy of France," they proclaimed, "it must, without delay, be put to an end" (201). Patients from France's overseas territories must be repatriated immediately, they insisted, and these other recommendations should likewise be taken up with haste; such changes, they noted, were long overdue.

Despite the gravity of the 1912 report offered by Reboul and Régis, the treaty ordering the transfer of patients from *l'Hôpital Civil de St-Louis* to *l'Asile de Saint-Pierre* in Marseille was not suspended until the dawning of the Great War, when travel by ship from the colonies to the Metropole was severely restricted and beds in French hospitals were set aside for soldiers injured in combat. The treaty was officially revoked by the minister of the colonies in 1918, but without any significant infrastructural improvements having been made within Senegal or French West Africa in the meantime, save a small military hospital that was built in Thiaroye (approx. 50 km outside of Dakar) in 1917 to offer psychiatric treatment and custodial care to Senegalese soldiers—the *tirailleurs sénégalais*—returning from the Great War. According to all accounts, Thiaroye quickly became overcrowded as well (Cheneveau 1938; Collignon 2002). *L'Hôpital Civil de St-Louis* remained an important center in the colony for *les aliénés*, and in Dakar, mental patients were held in specially cordoned off sections of either *l'Hôpital Principal* or *l'Hôpital des Indigenes*, which was renamed *l'Hôpital Le Dantec* in 1932.

"GET IT DONE!"—CHENEVEAU, 1938

By far the most candid document to be housed within the ANS (*Archives Nationales du Sénégal*) regarding the state of psychiatric care in colonial Senegal is a 1938 report written by Dr. Roger Cheneveau, a military doctor who held the high rank of *Médecin-commandant des troupes colonials*. Written a full two decades after the revocation of the treaty that sent West African "lunatics" to Marseille, Cheneveau's report expressed scorn and frustration about what he saw to be the colonial administration's systematic failure to address the sorry state of colonial psychiatry in the region. A number of reasonable and well-conceived proposals for reform had been put forth since the Great War and even earlier, Cheneveau asserted; while some of these had advocated the construction of regional asylums, many more had attested to the urgent need for a federal asylum that would serve the whole of French West Africa. Several of these recommendations had included detailed plans for the proposed asylum that were based on intensive site studies and analyses of data gathered from the far reaches of the federation. So detailed and extensive were these reports, Cheneveau insisted, that instead of simply repeating what had already been said or adding yet another proposal to the mix, he could only write his own report if he first took pause to consider why none of the prior recommendations had been actualized.

As Ann Stoler (2002: 87) notes, "the archive was the supreme technology of the . . . imperial state, a repository of codified beliefs that clustered around (and bore witness to) connections between secrecy, law, and power." Far from affirming the authority of the French colonial apparatus in Senegal, however, the reflexive nature of Cheneveau's report interjects doubt into its very claims of legitimacy; it intervenes as a critique of archival accretion, repetition, and purposeless accumulation. It also points to a certain discord between colonial officials at different levels—between those working "on the ground" in Senegal, for example, and the minister of colonies in Paris. Cheneveau's harsh critique of the unsatisfactory state of colonial psychiatry in Senegal (together with all of the unheeded recommendations that had been made prior) paints a picture of an impotent colonial apparatus, mired in such bureaucratic back-and-forth that it simply could not get things done.

Why, in Cheneveau's view, had none of the recommendations been acted upon? He believed that idealism had gotten in the way of practicality—many of the plans that had been put forth had been too extravagant and too costly. "One [had] wanted to build a grand and modern asylum, comparable to the large psychiatric hospitals of the Metropole. Such a clinic would certainly [have been] desirable," Cheneveau (1938: 5) wrote, but it was simply outside the realm of financial possibility for the colony. The documents also revealed "petty squabbles" (7) regarding how a federal asylum would be financed and where exactly it would be constructed, not to mention concerns related to transportation and accessibility from the various regions of the federation.

Others, Cheneveau remarked, had expressed a desire to "build an asylum that was exactly proportional with the needs of the local population" (6), but it was exceedingly difficult to figure out what those needs actually were. In any case, Cheneveau explained, quoting Reboul and Régis (1912: 114), "we must insist upon the fact that it is necessary to build too big and too ample a lunatic asylum" in the colonies because whatever is built will "become fatally and quickly too cramped and narrow" (Cheneveau 1938: 6). A case in point noted by Reboul and Régis was the recently built Ambohidatrimo asylum in Madagascar, which, from the moment its doors were opened, was already too small to accommodate the needs of the local population. In their eyes and in Cheneveau's opinion alike, madness affected many more "natives" within the colonies than the administration had acknowledged, and this was a serious problem that needed to be addressed. Put simply, if large asylums were built, the colony would have no trouble finding patients to fill them.

But how prevalent, really, was "native" madness? The question certainly preoccupied French and British colonial psychiatrists across the African continent during the first half of the twentieth century. With it came much speculation about both the "normal" state of the African mind and the role played by a too-abrupt exposure to colonial "civilization" in causing "natives" to go mad. In this, Megan Vaughan (1991: 107) draws insightful parallels between the way the "African in the 20th century" and the "European woman in the 19th century" figured into and were produced within the psychiatric imagination as being "unequipped to cope with civilization." Certainly by the 1930s, there was a widespread belief among colonial psychiatrists that madness was becoming more common among "natives" due to their inability to successfully adapt to the new conditions of colonial modernity—to become "sufficiently civilized." It is worth stressing that these theories did not condemn colonialism for driving people mad; instead, they tended to center upon the weakness and inadequacy of the underdeveloped African mind to grasp and assimilate to a way of life that was quite obviously more evolved. Perhaps the most well-known colonial psychiatrist to take this view was the South African–born J. C. Carothers, who worked from 1938–50 as head of the Mathari Mental Hospital in Kenya. Carothers (1951: 12) very famously drew parallels "between African thinking and that of leucotomized Europeans," and compared the mental functioning of adult Africans to that of European children. Throughout his career, he remained consistent in his belief in the racial inferiority of Africans, although his explanations regarding the origins of this inferiority shifted from biological and organic to social and cultural. Carothers argued that the childlike African living in a "traditional," pre-contact state rarely experienced madness at all, and that acculturation—especially the forces of Western education and migrant labor—could cause "native" madness; African men living in colonial cities were, in his eyes, especially prone, as they were the most often exposed to forces of colonial modernity.

Cheneveau, like Reboul and Régis before him, similarly viewed "native" madness as a critical problem that was only getting worse. Stressing the dire need for an asylum solution, he noted the formidable proposal for a federal asylum that was put forth by Dr. Frank Cazanove in 1931, entitled "*Rapport sur le projet d'un asile d'aliénés.*" As a high-ranking colonial military doctor, Cazanove had contributed to numerous such reports during his more than twenty years of service, but this iteration was perhaps his most developed. Here he recommended that a large institution be built in the small town of Mbaba, between the cities of St. Louis and Dakar; it would serve as a federal asylum for the whole of French West Africa. Drawing on a careful study of census data that had been collected the year before, Cazanove estimated that the asylum should be large enough to hold three hundred patients. Reflecting on what the appropriate structure and organization of the asylum should look like, he dismissed outright the idea that *les aliénés* needed to be kept in locked and guarded cells, and instead proposed a more open plan. In reality, Cazanove wrote, not all mentally disturbed persons are violent, and judging from the patients he had observed in Dakar, those who could be considered dangerous represented only a small portion. Cazanove's recommendation in this regard ran counter to what remained, in practice, a relatively standard carceral model for dealing with madness in colonial Senegal's hospitals. Under normal circumstances, Cazanove wrote, confinement was as unnecessary as it was inhumane. "Keep in mind," Cazanove (1931: 3) noted seriously, as if the bit of information he was about to relay was somehow easy to forget, "that mad natives (*les aliénés indigenes*) placed in small huts or cells die quickly in there."

Although Cazanove advocated against unnecessary confinement, his vision for Mbaba was based on principles of segregation that separated patients by ethnicity and country of origin as well as by degree and type of mental illness. The patients' quarters of the asylum he proposed were to comprise one large building, one small building adjacent to the larger building, and a series of "native style" huts. The large building would be reserved for "Europeans and *les assimilés* (Syrians, Moroccans, Indians)" as well as the more "evolved natives" and those who could provide payment; in this way, Mbaba would be modeled after the asylums in Bien-Hoa (French Indochina) and Anjanamasina (Madagascar), Cazanove pointed out (1931: 3). The small building would contain twelve rooms reserved for patients who did prove to be a danger to the other patients and the asylum staff. The "native style" huts would be reserved for the rest of the patients, Cazanove explained, including those non-Europeans who were "unassimilated" or "unevolved" and those who could not afford to pay their way. One is led to wonder, in fact, about the extent to which a patient's ability and willingness to pay was itself taken as proof of his or her "evolved" status, and inversely, if being unable to pay was a clear sign that one had not yet evolved.

In Cazanove's view, the "native style" huts had several advantages. First, they were easy and relatively cheap to build; if the need was there, new huts could be constructed in the courtyard without too much fuss. Second, the huts would each be large enough to sleep 8–10 patients, but their use remained flexible. In order to prevent discord and maintain order, Cazanove explained, patients might be grouped in the huts by ethnicity, or they might also be separated by malady; those suffering from problems that were thought to be of an organic nature, for example, would be assigned to a specific area, while those who had contagious diseases would be kept in yet another. Lastly, the huts were assumed to be better suited to the needs of the "unassimilated" patients than the brick-and-mortar buildings because they more closely resembled the thatched-roof dwellings typically found in villages across the region. In terms of its separation and segregation of persons assumed to be at different civilizational "stages," Cazanove's proposal certainly reflected France's then-current policy of colonial association rather than its past policy of assimilation.

Cazanove recommended that patients be admitted under close observation within a specially designated pavilion; this would give doctors and staff the time to properly assess the condition of each patient and it would limit unnecessary internments. He anticipated that many patients—from those suffering from mental confusion brought about by intestinal parasites to those afflicted with "melancholic depression due to their expatriation in France or Morocco" (1931: 4)—would respond quickly to rest and proper treatment during this initial stage, and they could be released without an extended stay. In the other cases, Cazanove wrote, the period of observation would allow patients to be properly diagnosed and assigned to the section of the asylum that best suited their needs. Patients could also be assessed at this point according to whether they could be "put to work, and what type of work they could be asked to do" (5).

Indeed, a key feature of Cazanove's proposal had to do with what he described as "*l'utilisation des aliénés*" (the "use" of lunatics); here again he drew on the French colonial asylums in Bien-Hoa and Anjanamasina for inspiration. Cazanove noted that native patients (*les aliénés indigenes*) could be enlisted to do many different kinds of labor: agricultural work and food production, maintenance work, laundry, and so on. He made no mention of putting European or "assimilated" patients to work in the same capacity, however. While Cazanove did not devote much space to the details of the plan, it was evident that he expected this "free" source of "native" labor to keep the day-to-day operating costs of the asylum relatively low. A secondary justification might have been that assigning patients productive tasks would both deter idleness and serve as a basis for moral and occupational rehabilitation. European labor, we might assume, was not seen to be ripe for extraction in the same way, not as likely to benefit from the rehabilitative potential of productive labor.

Cazanove envisioned that the Mbaba asylum would be important not just for its capacity to contain and treat madness in West Africa, but also as a center for the research of African psychopathology. To this end, the asylum would have its own on-site surgical theater, laboratory, pharmacy, archive center, and library. When the proposal was submitted to the IGSSM (*Inspection Général des Services Sanitaires et Médicaux*), however, it was rejected as unnecessarily luxurious and far beyond the means of the federation. In 1932, Cheneveau explained, the governor general of French West Africa ordered Cazanove to return to his 1931 plans and make revisions, which he did with the help of Médecin Général Sorel, but this new iteration was still deemed too costly.

The following year, the colonial administration changed course, taking a more decentralized approach. Shelving plans of a federal asylum that would serve the whole of French West Africa, the governor general requested that the lieutenant governor of each colony in the federation draw up plans for a medical annex that would be designated for "incurable or violent lunatics" and that could be connected to each regional hospital (Cheneveau 1938: 11). At this point, specific recommendations were made for sites in Niamey, Abidjan, Porto Novo, and either Sebikotane or Gorée in Senegal. Cheneveau notes with frustration, however, that communication on the matter then went silent for three years—there was no record of any action having been taken. When the discussion was finally picked up again in 1937, the question of whether to build a federal asylum or a series of regional hospital annexes was debated anew. In March of that year, the governor general requested financial assistance from the minister of colonies in Paris to proceed with the construction of regional annexes. The request was denied, but after a series of exchanges between colonial officials at different levels, the governor general notified the lieutenant governor of Senegal in August 1937 that he intended to move forward with a heavily revised version of Cazanove's plans for the Mbaba asylum. He requested that appropriate studies be done to investigate whether the town of Thiès (also between Dakar and St. Louis, but closer to Dakar) might be a better choice for the institution, and while he acknowledged that many modifications would have to be made to the original plans due to budgetary constraints, he optimistically assured the governor of Senegal that work could begin on the project as soon as the next cycle of loans from the administrative budget had come through (12).

It was at this point that Cheneveau's own report, itself destined for the IGSSM, became part of the story, for the central task of the report was to put forth a final set of recommendations regarding the future of a West African asylum. Cheneveau's report was submitted in May 1938. Just one month prior, the *Congrès des aliénistes et neurologistes de langue française* had convened for the forty-second time, this time in Algiers. Among other key points, the final report of the conference stressed once again that appropriate psychiatric facilities should be constructed in the French colonies, without delay (Aubin 1938; Collignon 1978). In the last section of Cheneveau's report, he proposed that a two-tiered system of psychiatric care be put into place. At the regional level, specially designed and staffed annexes should be established and administrated by the large, urban hospitals in each of the different colonies that comprise French West Africa. On the federal level, Cheneveau confirmed that the best plan of action should be to build a toned-down version of Cazanove's Mbaba asylum in Thiès. The plan was adopted at the end of June, and in early July, the governor general of French West Africa, Jules Marcel de Coppet, signed a decree creating a federal Psychiatric Assistance Service (*Service d'Assistance psychiatrique*) that would be charged with the tasks of outlining the conditions for placement and care—and also overseeing—the newly ordained facilities. As Collignon (2002: 463) notes, the decree, which was "signed 26 years after Reboul and Régis' report and exactly 100 years after the French law of 1838 went into effect, filled a long-standing legal void."

The year 1938 was all set to be a turning point, a moment of long-awaited action vis-à-vis the advancement of colonial psychiatry in French West Africa. It was imagined in these documents as the beginning of a new era—optimistic and future-oriented—that would put a definitive end to years of unheeded recommendations for amelioration. Cheneveau's report, highly self-conscious and extremely critical of this history of inaction, was itself positioned as a distinct break from the past. But alas, while minor action was taken to establish and maintain regional psychiatric annexes affiliated with urban hospitals, Cheneveau's recommendations for the federal asylum in Thiès were never realized—the proposal itself was fated to become yet another repetition of the same. As World Was II loomed, the proposal was shelved alongside all the others, and all plans for building the federal asylum were once again pushed to the back burner. Here once again was a vision for a particular future that never came into being.

CAP MANUEL AND COLONIAL VIOLENCE

Cap Manuel, the annex of *l'Hôpital Le Dantec* (formerly known as *l'Hôpital des Indigènes*) in Dakar that featured at the start of this chapter, contained around 90 beds—60 of which were reserved for patients with infectious diseases such as tuberculosis and leprosy, and 30 of which were reserved for psychiatric patients (Diouf and Mbodj 1997). Although far from expansive, in the absence of Cheneveau's proposal being realized, the annex would become the largest and most important psychiatric service in all of French West Africa during the 1940s and early 1950s. While the other general, civil, and military hospitals in the colony still had quarters set aside for psychiatric patients, none claimed the capacity of *Cap Manuel*.

Cap Manuel was not a progressive institution by any stretch of the imagination. The common trait shared by the motley group of men and women interred there was that they were seen to "constitute a danger to the [general] population" (Rainaut 1981: 431). Many of the mental patients in *Cap Manuel* had come onto the radar of the colonial police and medical authorities—and were subsequently locked away—because they had committed acts of violence or disregarded the law. Cazanove's 1931 assertion that not all mentally disturbed persons should be treated as violent and dangerous appeared to hold little sway here; instead, it seemed a rather quaint—albeit misplaced—relic of liberal paternalism. Up until just a few years before *Cap Manuel* was closed, in fact, there had been armed guards—*tirailleurs* holding bayonets—assigned to stand guard at the hospital's entrance, not to protect the patients within, but to protect the people on the outside. This carceral model of psychiatric care was far from exceptional across sub-Saharan Africa during the late colonial era. In his 1950 monograph about mental illness in the Gold Coast (Ghana), for example, British colonial psychiatrist G. H. Tooth (1950: 110) similarly noted that "the primary function of [the Colonial Mental Hospital in Accra] has been *to protect the public from dangerous and criminal lunatics.*" Lunatics who were not perceived to be a threat to others, he explained, were almost never institutionalized.

While colonial psychiatry's preoccupation with "native" madness had always been closely intertwined with the colonial imperative to maintain order, the relationship between madness, violence, and colonialism came to be articulated in radically different ways and for vastly different purposes during the 1950s. At one end of the spectrum were the colonial doctors and administrators who viewed violent acts of "natives" within their colonies as either a sign of natural inferiority—their "normal abnormality," as Lynette Jackson (2005: 101) has argued after Megan Vaughan (1991)—or as a symptom of mental illness. J. C. Carothers (1953: 123), for example, insisted that within the colonies, "violence is often a symptom of psychiatric conditions and, if search be made in prisons of very underdeveloped countries, mentally deranged and defective persons will certainly be found." At a time when the colonial apparatus was being challenged throughout sub-Saharan Africa, such views of violence—as evidence of either the natural inferiority of Africans or as a symptom of the madness that had resulted from their inability to assimilate to colonial modernity—recast the violent "native" as a madman and reframed anticolonial violence as proof that local populations needed the paternalistic arm of colonial rule for support and guidance, thus justifying the containment and medicalization of those who actively fought colonial authority. On the other end of the spectrum was Frantz Fanon's (1952) scathing critique of racism and the psychological damage inflicted upon subjugated peoples. Colonial oppression, Fanon would write in *Les Damnés de la Terre* (1961), drove people mad, and catharsis (not to mention independence) could only come through liberation struggles that would bring colonized peoples into violent conflict with their colonizers. "Armed conflict alone," wrote Fanon, "can ... drive out these falsehoods created in man which force into inferiority the most lively of minds" ([1961] 1963: 294).

Unlike so many other parts of the continent, however, Senegal was not a place of armed conflict or violent liberation struggles during the 1950s. In fact, as its grasp on its West African territories began to weaken in the aftermath of World War II, France asserted its legitimacy not by force or through the exercise of military power, but by reforming its colonial institutions and implementing new modernization projects that would lead to a continued (and even stepped-up) French presence. This was an era of enhanced welfare colonialism. Within Senegal and in Dakar in particular, a French development fund known as FIDES (*Fonds d'Investissements pour le Developpement Économique et Social des territoires d'outre-mer*) earmarked significant expenditures for modernization and development projects between 1948–59 (Gautron 1964). It is within this context that the 1956 closure of *Cap Manuel*—and the establishment of the new Fann Psychiatric Clinic—is best understood.

In 1950, an American medical researcher by the name of Dr. Eric Berne traveled to Dakar to collect information for a project about psychiatric services throughout the world. Tucked among yellowed archival documents in the ANS is a letter he wrote to the director of public health in French West Africa in 1955—the same year that Rainaut took over as director of *Cap Manuel*; Berne described the evolution of his project and explained that he was finally in the process of writing up his results.[15] The letter asked for an update on any changes in psychiatric care that had taken place in Senegal since his 1950 visit. Berne recalled in his letter that a third of the *Cap Manuel* annex had been reserved for psychiatric patients and that several beds were also set aside for the more agitated or aggressive patients, but in what was perhaps an act of diplomacy, he made no mention of the prison-like feel of the place, or the horrid conditions in which patients were kept. Instead, he noted that most of the patients within *Cap Manuel* were male and almost all were of West African—and not European—descent. It seemed to be standard procedure, Berne noted in his letter, to repatriate European patients whenever possible. Berne had also noticed that, by and large, doctors had a great deal of difficulty understanding and being understood by the patients; only about 30–40 percent of the patients spoke any French at all, while the remainder spoke "only the dozens of indigenous dialects" of the region.

Berne's letter also mentioned the rumors that had been circulating at the time of his 1950 visit regarding an American company that had wanted to buy *Cap Manuel* and turn it into a fancy hotel. Had there been any more talk of this? And what, Berne asked, had become of the plan to construct a 320-bed psychiatric hospital and consultation center near the city of Thiès that would serve the entire region of French West Africa? The ambitious plan, Berne noted, had been highly anticipated, and had included detailed blueprints for the layout of the hospital. It had even described some of the "state of the art" treatments that would be offered in the new hospital, such as electroshock therapy, drug-induced sleep therapy, chemical restraints, insulin treatments, and occupational therapy. Although it had then been twelve years since Cheneveau filed his report that condemned the inaction of the colonial administration and recommended immediate construction of the Thiès asylum, the plans still appear to have been fresh in people's minds.

A response to Berne's letter, dated March 3, 1955, from General Inspector Talec, also appears in the archives.[16] The letter outlines the substantial changes that had taken place since Berne's visit. *Cap Manuel*, the general inspector explained, was no longer able to meet the needs of Dakar's growing population and had been scheduled for demolition. Plans for the Thiès hospital had been definitively abandoned. The colonial administration had decided to build smaller psychiatric services in each region of French West Africa instead of a single, large hospital to serve the entire federation. Ground had already been broken for Senegal's hospital. Located but a few kilometers from downtown Dakar, it would be funded partly by way of the General

Budget of the Colony, and partly by FIDES. The new hospital would be situated alongside several other specialized medical facilities and affiliated with the University of Dakar.[17] The Fann Psychiatric Clinic was thus in its early stages of development. According to General Inspector Talec, plans for the clinic had been reviewed and refined by experts from Paris as well as Dakar. Designed according to "ultra-modern" European standards, it would be an enlightened contrast to the dark, prison-like asylums of the past.

PAJAMAS AND THE MAKING OF PATIENTS

In early 1956, several months before patients and staff were transitioned to Fann, Jean Rainaut attended a conference of psychiatrists in Côte d'Ivoire. While he was there, he writes, he was absolutely overwhelmed by the interest his colleagues showed regarding the newly constructed facility. News of Fann had already traveled far and wide. Rainaut writes, however, that responses to the Fann plans were less enthusiastic in the Metropole, where critics judged this new face of African psychiatry as radical and superfluous. Why spend so much time, effort, and money on building a state-of-the-art facility in the colonies? Rainaut (1981: 432–33) writes that he and his colleagues were even scolded by a handful of critics for being "dangerous innovators" in the field of colonial psychiatry who did not know their limits. In his recollections of the era, he depicts himself as something of a maverick. His critique of the ongoing use of carceral psychiatry in late colonial Senegal, it should be noted, was directed at the fact that it was an outmoded and inhumane model of psychiatric care, but he did not go so far as to launch an explicit critique of the colonial apparatus.

Despite decades of recommendations made by colonial doctors and administrators that the federation of French West Africa take charge of its mental patients in a comprehensive way, the "productive" power of a paternalistic welfare colonialism did not touch the domain of psychiatric assistance in Senegal until the 1950s. The establishment of Fann certainly marked a dramatic shift in colonial psychiatry in Senegal, and because the founding of the clinic signaled a new approach to psychiatry and the psychiatric institution in sub-Saharan Africa, some have since situated Fann within narratives of decolonization and Senegalese independence (Rainaut 1981; Collignon 1976). Others, however, have taken an altogether different view, arguing that the construction of Fann should be seen as an attempt to maintain colonial legitimacy at the very moment that France's future in West Africa was being called into question. From this perspective, the idea of Fann offered a progressive new face of colonial benevolence and care that could stand as a justification for continued colonial intervention in Senegal. Taking a note from Foucault, Diouf and Mbodj (1997) even suggest that the more humane model of psychiatric assistance offered by Fann, which was such a clear departure from the penal model that had come before it, marked an even more highly refined means of social control through the implementation of new techniques of care, discipline, and resocialization.

In describing the first round of patients to arrive at Fann from *Cap Manuel*, Rainaut (1981: 433) wrote the following: "Pajamas were waiting for [the patients] on every bed. Pajamas are not traditionally Wolof, Serer, Lébou, or Toucouleur, but symbolically, the pajamas said a lot. Quite simply, they represented a new era in which the mentally ill patient in a hospital would recover his status as a socialized human being" (my translation). While it seems a wholly benevolent act, one might argue that giving a patient pajamas that are "not traditionally Wolof, Serer, Lébou, or Toucouleur" does not help him "recover his status as a socialized human being" but actually neutralize his social and ethnic identity in an attempt to socialize him according to a universal (read: Western) model of what a patient—and a person—should be. Although it was a far cry from the carceral violence of earlier colonial psychiatric interventions, this new and "progressive" model of care at Fann enacted a form of violence even more subtle and intimate. Care, in these new terms, was necessarily the unmaking of the subject. Pajamas not only mark but *make* patients, just as "sleeping in beds made with fresh linens" and eating at a table with a fork, a spoon, and a knife creates a certain kind of social person and establishes a certain kind of institutional order. The *humane* treatment that was to be offered at Fann, highly touted by Rainaut, was premised upon a very specific idea of what a *human* was and how a *human* should behave. Much more than about restoring patients to baseline mental health, this new brand of psychiatric assistance and rehabilitation would mold new subjectivities, teach new habits, and affect new orientations in the world, and it would do so by socializing patients to the moral and material accouterments of French civilization. To emerge as "cured" from this new colonial psychiatric institution was to be transformed into a new kind of social person.

The legitimacy of the new Fann Psychiatric Clinic hinged upon its break from the violent psychiatric interventions of the colonial past—interventions that were themselves framed as forms of care. As a product of the late colonial regime, however, this was a past that nevertheless haunted Fann, and from which Fann could never be fully disentangled. This colonial legacy, present yet also disavowed, was Fann's very first "impossible inheritance."

Many Battles

"I WAS BORN ON GORÉE ISLAND," Demba said, "but no, I didn't grow up there. Right after I was born, it was *le débarquement*, you know. My father worked at *l'Imprimerie Nationale*, but when the bombardment happened . . . DEET! DEET! DEET! . . . we all had to leave. Gorée ended up being a strategic military site during the war. We had to evacuate. My father's work was moved to Rufisque so that's where we went . . ."

"Wait . . . what?" I interrupted. "Who landed on Gorée in 1940? Who was doing the bombing?" This was one of my first recorded conversations with Demba. I had just asked him about what things were like for him—and what Senegal was like—when he was a kid.

"You know, the French *came under attack*," Demba said in an exasperated tone, and with an expression to match. "It was *the war*." And then he quickly moved on to another topic.

It was not until recently, when I went back and listened to some of these conversations with Demba, that I became aware of the extent to which the motifs of *battle* and *war* pervaded his stories. Most often, the battles he spoke of were spiritual, existential, economic, or familial. Here, though, Demba was making reference to a "real" battle—a military confrontation—that, in a sense, set his life in motion. The reference was admittedly lost on me at the time. Although I know next to nothing about military history, I could not conceive of a scenario in which Gorée Island would have been a World War II battle site.

But this military battle really did happen. The French (and of course, the Senegalese population whose lands were occupied by the French) came under attack on Gorée Island and the Dakar (Cap-Vert) peninsula. Who led the attack? Also the French. The federation of French West Africa was controlled by the Vichy government after the 1940 armistice. In September 1940, the Free French troops, led by General de Gaulle from his London headquarters, carried out a military operation designed to persuade the Vichy-led French West African colonial administration to switch sides and join the Free forces. As the story goes, however, de Gaulle "grossly overestimated sentiment for his cause, and his naïve attempts to subvert the colony's loyalty failed absolutely" (O'Hara 2013: 54). With his hopes for a peaceful resolution dashed, de Gaulle ordered the Free French troops to take the colony by force. As they tried to secure landing for their ships, they were fired upon by cannons from Gorée and the mainland, as well as a Vichy French fleet. The battle, known as the Battle of Dakar or *Opération Menace,* lasted for three days and led to eighty-four fatalities and the destruction of several battleships, torpedo planes, and submarines (55). It ended in de Gaulle's defeat and humiliation—he had no choice but to withdraw his forces and leave French West Africa in the hands of the Vichy government. He could not, he said, "shed the blood of Frenchmen for Frenchmen" (Humbert and Mellor 2009: 33). It was this battle that had led Demba's family to evacuate the island when he was an infant.

There were other battles, too. During another conversation, Demba said to me: "Last year—all of last year—I was *in battle.* It was *a battle of titans!* 'A battle of titans', ehm—I read that in a book once . . . what was it called? I used to have lots of books, you know; I would read and read. But most of my books took water during the rains one year and were beyond repair. Ah yes—it was *l'Espoir* by André Malraux. Have you read it?" I shook my head, no, I hadn't read it.[1] More evidence, for Demba, of my hopeless ignorance. "You know," he said impatiently, "Spain, the war, *Guernica,* Picasso . . . ?"

Demba waged his titanic war against a many-headed beast. Things had gotten much worse with his brothers again in recent months. They tormented and persecuted him, he said; they never gave him his fair share. "The walls of my room have started to crumble," Demba said. "I can't really sleep there now, and my brothers refuse to help. I have been moving around a lot, sleeping here and there. To repair my room I'm going to need plaster, cement, and paint. I am looking for money, and when I find some I will go back and work on it more. I'll stay in my room tonight."

"Your room here at the hospital?" I asked.

"No, my room in Rufisque! I CANNOT STAY HERE ALL THE TIME!" Demba was shouting at me now. "This is NOT MY PLACE! I am just here to rest a little until I feel better and then I'll go back. I don't want to stay here so I am not going to stay long. But I don't have any money. I don't have anything to eat. That's why I come here and eat in the cafeteria. Otherwise I would just go back. I don't have any business here! Nothing can cure me here—I am not sick! I am sick with other things."

"What other things?" I asked.

"It's complicated. I am tired, and they say I should stay here a spell to rest. I have other problems. I have these things here on my body [he motions to his lower body] that hurt sometimes and itch. It isn't AIDS or anything like that, they've reassured me. I try to take care of it, but these things bother me all the time. And all the time, it is a question of money (*xaalis*). There is no such thing as madness, really. It's just what happens when you don't have any money! I paint, I write, I am an artist! But I have nothing at all, nothing. Nothing. Look. [He reaches into his right pocket and pulls out a fistful of cigarette butts that he has most likely retrieved from the street.] See this? This is what I have to smoke. I have to eat, too. And I have nothing. See my pants? These are my only pair. See how dirty they are? It isn't normal. Here, it's not my place."

And there was more still. "I'm being troubled by the *djinné* (jinn) again," Demba confided. "This itching, this impotence—that's what this is about. A *djinné* said to me: 'You're going to marry me. Every Friday I will come to you.' So, Friday is the day of my *djinné*. This means that I have to say [to human women]: Adja, be careful, you shouldn't come to my room. And this *femme-djinné* (jinn wife / woman), I can't meet her expectations, so she brings me problems. She says to me: 'All that you want, you will have. Money, every-thing, only you can't take a [human] wife.' And I refuse. And so I have prob-lems. The *djinné*, they want me to drink alcohol, and to smoke *le chanvre* (marijuana), but I don't. You have to choose worlds. It's like *les Al Capones* or the mafia, or *les libre-penseurs* (Free-Thinkers). You have to choose worlds. And then, well, there are always problems."

TWO

Origin Stories

COLLOMB'S FANN AND SENGHOR'S SENEGAL

SHORTLY AFTER THE 1979 DEATH OF DR. HENRI COLLOMB, the French military psychiatrist who had acted as director of the Fann Psychiatric Clinic in Dakar from 1959–78, Senegal's president Léopold Sédar Senghor penned an obituary for the journal *Psychopathologie africaine.*[1] Titled "Henri Collomb (1913–1979) ou l'Art de mourir aux préjugés," the three-page obituary applauded Collomb and his colleagues at Fann for creating an institution that was as uniquely Senegalese as it was distinctively modern (Senghor 1979). In Senghor's view, Fann was nothing less than an exemplary institution of the nascent Senegalese state.

Senghor and others understood the Fann clinic to be innovative in at least two ways. First, Fann represented a departure from the carceral colonial psychiatric practices that had come before it. Second, under Collomb's directorship specifically, Fann's distinct approach to treatment posed a challenge to many of the more conventional Western psychiatric practices of the day. However, it was not simply Fann's divergence from colonial practices or conventional psychiatry that made Senghor take interest in Fann during his presidency. Rather, Senghor hailed Collomb's Fann as an exemplary institution because it embodied and symbolized the new national aesthetic, rooted in Negritude and actualized by *l'Ecole de Dakar* [The Dakar School], thereby demonstrating Senghor's vision of a new kind of Senegalese modernity.

HENRI COLLOMB AND *L'ECOLE DE FANN*

In January 1959, French military doctor and professor Henri Collomb, then 45 years old, was appointed to the Faculty of Medicine of the University of

Dakar. Although he had only just arrived in Senegal, Collomb had worked in sub-Saharan Africa for years. As a member of the Free French Forces, he had begun his oversees career as a military doctor in 1939, first in Djibouti and then in Somalia. He had also worked in Ethiopia, where he served as a doctor for Haile Selassie and his court (as well as for the general population) from 1943–48 (Arnaut 2006; Bullard 2005a). During the early 1950s, Collomb had been stationed in French Indochina.[2] As *professeur agrégé*, Collomb replaced Dr. Jean Rainaut as the director of the Fann Psychiatric Clinic, then known as the *Service de Neuro-Psychiatrie de Fann* because of its joint affiliation with the nearby divisions of neurology and neurosurgery.[3]

Upon his arrival at Fann, Collomb found a relatively conventional psychiatric clinic, by Western standards; this alone was hugely innovative for the colonies. From the layout of the building to its administrative structure and patient care procedures, Fann looked very much like a psychiatric clinic might have looked in France at that time (Martino 1968: 10). Each of the clinic's five divisions was headed by a European doctor and closely monitored by a team of nurses. Doctors examined patients weekly to check their progress. Patients were not permitted to move about the halls unless supervised, and the doors on their rooms were locked from the outside. The clinic was also closed to the exterior, and patients' families and friends had to adhere to strict visiting hours.

Over the next two decades, many changes would take place at Fann. It is fair to say that Collomb and his colleagues' innovative approach to mental health care would prove to be as different from conventional Western psychiatric models as Fann itself had been from *Cap Manuel* and the other colonial psychiatric facilities that had come before it. Reflecting on his first few years at the clinic, Collomb (1976: 11) confided to a Parisian audience at a 1976 conference that "we began [at Fann] with Western psychiatry as it was practiced in Europe during the 1950's and 1960's. The director of the clinic and his colleagues in white examined a patient without worrying too much about the patient's own words, and estimated from his symptoms . . . the degree of his illness."

The approach to mental illness he first brought to Fann, Collomb says, privileged physical symptoms over words, and over the meanings patients attributed to their distress. The patient was more or less treated as a biological organism whose social and cultural environment, interpersonal relationships, and past experiences had little to do with the diagnosis and treatment he or she received. Looking back, Sarr, Seck, and Ba (1997) call this the "organic phase" (*la phase organiciste*) of psychiatry at Fann. Of the articles published by Fann doctors during this time, many included references to mental disorders caused by disease, trauma, or neurological impairment. For example, out of sixteen articles co-authored by Collomb (in collaboration with other psychiatrists and neurologists working at Fann) between 1958 and 1961, seven deal with the effects of epilepsy, lymphatic filariasis, myocardial infarctus, tuberculosis, and alcoholism on mental health. Another two describe the nature of tropical pathologies more generally, and two more deal with the "problems in African psychiatry" and psychiatry in Senegal. Yet another discusses the use of tranquillizers in overseas (*outre-mer*) medical practices. The remaining articles touch on topics like postpartum psychosis and mitral stenosis, acute deliria, homosexuality among Black African Muslims, and the mental problems that affect colonial armies in tropical regions.

For patients at Fann during these early years, the clinic environment—though a far cry from the carceral horror that had been *Cap Manuel*—was sterile and alienating. Aissatou, who began working as a nurse at Fann in 1962 at the age of 23 and has been retired since 1992, recalled that when she first started at the clinic, "patients were still shut up in their rooms. They only got to go outside once or twice each week, and even then, it was only so the rooms could be cleaned." This, however, was all about to change. She continued:

> But then, one day, not long after I began working at Fann, Collomb went down to Casamance [a region in southern Senegal] for the first time to visit with a healer (*guérisseur*). This healer had many [mentally ill] patients in his care, and he let them move about freely. Collomb saw this, and asked the healer, "Why do you let them roam about as they wish?" The healer told Collomb, "If one wants to treat a mentally ill person, one must consider him as one would consider oneself. He should not be isolated. If he is, he will withdraw, pull away. It will be impossible to help him."
>
> As soon as Collomb returned to Fann, he changed everything. He gave the patients their freedom! All at once, he opened the doors, took off the locks, and allowed the patients to move about as they pleased. They were able to go anywhere they wanted; they were able to sit outside, walk around, and talk to each other.

Aissatou admitted that, at first, clinic personnel (herself included) were apprehensive about Collomb's decision to change the clinic in this way. "It was hard for us, at first. We were scared. And yes, there were incidents every now and then. Once a patient hit me over the head with a brick and I lost consciousness. When I opened my eyes, there was blood all over me!" Despite her gruesome story, she insisted that it was much better for the patients to be able to move as they pleased rather than "to be locked in their cells." According to her, Collomb realized just how important this freedom was for his patients. It kept them from feeling too isolated, and in turn, they seemed to recover faster. Notably, Collomb's early visits with healers across Senegal marked the beginning of a long-term collaboration. Collomb paid visits to these healers frequently, and likewise welcomed them to visit the clinic. These were the origin stories upon which the new Fann came to be built.

In 1967, just a few years after Collomb began instituting the abovementioned changes, a Fann psychiatrist named Dr. Daniel Bartoli (1968: 21) wrote that the conventional psychiatric model had not been successful because it was too different from what patients were accustomed to in their everyday lives: "The individual [was] . . . isolated by this structure that was foreign to him. Coming from a collective life, he enter[ed] a world of individual existence. Coming from traditional society, he [was] confronted with a Western way of life." As such, Bartoli explained, hospitalization may itself have been a traumatic experience for many patients—and thus completely counterproductive to the therapeutic process. He contrasted the old model with the way Fann was organized in 1968:

> The hospital is largely open to the exterior, and also on the interior between divisions. Patients go freely throughout the hospital; they come and go as they please. They have constant access to the doctor's offices. Their families almost always have access to the hospital, as well. There are no longer any "visiting hours"; some patients' families spend entire days, and sometimes even nights, with them (23).

According to Bartoli, this new model allowed patients to remain connected (or helped them to reestablish connections) to their social worlds. This, he said, was crucial for the establishment of an effective psychiatric practice in Senegal. Collomb wholeheartedly agreed, writing that "psychiatric care . . . must be inspired by the sociocultural conditions specific to each country" (1965a: 72); therefore, psychiatry in Africa should be "adapted to the realities of African societies" (1967b: 173; see also Collomb 1968).

The trope of African collective life, which was depicted in sharp contrast to the individualization and atomization of life in the West, would become central to Collomb's project at Fann. A key concept that was elaborated upon by Collomb and *l'Ecole de Fann* during the 1960s—but that was also fiercely contested by some members of the group, a point to which I shall return—was that of *le moil de groupe*, or the "group ego," which extended Freud's concept of the ego beyond the individual to include his / her kin and community (Bartoli 1968; see also Parin et al. 1967). Expounding upon this idea, Bartoli (1968: 20) writes that in traditional Senegal, "the individual is part of a group in which he has his place, his role, and his status. His personal history is profoundly affected by this arrangement. The organization of personality and the forms that illness takes are determined by this situation."

Views of an essentialized—and often idealized—"traditional" African life informed Collomb's restructuring of the clinic and guided his reconceptualization of psychiatric care in Senegal.[4] "African existence," Collomb (1967b: 1731) wrote, "is collective; it has not yet submitted to the laws of efficiency and productivity. It is animated by speech, dance and rhythm, communal meals." This essentialist view was reflected in many ethnological accounts of Africa. It was likewise celebrated as both a national aesthetic based on the valorization of Negritude and a state ideology by President Senghor, a point to which I shall return in the last part of the chapter.[5] Crucially, the way "traditional African values and lifeways" were imagined both within Senghor's project and by *l'Ecole de Fann* tended to downplay Islam and its influence as constitutive of "tradition," despite the fact that Islam has been present in the region since the eleventh century, and an estimated 92 percent of Senegal's current population identifies as Muslim.

By the early 1960s, Collomb was calling for a reassessment of the validity and efficacy of Western psychiatric models in non-Western places. The Fann group advocated a new and highly localized kind of psychiatry that not only took patients' social and cultural worlds into account, but allowed itself to be modified by these "other" worlds. The "Western psychiatrist necessarily experiences acculturation," Collomb points out in a 1967 article, and "the observer is modified by his observation. A better approach [to psychiatry in Africa] supposes the abandonment—or at the very least, the modification—of Western frameworks" (1967b: 1723). Below I examine two key facets of the Fann School's innovative approach. I first consider the group's commitment to understanding local exegeses of madness and its cure as the key to building a robust and effective clinical practice at Fann. Here I also discuss the progressive demedicalization of Fann's approach, as well as the group's turn toward psychodynamic methods and psychoanalysis. I then move on to detail the group's efforts to create a culturally informed therapeutic community at Fann.

The Place of Culture in Collomb's Fann: Understanding Local Exegeses of Madness and Suffering

Insisting that mental health research "in very different cultures . . . must include psychosociologists and ethnologists in addition to psychiatrists," Collomb (1967b: 18) began assembling a multidisciplinary team of researchers and specialists at Fann as early as 1962. The predominantly European group, which included anthropologist András Zempléni,[6] psychologist Jacqueline Rabain, psychoanalyst Marie-Cecile Ortigues and her philosopher husband Edmond, Norbert Le Guérinel, Paul Martino, Marie-Thérèse Montagnier, Danielle Storper-Perez, Simone Valantin, and Jacques Zwingelstein, to name but a few, came to be known as *l'Ecole de Fann*. Together, they worked at the interstices of clinical psychiatry, psychoanalysis, ethnography, and the social sciences to pioneer a new approach to mental illness.

René Collignon, a social historian who worked with Collomb at Fann during the 1970s and who has published extensively on the history of psychiatry in Senegal, notes:

> What developed during the 1960's, amongst the analytically-inspired clinicians working Fann, was the realization that . . . the patient was speaking to the foreign doctor through his own culture, and because of this, it was necessary to try to understand the subject's place in what he was saying and in the way he was making use of traditional references (Collignon 2000: 287).

Collomb (1967a: 18) came to believe that "every symptom assumes its true significance only in relationship to a cultural system." Likewise, *l'Ecole de Fann* took the concept of "culture" as its point of departure and sought both to understand local exegeses of mental illness and to integrate these into the clinical experience at Fann. Although Collomb and his colleagues never denied the significance of organic and biological causes of mental problems— Collomb (1967b: 1723) wrote, for example, that "the organic dimension of psychiatry remains very important; this is one of the points that we cannot stress enough"—and always sought to rule these out first, the group focused their attention on the social and cultural dimensions of illness and therapy. Their motivation in this regard was as much philosophical and documentary / archival as it was practical; note the "not yet" in Collomb's statement that "African existence has *not yet* submitted to the laws of efficiency and productivity" (1731; my italics). The Fann group most certainly understood "traditional" culture to be threatened by the rapid social transformation that accompanied modernization, and modernization to be a key contributor to mental distress. Collomb (1976: 11) likewise feared that what he called "traditional psychiatry"—meaning the local explanatory models for mental disturbance and the therapeutic practices in place to cure them—was "at risk of disappearing in favor of modern scientific psychiatry." Motivated by something of a "salvage paradigm" (Baker 1996; Clifford 1989; Russell 1999), the Fann project was committed to the "preservation of negritude values, particularly to the profound and rich humanism that characterizes traditional psychiatry" (Collomb 1976: 11).[7]

Anthropologist András Zempléni, a key figure at Fann from 1962 until 1968, carried out extensive ethnopsychiatric research into local (primarily Wolof and Lebu) interpretations of mental disturbance and suffering. His studies in the domain of ethnopsychiatry, which stand as a hallmark of the Fann School and remain an enduring contribution to anthropology and cross-cultural psychiatry even today, focused primarily upon

> the image that [culture] gives to mental disorders, on the categories of pathology it distinguishes, on the etiology it puts forward, on the relationships it establishes between the phenomena of mental pathology and magico-religious systems, social organization, types of activities, situations it finds traumatizing . . . In short, it [was] about showing what illness and therapy mean within the culture (Zempléni 1968:49).

The term "ethnopsychiatry," first used by Haitian psychiatric Louis Mars (1947; see also Paul Farmer 1992) but popularized by anthropologist / psychoanalysis Georges Devereux in the 1950s and 1960s, refers in part to "the systematic study of the psychiatric theories and practices" of a cultural group—a study of the "folk psychology" of a people (Devereux 1961: 1).[8] In recent years, it should be noted, the term "ethnopsychiatry" has fallen out of favor in most circles. Indeed, "ethnopsychiatry" is today most often equated with: (1) the strand of racist colonial psychiatric research that affirms theories of "primitive mentality" (Lévy-Bruhl 1922) and the "African mind," best typified by J. C. Carothers, or (2) a form of relativistic thinking about culture and madness that fetishizes difference to such an extent that it fails to account for the colonial relations that produced difference in the first place (and in so doing, serves to enforce rather than complicate ideas about cultural otherness and marginalization). As I shall discuss at length in chapter 5, contemporary ethnopsychiatric practice has also found itself at the center of debates about immigration, recognition, difference, and the appropriate provision of mental health care in France (cf. Fassin 1999, 2000; Fassin and Rechtman 2005; Nathan 1994). In spite of these recent debates surrounding the term, however, Zempléni's research is correctly called ethnopsychiatric in that he worked with healers in the Senegambian region to document the locally understood sources and symptoms of mental disorder, as well as the therapeutic techniques healers used to cure the afflicted. Working as part of the Fann group, he explained:

> [M]y task was twofold. First, I was to provide the clinician with whatever useful information I could find concerning those concepts of illness, etiological representations, and therapeutic rites that he encountered in his daily practice [in the Fann clinic] and could not understand. Second, I planned to undertake a monographic study of the traditional system of interpretation of mental disorder among the Wolof and the Lebou (1977: 90).

Zempléni's research into local exegeses of mental affliction played an important role in helping Fann doctors to better understand how patients and their families conceptualized the sources of their suffering. Collomb and the other Fann doctors leaned heavily on the ethnopsychiatric research carried out by Zempléni; they collaborated with him frequently and cited him often. These studies articulated four main locally defined sources of mental disturbance, including *liggeey* (sorcery, spell-casting; French: *maraboutage*), attacks by *dëmm* (witches), possession by *rab* and *tuur* (wild spirits and domesticated spirits, linked to one's lineage), and persecution by *djinné* (or *jinn*, invisible beings or spirits of the Islamic tradition).

Liggeey, a Wolof word meaning "work" (noun) or "to work" (verb) and that is used interchangeably with the words *maraboutage / marabouter* in French, refers to an enchantment that can disturb or harm a person, or make him / her behave in an uncharacteristic manner. Effects of *liggeey* might be physical, mental, or social; a person who falls victim to *liggeey* might suffer any of a number of problems: depression and anxiety, social withdrawal, sterility, sleeplessness, money problems, failed exams, relationship trouble, or—as brilliantly captured by Ousmane Sembene in his 1975 film, *Xala*—impotence. *Liggeey* is performed and can only be cured by a specialist, generally referred to as a *fajkat* or a *marabout*,[9] who usually does so at the request of someone who has sought their services, and typically receives compensation in the form of money or goods (Diop et al. 1966; Martino 1968; Zempléni 1966).

Dëmm (witches, or *sorciers* in French) are described as human men and women who are said to possess extraordinary powers that allow them to fly through the night. They do this, it is said, to prey on people while they sleep and to feed on their vital energy (*fit*), which is located in the liver, or sometimes in the heart, of their victims. It is also said that *dëmm* are impossible to distinguish from friends and neighbors, but they live a secret double life. Depicted as devourers of human flesh, some people say *dëmm* magically but very literally extract and devour human organs. Others insist that their action is purely symbolic—but no less real. Some say that being a *dëmm* is an inherited status, usually passing from one generation to the next on the mother's side; one might be a *dëmm* but not know it. Although some people say that *dëmm* work alone, others insist that they form brotherhoods or secret societies (Martino et at. 1968; Zempléni 1966). When a *dëmm* attacks, the physical symptoms are serious and may even lead to death (Collomb et al. 1964; Martino et al. 1965). According to Dr. Paul Martino (1968: 14), who worked as a psychiatrist at Fann from 1962–69, a person attacked by a *dëmm* is likely to present what looks like an "acute anxiety attack, with or without elements of delirium or confusion." Traditionally, the only person equipped with the power and knowledge to undo such an attack is a *bilejo,* also an inherited role, whose primary function is to expel witches.

The third locally acknowledged source of mental disturbance addressed by Zempléni—and the source that he spent the bulk of his time in Senegal researching and describing—are *tuur. Tuur* are spirits that have been affiliated with a family, usually for many generations. *Tuur* can be benevolent and protective, but if neglected, they can wreak havoc on the human who has failed to properly recognize them, causing illness, miscarriages, and madness. If this happens, the alliance between *tuur* and person (and thus, the lineage) must be reaffirmed. *Tuur* are a subclass of *rab* spirits; that is, all *tuur* are *rab,* but not all *rab* are *tuur.*[10] *Rab* spirits—the Wolof word *rab* means "animal" in English—are usually thought to be wild or untamed, compared to the domesticated *tuur.* A person attacked by a *rab* might fall ill or exhibit uncharacteristic behavior. Symptoms may include impaired motor skills, refusal to eat, unusual bodily pains or sensations, hallucinations, a desire to be alone, or partial paralysis, and may worsen over time if ignored. In order for a person who is being afflicted by a *rab* to regain his or her health, he or she must acknowledge the spirit and establish an alliance with it, not try to exorcise it. The ceremony in which this alliance is forged is called a *ndëpp,* an intensive and complex therapeutic process that lasts for up to seven days and nights.

During the *ndëpp,* the afflicting *rab* is named, affirmed, and praised. Sacrifices are made, and in the end, a type of domestic altar, or *xamb,* is built in which the *rab* (now considered a *tuur*) will reside. From that time on, the afflicted must regularly visit the *xamb* to make sacrifices to his or her *tuur. Ndëpp* ceremonies are always officiated by a *ndëppkat,* or a spirit medium, and attended by family members and others who have gone through the same procedure and are themselves in alliance with one or more *rab* or *tuur.* Members of the community are also invited to attend parts of the ceremony. The *ndëpp* and its attendant rituals and consultations, as Zempléni describes them (e.g., Zempléni 1966, 1967, 1968, 1977) take the form of a complex psychodrama; it is rich in symbolic action, and has the capacity to both transform the afflicted and affirm his or her social and familial relationships.[11]

Djinné (as is often written in Senegal) or *jinn,* are also invisible beings or spirits, but of the Islamic tradition. The extent to which *djinné* are operationally defined by people in and around Dakar as a class of spirits wholly separate from *rab* and *tuur,* however, is a matter of debate. As I was sitting with Demba one day, trying to find clarity with all of this, he grew increasingly frustrated with me. "No!" he said. "You haven't understood a thing! The *rab* are the *djinné,* and the *djinné* are the *rab*! They are the same!" Other friends of mine in Dakar guessed that *rab* was a larger category of invisible beings, and *djinné* were a subgroup. According to the Qur'an, *jinn* are spirits that occupy the world alongside and among humans, often preferring to live near trees or water. Some *jinn* are thought to be kind and sociable, while others are ambivalent to humans. Others still are thought to be malevolent, cruel, and vengeful. In Senegal, *djinné* are thought to have the capacity to transform into animals or to take on human-like form; "some among them derive a delightful pleasure in appearing before humans in a terrifying form," thus provoking fear and mental distress (Diop et al. 1966: 115). They are sometimes described as capricious and they are understood to be attracted to all that is beautiful, flashy, or new— *djinné,* it is said, might fix upon babies or children, material goods, animals, beauty itself, money, a special talent, or a husband or wife, and might try to take these objects of desire as their own. Some *djinné* are even thought to be able to "penetrate humans by way of their orifices and act on them from within" (115). According to Martino (1968: 13), patients persecuted by *djinné* who are seen at Fann present acute episodes of confusion and delirium, often accompanied by disordered behavior. Traditionally, such patients would seek care from *marabouts* who work exclusively with the Qur'an (writing verses of the Qur'an, reciting verses and prayers).

Research into local exegeses of mental disturbance became the backbone of the Fann School's clinical orientation under Collomb's directorship. Importantly, the Fann group did not view these local explanations of madness as mere cultural representations of universally occurring (let alone biomedically defined) mental illnesses that existed underneath it all; their primary objective was not to translate or "make sense" of these manifestations according to a universal (read: Western) psychiatric nosology. From early on at Fann, in fact, Collomb identified such an endeavor as misguided, even fruitless. It was not simply that explanatory models for mental affliction in Senegal differed radically from conventional Western psychiatric understandings, but that clinical presentations of mental distress at Fann—and in the African context more generally—also tended to look very different. What claims to universality could thus be made, and for whose benefit? We can better understand Fann's position vis-à-vis the use of Western psychiatric diagnoses in non-Western contexts by taking a closer look at the group's approach to schizophrenia.

Collomb made frequent note of the absurdly large variation reported in the rate of schizophrenia across the African continent, which ranged "from 15% to 70%, according the period and the diagnosing psychiatrists, for similar populations" (Collomb and Ayats 1962: 592). In Collomb's view, schizophrenia was dramatically overdiagnosed in most African psychiatric hospitals. The reason for this, according to Collomb (1965b), was because patients seen at African psychiatric clinics were more likely to report delusions and hallucinations than their European or North American counterparts, and Western doctors tended to assume these to be indicators of schizophrenia. To Collomb and the Fann doctors, this was a grave mistake; the diagnosis was used sparingly at Fann, and the clinic's rates consistently fell at the lower end of the spectrum.[12]

In the African psychiatric context, Collomb wrote (1965b; see also Ortigues et al. 1967), delusions and hallucinations were common and usually temporary symptoms—they were rarely indicative of psychosis, and patients tended to recover quickly and fully. Collomb and the Fann team leaned heavily on the diagnosis of *bouffées délirantes* [temporary or transitory delusional states] to distinguish these from schizophrenia. *Bouffées délirantes* were described as sudden states of delirium not preceded by other symptoms, but that usually occurred after a traumatic or stressful event, such as an accident or the death of a loved one (Collomb 1965b). Delusions and hallucinations commonly accompanied these states of heightened anxiety, but importantly, patients experiencing them "were often conscious of their troubles and sought quick assistance" (Collomb and Ayats 1962: 592). To Collomb and his team, it was clear that conventional categorical distinctions in Western psychiatry between neurosis and psychosis simply did not hold up in this context. "True" schizophrenia did exist—and Fann doctors tended to link the presentation of "true" schizophrenia to rapid modernization, urbanization, and social change (Centre Hospitalier 1968; see also Corin and Murphy 1979)—but, they insisted, it tended to present as "autism, a progressive withering of social contacts, and an eventual vegetative inertia" (Collomb and Ayats 1962: 591). Other "atypical" symptom presentations at Fann included what Collomb and Ayats described as "anxiety states accompanied by severe somatic or vegetative phenomenon" (591). Delusions of persecution were common; melancholic depression was seen to be rare. For Collomb and *L'Ecole de Fann*, the key to creating a valid and effective psychiatric practice in Senegal—and especially, to relieving the suffering of their patients and reintegrating them into their social worlds—rested less on the establishment of a symptom-based diagnosis that was in accordance with, or could be translated into, a Western psychiatric nosology than it did on understanding the local explanations for mental distress that informed and shaped their patients' suffering, and also taking seriously the therapeutic approaches that could treat them.

The Demedicalization of Fann's Approach and the Turn toward Psychodynamics

In the 1975 article "Histoire de la Psychiatrie en Afrique Noire Francophone," Collomb wrote that Fann's reconceptualization of psychiatry was under way even before it was phrased as such. A significant part of this move, explained Collomb, was the demedicalization of Fann's theoretical approach—he asserts, for example, that "African psychiatry . . . is liberating itself from the influence of biomedicine and taking its place among the human sciences" (Collomb 1975: 100). Throughout the 1960s, Collomb and others lobbied for the formal separation of Fann's psychiatric services from those of neurology; in 1970, the clinics were finally divided in two. According to Couloubaly (1997: 217), this marked the moment psychiatry in Senegal formally and definitively "disengage[d] itself from the medical model."

There were other important innovators working in the domain of psychiatry during the early post-independence years in sub-Saharan Africa, including T. Adeoye Lambo and his colleagues at the Aro psychiatric hospital in Abeokuta, Nigeria. Like Collomb and the Fann School, they were also key figures in the emergence of transcultural psychiatry. Importantly, however, Lambo would come to reject psychodynamic approaches (and especially psychoanalysis) as unsuitable—even suspect—for use within African contexts (Heaton 2013). Instead, he and his colleagues firmly embraced the medical model—and with it, psychiatry's claim to universality—in an effort to depathologize the African psyche and decolonize psychiatric thought itself. It was by taking up the medical model and amending psychiatric thought and practice from within that Lambo and his colleagues strove to make it a *truly* universal medico-scientific endeavor.

In contrast, a key innovation of the Fann School was its centering of the psychodynamic approach. Already in the early 1960s, the Fann group was emphasizing the importance of determining the cultural meaning and structural significance of a given linguistic sign (Collomb 1975) as the group's members strove to integrate the lived cultural realities of their patients— socialization processes, family structure and relational dynamics, belief in the existence of spirits that affect the everyday lives of the living—into their everyday practice. The group also experimented with psychoanalysis. To illustrate how spirits and spirit possession were refracted through psychoanalysis, I turn now to a discussion of *Oedipe Africain* (1966), a psychoanalytic study published by French psychologist Marie-Cécile and her philosopher husband, Edmond Ortigues, based on Marie-Cécile's clinical experiences working as an analyst at Fann from 1962–66.

Oedipe Africain reflects the Ortigues' concern with the effects of modernization and acculturation on the psyches and subjectivities of Marie-Cécile's African analysands, which was a topic of shared preoccupation among many members of the Fann School. Their work, however, rejected any notion of a "moi de groupe" or group ego (e.g., Parin et al. 1967)—a point which set them apart from some of their colleagues at Fann—and demonstrated a "dedication to hearing and to helping emerge the voices of individuals" in consultation (Bullard 2005b: 178). In *Oedipe Africain,* the central theoretical task of the pair was to engage with and reformulate the way that Freud (and psychoanalytic theory more generally) had conceptualized the Oedipus complex, and also test the presumed universality of the complex. Critical of the fact that it suggested a belief in the universal attitudes of real persons in real situations, the Ortigues took a Lacanian-inspired approach and instead considered the Oedipus complex in structural terms.[13] From this perspective, things do not have or produce meaning in themselves but through their relationships with other things; it is therefore the structure—not the variables that occupy the structure—that determines meaning. The Ortigues, following Lacan, asserted that the Oedipus complex must be approached not as a negotiation between three real people [mother-father-child], but as a structure of intersecting relationships in which the loci are empty spaces. By shifting the center of meaning to a "fourth term" [the structure itself], the Oedipus complex could thus be approached as a system in which the person [the father] comes to be replaced by the function of the sign [the phallus] (M.-C. Ortigues and E. Ortigues 1966: 72). Viewing the Oedipus complex thus—in terms of the function of the phallus and the Symbolic "law of the father" that extends beyond the relationship of one individual to another and prescribes relationships of power, authority, and recognition within a society—the Ortigues postulated that the Oedipus structure reveals itself in Senegal through its "explicit, central, and incontestable" reference to a Symbolic father that is quite different than that which they had encountered in Europe (57). The position of the Symbolic father in Senegal, wrote the Ortigues, is marked by ancestors and spirits (151). The father is, in effect, subsumed into and part of this order, himself taking his place as an *"ancêtre inégalable"* (an unchallengeable ancestor). In this context, the resolution of the Oedipal conflict is a negative one: rivalry, aggression, and competition between son and father are displaced horizontally onto the brothers, but this aggression is then overcompensated by a powerful solidarity.

It is from this perspective that the Ortigues sought to understand spirit possession and its link to mental illness in Senegal. Ancestors and spirits obviously played an important role in everyday life in Senegal; their existence was not a matter of debate. Belief in the earthly presence of spirits, the Ortigues repeatedly asserted, was obviously not pathological in Senegal. Spirit sickness, however—the physical and emotional manifestation of symptoms that are attributed to a spirit—does signal a problem. According to the Ortigues, because ancestors and spirits mark the position of the Symbolic father, a problem in one's relationship with these ancestors or spirits signals a problem in one's ability to integrate oneself into the Symbolic Order. Spirit possession thus marks the subject's struggle to come to terms with the "law of the father" (M.-C. Ortigues and E. Ortigues 1966: 193).

One of the cases of spirit possession presented by the Ortigues in *Oedipe Africain* is that of a 14-year-old boy named Talla. Talla's possession experience is described in detail, from the violent onset of symptoms and his profound fear of the visions, dreams, and hallucinations he was having, to the identification and naming of the *rab* who possessed him, the sacrifices offered to the *rab*, the building of a domestic shrine (*xamb*), and finally, to his recovery. By accepting his possession, identifying the spirits responsible for the attack, affirming his place within his lineage, and securing an alliance with those spirits, the Ortigues write, Talla was able to integrate himself into the Symbolic Order and thus return to a state of good health. Thirty-four-year-old Omar, however, was not so lucky. For him, spirits referencing the position of the father remained unnamable and unknowable. Omar's hallucinations of a nameless, human-like form trying to enter his body soon gave way to images of his own *corps morcelé*. Unable to integrate himself into the Symbolic Order, he was described by the Ortigues as manifesting severe psychosis (M.-C. Ortigues and E. Ortigues 1966: 198–223).

A key point made by the Ortigues in *Oedipe Africain*, then, was that psychoanalysis "had to be stripped down to its barest structural formulation in order to give a convincing account of a universal psychic structure in the face of manifest cultural differences"; as a theoretical formulation, it was more helpful as a map that could "guide psychoanalytic practice with individual patients" than as an anchor with which "to ground the idea of a universal human psyche" (Lock and Nguyen 2010: 172–73). Beyond this, the study also offered rich commentary on the difficulties of cross-cultural psychoanalysis—especially in postcolonial settings. Bullard (2005b: 175), in fact, has noted that a lasting contribution of *Oedipe Africain* is its "honest confrontation with the strains and difficulties of providing therapy in this post-colonial and transcultural situation—a situation in which language, social structure and race created obstacles to transparent therapist-client relationships."

Creating a New Kind of Therapeutic Community at Fann

As Collomb and *l'Ecole de Dakar* modified the physical space of the clinic and opened new lines of theoretical inquiry about mental illness in Senegal, they also transformed their practical approach to treatment and therapy, implementing several innovative practices into Fann's repertoire. According to Fann psychiatrist Momar Guèye (1984: 2), "Opening the doors of the clinic," along with "introducing patient's families, and instating group therapy sessions that resembled village meetings . . . allowed for the possibility of having human relationships within the psychiatric hospital." In the mid-1960s, Collomb and his colleagues instituted weekly group therapy sessions, called *pénc* meetings. In 1971, the clinic began requiring patients to have a family member or friend (*un accompagnant*) stay with them for the period of their hospitalization. These practices, along with the introduction of frequent communal meals and tea (*attaya*) sessions, doll crafting, games, theater productions, a monthly newspaper initiated by patients, art therapy, and a number of other activities, laid the foundation for the creation of a new kind of therapeutic community at Fann (Dorès and Tourame 1975; Sylla et al. 2002; Tripet 1968).

Notable was the group's effort to integrate locally recognizable and ordinary ("African") cultural practices into this clinical setting, amidst an array of other creative and occupational activities that emphasized creative self-expression, especially through art and writing. While this integration was certainly motivated by a desire to bring culturally familiar elements into the clinic in a way that would keep patients (and their family members) from feeling alienated or isolated, one could also argue that the decontextualization and rescripting of local forms as "craft" or "hobby" and "authentically African ways of being" (always amidst other possibilities) played an important role in transforming the subjectivities and sensibilities of Fann patients, and that Fann's emphasis on creative self-expression privileged a very historically and culturally specific version of the "self"—autonomous, individualized, and equipped with rational self-awareness and the power of reflection—that was crucial to Fann's rising psychotherapeutic orientation.

Pénc *Meetings and the* Accompagnant *Policy*

Named *pénc* after the Wolof word meaning "village meeting or gathering," the town hall–type meetings were designed to create a village-like sense of community within the clinic. Here again the notion of collective African life was invoked; *pénc* meetings were described as having been designed "in the image of the traditional African village" (Dia 1977: 373). The intention of these meetings was to allow patients a forum in which they might come together and share their stories, problems, complaints, and experiences. Patients' family members, guests, psychiatrists, psychologists, nurses, social workers, researchers, and visitors were invited to attend and participate, for at this time, destigmatizing mental illness and helping patients reestablish connections to their social worlds was deemed crucial to an effective therapy at Fann.

At *pénc* gatherings, patients were encouraged to speak up and out—at the doctors, about each other, about Fann, or about the world outside. From the beginning, the desired result of the *pénc* was to foster a collective affirmation, validation, and sense of liberatory speech (Dia 1976, 1977; Dia et al. 1976; Collomb 1975). What remained more or less uninterrogated as the *pénc* concept was folded into the clinic, however, was the fact that the village gatherings upon which the meetings were modeled were, at their origin, far from egalitarian affairs. Participation (and power relations more generally) reflected a gendered and generational divide that allowed some voices (older male voices, in particular) to speak and be heard while others were silenced. I shall elaborate upon this contradiction and its practical consequences in chapter 6, when I discuss the clinic's *pénc* meetings in greater ethnographic and analytic detail.

While *pénc* gatherings were described by many at Fann as a unique and distinctly Senegalese addition to the clinic, it should be noted that meetings following a similar format—and also aimed at egalitarian participation and liberatory speech—did exist elsewhere. In Gorizia, Italy, for example, radical Italian psychiatrist Franco Basaglia also instituted "town meetings" during the 1960s.[14] Although never formally aligned with Basaglia's radical psychiatry in Italy or with the anti-psychiatry movement[15] that was gaining momentum in Europe and the United States during the same time, Collomb's position vis-à-vis conventional psychiatry—as well as some of the changes that he instituted at Fann—intersected with such ideas and movements in a number of ways, leading famed contemporary ethnopsychiatrist Tobie Nathan (1997: 11) to surmise that the philosophical and practical approach espoused by the Fann School "oscillated . . . between . . . antipsychiatry on the one hand (represented more or less by Collomb), and Lacanian psychoanalysis on the other." Although my own analysis of the clinic's past has led me to envisage a more complex—and less dramatic or extreme—picture than Nathan's, his work nevertheless gestures toward the uniqueness of the Fann project.

In addition to instituting weekly *pénc* sessions, Collomb and his colleagues believed that patients had a better chance of recovery—and were more likely to be reintegrated into their communities after their hospitalization—when they were accompanied by a family member or friend for the duration of their stay at Fann. The *accompagnant* policy was formalized at Fann in 1972; from that time, patients were required to have a family member or close friend stay with them during their hospitalization, which at that time tended to be between one and three months. At its inception, the *accompagnant* policy attempted to institutionalize a moral economy of family caretaking and therapy management in the clinic, which doctors justified by claiming the policy's genesis in "traditional" African ways of life. The policy emphasized the need for an active family presence in the clinic, and demanded the full-time attention of one family member to *the work of care*. This caretaking was, of course, unremunerated; it was a sacrifice the family was expected to make on behalf of the patient.

The two earliest and most comprehensive articles about the *accompagnant* policy (Diop and Dorès 1976; Gbikpi and Auguin 1978) were written by specialists who worked at Fann in the years after its implementation. Diop and Dorès (1976) note that from the policy's inception, female patients were required to have female *accompagnants*; male patients could have either a female or male *accompagnant*. In practice, though, *accompagnants* were usually women, and Diop and Dorès offer several reasons for this. In a way that thoroughly reflected their own culturally informed assumptions about gender, work, kinship, and family life, they assert that female family members were more likely to be available because they were less likely to be working outside the home. Women, they explain, could usually leave their homes in the hands of co-spouses, sisters, or daughters while they were away. In any case, Diop and Dorès tell us, doctors preferred women over men because they were perceived as being cleaner, more skilled at caretaking, and better able to contribute readily to the ambiance of the clinic. They were also more willing and able to perform light domestic duties, such as laundry and cooking (1976: 360).

An important question, however, is why *accompagnants* were deemed necessary in the first place. First, doctors thought that the full-time presence of a family member would keep patients from feeling isolated and estranged; the *accompagnant* would act as a touchstone of sorts. Keeping the patient connected to her social world meant that she would be less likely to experience her stay at Fann as an additional trauma of institutionalization. An interesting point made by Diop and Dorès (1976: 360) is that *accompagnants* comprised an important third group in the clinic—a group whom they call *"non-soignants non-fous"*—that consisted of neither caregivers nor patients. This was crucially important, as it meant that they brought the attitudes and habits of everyday life into the institution. As Gbikpi and Auguin (1978: 8) note, the presence of *accompagnants* helped transform the clinic from a community of patients into one that more closely resembled the world outside. *Accompagnants* spent time not only with the patients but with each other; their presence at the clinic created a more relaxed atmosphere. As the *accompagnants* formed relationships among themselves, helped one another, told stories, and simply went about their daily tasks, their actions modeled "normal" behavior to the patients and contributed to a sense of community in which the patients could also participate (Diop and Dorès 1976: 361).

The *accompagnant* also played a central role in the treatment of her patient. Not only did she bear witness to and support the process of recovery, she also helped the patient accept her hospitalization as well as the course of therapy prescribed by doctors. Further, the *accompagnant* made sure the patient was eating and sleeping properly and taking her medication as directed; she even administered dosages and helped the patient to bathe, get dressed, clean their room, and use the restroom (Diop and Dorès 1976: 360). The *accompagnant* was able to monitor the patient's day-to-day progress and report any problems that might arise. "Things that happen when the staff is not around, especially at night, do not escape [the *accompagnant*]. He can, therefore, intervene to end a dispute, calm an anxious patient, call a nurse or guard" (361). In this sense, the *accompagnant* acted as both an advocate for the patient and an assistant to the staff. And because *accompagnant*s took charge of many of the quotidian responsibilities of the nurses and other staff, the latter were, in theory, better able to devote their time to the more critical problems that arose in the clinic (Gbikpi and Auguin 1978: 13).

Another important role played by the *accompagnant* at Fann was that of liaison between the clinic and the family. As a translator of sorts, the *accompagnant* was charged with the duty of making sure the rest of the family understood both the terms of the patient's psychiatric diagnosis and also the measures taken to bring about her recovery. The *accompagnant* kept the family involved and aware of the patient's condition; her familiarity with the clinic helped to demystify both psychiatry and Fann itself. Further, patients' families tended to visit more often when an *accompagnant* was on site (Diop and Dorès 1976; Gbikpi and Auguin 1978).

For the psychodynamically oriented Fann clinic of the 1970s, the constant presence of *accompagnant*s brought another important benefit as well. Above all, Fann doctors thought that the careful observation of the patient-*accompagnant* relationship could elicit valuable information about the relational dynamics that existed between patient and family (Diop and Dorès 1976: 362). Most notably, in cases where the patient's *accompagnant* was his mother or father, Diop and Dorès write that there was a "strong temptation to privilege the study of early childhood, and in particular, problems of identification" (363). From the doctors' perspective, issues arising during the early psychosexual development of the child were a significant factor in the patient's manifestation of neurosis. Displaying an interesting choice of words given the context of their discussion, Diop and Dorès note that, by way of the *accompagnant*, Fann staff were able to "penetrate" family life (*"Par son intermédiare, il pénètre dans les familles"*) (362). Likewise, Gbikpi and Auguin (1978:13) write that the presence of the *accompagnant* allowed the doctors to "penetrate the patient's environment in order to better understand the origins of his illness" (*"Pénétrer l'environnement du malade afin de mieux saisir la genèse de la maladie"*). From this perspective, the presence of the *accompagnant* offered a privileged window into the patient's primary relationships and furnished clues about the very source of the patient's suffering, thus the *accompagnant* could and should be used as a "therapeutic tool" (67).

Although the general consensus among doctors and staff regarding the *accompagnant* policy was favorable from the start, relationships between *accompagnants* and their patients—as well as between *accompagnants* and staff—were not without problems (Diop and Dorès 1976: 361). Gbikpi and Auguin (1978) relate that many unforeseen difficulties had already arisen in the seven years since the policy had been instated. In cases where the *accompagnant's* relationship with the patient was a central source of conflict (as when the *accompagnant* was the patient's abusive parent) or when the *accompagnant* was subjected to the same sources of family conflict as the patient (as siblings often were), treatment was all the more difficult to navigate because doctors and staff had to intervene in these relationships and take care not to exacerbate existing conflicts. Having these relationships present at the hospital was useful but also dangerous. At the clinic, Gbikpi and Auguin relate, "the *accompagnant* is still too often perceived as a *sane* representative of the family who has come to help the *patient* . . . get better" (67). In that mental illness likely stems from these troubled relations, they explain, Fann doctors and staff should concentrate on these relationships, rather than on the patients themselves, as the site of illness.

Other challenges arose from the new practice as well. *Accompagnants* sometimes experienced difficulties adapting to life in the hospital. In some cases, they clashed with the staff, making the latter's work all the more difficult (Diop and Dorès 1976: 362). Sometimes, the *accompagnants* would just leave. Most notably, Gbikpi and Auguin (1978: 56) relate that an unexpectedly high number of *accompagnants* themselves suffered from serious mental disturbances that were revealed during the period of their stay at Fann, and a few even required treatment. *Accompagnants* often voiced somatic complaints and suffered from insomnia (Diop and Dorès 1976: 362). If not approached with care, Gbikpi and Auguin (1978: 67) warned, the practice could result in making manifest a psychiatric condition within the *accompagnant* herself and "sending two ill people (*malades*) back to the family instead of one."

Despite these issues and problems, the *accompagnant* policy became—and continues to be recognized as—one of the trademark innovations of Collomb's Fann. According to Diop and Dorès, there was a substantial difference between the patients who were hospitalized alone and those who were interned alongside an *accompagnant*. For the latter, clinic stays tended to be shorter, relapses occurred much less frequently and outpatient check-up appointments were kept more often (Diop and Dorès 1976: 362).

Art Therapy and Pinthioum Fann, *the Patients' Newspaper*

In a 1968 paper, Swiss psychoanalyst Lise Tripet described the work she had recently concluded at Fann in the domain of art therapy. During a three-month period, she had explored artistic expression—especially painting—with a dozen or so patients. In an effort to build a new kind of therapeutic community at Fann during the 1960s, the Fann group had integrated art into the repertoire of activities offered to patients. Importantly, however, art therapy was not imagined by the Fann group as a simple occupational exercise, but rather as a therapeutic technique with rich psychoanalytic potential. Tripet (1968: 420) reflected on what motivated patients to choose painting over these other activities at Fann, noting that while "the need for company, and to get cigarettes" was certainly a factor, most patients also seemed to be in search of something more; pictorial expression, she suggested, may offer patients a means to and a pathway for expressing that which they are not able to express otherwise. In her paper, Tripet presents an in-depth exploration of the illness stories and artwork of five patients; in so doing, she comes to two conclusions. On the one hand, she writes, "messages transmitted by way of pictorial expression are of a universal character" and tend to "reveal basic existential needs" (447). On the other hand, she insists, it is imperative to be familiar with the "cultural references" made by patients in order to truly grasp the works of art that they produce. Maintaining this dialectic and keeping both of these principles in sight at once, she explains, is crucial to the therapeutic endeavor (448). During her time working at the Fann clinic, Tripet also organized an exhibit of artistic works produced by Fann patients; the exhibit was displayed for the occasion of the second Pan-African Psychiatry Congress in Dakar in 1968.[16]

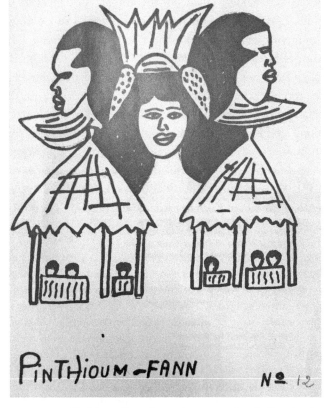

FIGURE 5. *Pinthioum Fann* (journal cover, undated). Drawing by Demba / Magatte Ndiaye.

Another remarkable initiative taken up at the clinic during the 1960s was *Pinthioum Fann,* a newspaper produced by patients and, for a time, circulated on a monthly basis. In *Pinthioum Fann,* poetry, prose, and cartoons took their place alongside news stories and reports on current events—almost exclusively written by patients. Articles and features covered topics ranging from philosophy and culture to politics, to daily life within the clinic, and to details of the clinic's weekly *pénc* meetings. Patients and staff alike made up the paper's editorial board; the renowned Senegalese author and playwright Abdou Anta Ka, who had himself been an inpatient at Fann during the mid-1960s, served as its editor for a period.[17] The newspaper was sold in front of the hospital entrance for 200 fcfa (40 U. S. cents) and according to a retired nurse named Seynabou, it was even distributed to sites outside of Senegal, including psychiatric clinics in France and the United States. Yearly subscriptions were made available for the sum of 6,000 fcfa ($12 USD, for a regular subscription) or 10,000 fcfa ($20 USD, for a supporting subscription). The money generated from the sales of the *Pinthioum Fann* went toward the production of future issues.

Although I was not able to find information about the number of copies sold or the revenue generated by the newspaper, or even confirm the number of issues that were published as part of this initiative, several *Pinthioum Fann* publications have been preserved and archived in the Fann's small onsite document center. One of these preserved issues, dated from November 1970 (issue 19), leads with an unsigned editorial stating that the paper was starting up again after a period of involuntary suspension. The editorial reflects on the importance of *Pinthioum Fann* to patients, and describes the positive impact of the paper both within and outside of the clinic:

> [I]t took the involuntary suspension of *Pinthioum Fann* to realize how much our newspaper was appreciated by its readers, and how useful it has been both inside and outside of the Fann Hospital. The contents of *Pinthioum Fann* have significantly changed the way caregivers and stewards behave toward the sick / patients [*les malades*]. Because of *Pinthioum Fann*, patients no longer appear as beings rejected by society: beings apart, less than nothing, that one can rebuff at will, neglect, scorn, or flee, or treat as a source of entertainment, or of a laughter that wounds ... In terms of treatment, *Pinthioum Fann*'s articles on the socio-cultural aspects of African life allow the white doctors to better understand African beliefs. To this effect, *Pinthioum Fann* has even suggested in an editorial that a roundtable of psychiatrists and healers be held ... so that traditional methods of curing mental illness will not be lost with the disappearance of the healers. *Pinthioum Fann* also plays an important role within the psychiatric divisions. It is a form of entertainment for patients; it strengthens relationships between patients and staff ... This social dimension of *Pinthioum Fann* delivers the patient from his isolation. (*Pinthioum Fann* 1970: 2).

The same issue of *Pinthioum Fann* featured an obituary of a renowned healer, Demba Boudy Faye, written by Collomb. Collomb had attended Faye's funeral in Mauritania, he wrote, because he had owed it to this man who had been his friend for so many years, and who embodied, for him, a "completeness of being in harmony with the world" (3). The issue also featured a summary of a *pénc* session that had taken place in October, during which two attending healers from northern Senegal, Ousmane Ba and Abdoulaye Wane, praised Collomb and his colleagues for the work they were doing at Fann, and for the fact that patients moved about freely and lived "en famille." The healers noted that a clinic like Fann should be established in the North, and told the group that they were ready to commit their own resources to make it happen. Wane was quoted in the piece: "Your methods have seduced us, Professor Collomb. I am ready to make a large contribution to the construction of a clinic where we will collaborate together" (7). For his part, Ba noted that he would commit "10 heads of cattle, sheep" and likewise help "to dig a well, to weed the site where this clinic would be built, and to make sure it was maintained properly" (7). Ba said that he would contribute food and milk to feed the patients being cared for within the clinic.

According to Seynabou, *Pinthioum Fann* was only sporadically printed after the late 1970s because the money needed to keep it going was getting harder to come by, and also because patient and staff support had dwindled. Still, though, this publication is remarkable because it both describes and itself stands as an artifact of an extraordinary moment in Fann's history.

Living by Its Illusions (The Fronts and Backs of Things)

In a 1972 article, Collomb wrote:

> If modern psychiatry remains shut up within its own walls, it condemns itself to reclusion and to the impossibility of establishing contact between the caregiver, the patient and his environment. Modern psychiatry will then live by its illusions, by means of neuroleptics and electroshock, and will discover, in twenty or thirty years, that it has not made the least bit of progress..., that it has not accomplished its mission. (1972: 34)

The above statement is well aligned with the philosophy of care that was embraced and celebrated by the Fann group. It gestures toward the necessary demedicalization of psychiatry as well as the need to help patients reestablish connections to their social worlds; it speaks to the forms of attentiveness that were cultivated at Fann vis-à-vis the social and cultural dimensions of mental illness and therapy. Reading it, one might be led to believe that Collomb and his colleagues rejected the use of both psychopharmaceuticals and electroshock treatment outright. This was not the case, and it is crucial to complicate the narrative that has, up to this point, stressed the innovation, demedicalization, and cultural sensitivity of Fann's early approach. This is a point, then, where I must unsettle the very narrative that I am writing here.

In 1981, Georges Zeldine, who worked as a psychiatrist at Fann between 1972 and 1974, published an article titled "Un témoinage sur Fann" ("A

Testimony on Fann"). Although he had written the article back in 1974, he says in the introduction, he purposefully waited until after Collomb's death to publish it. The article stands as the most critical—even iconoclastic—piece written about the early years of the Fann clinic. It is clear that Zeldine intends to tell a different kind of story about Fann, one that might serve as a counterpoint to the unending praise the clinic had received over the years, both nationally and internationally. Perhaps Zeldine had a bone to pick with Collomb; perhaps he was disgruntled or disillusioned, or himself seeking attention. The feel of the piece oscillates between melancholic and vengeful. The article has made me reflect upon the fronts and backs of things—fronts that are meant for show and display, and backs that are just as central, just as important, but are meant to be hidden from view. Stories, too, have fronts and backs like this.

Zeldine criticizes the weight of Collomb's legacy, as well as what he perceives to be the misguided therapeutic ventures, like *pénc* sessions, undertaken by the Fann School. He notes the degraded conditions of the clinic. Above all, he criticizes the story that Fann had been telling about itself for so long—the story upon which its reputation was built and that Western audiences in particular loved to consume—about the liberation of madness and the successful adaptation of psychiatry to African realities at Fann. Zeldine points to the willful blindness of this view, insisting that while *pénc* sessions were celebrated as a key therapeutic tool (and a crowning achievement) of Collomb's Fann, neuroleptic medications and electroshock therapy were still very much a part of the clinic's therapeutic repertoire. "If the *pénc* sessions were weekly, dazzling, with cameras purring in the background . . . neuroleptic medication was daily and occurred in silence" (Zeldine 1981: 143). This is an important and valid critique. One need only cast a quick glance at Collignon's (1978) excellent annotated bibliography of works written and published by *l'Ecole de Fann* during the clinic's early years to see numerous notes regarding the use and study of neuroleptics, antidepressants, tranquilizers, and other psychotropic medications.

In his 1965 article on *bouffées délirantes*, Collomb himself mentions the use of both neuroleptics and electroshock therapy in the treatment of afflicted patients, touting the "remarkable efficacy" of electroshock treatment in particular: "The importance allotted to electroshock might come as a surprise. More than half of our patients are treated with electroshock therapy. Our positive daily outcomes with this procedure justify this course of treatment" (1965b: 214). In an interview with Hubert Fichte, a German ethnologist who visited Fann in 1974 with his photographer partner, Leonore Mau, Collomb goes even further to justify the treatment. While the clinic attempted to treat patients without the use of antipsychotic medications or electroshock therapy, Collomb notes, "sometimes electroshock treatment satisfies the desire for an initiatory death, like a symbolic death, something that in traditional African societies precedes every new phase of transformation or development, and that can take place at the start of a psychiatric illness as much as it can signify the healing of it" (Fichte 1980: 26, cited in Deliss 2011: 231). Here, Collomb makes recourse to a particular imaginary of the rituals and symbols of "traditional Africa" in order to depict Fann's use of electroshock therapy as culturally meaningful and thus appropriate, thereby justifying this very violent form of "care."

Leonore Mau photographed treatments during that visit. Many years later, in an interview for the art magazine *O32c*, the photographer was asked about her encounter with electroshock therapy at Fann. She responded: "I thought to myself, 'You have to photograph this.' This [electroshock treatment] is something that Collomb had actually declared inappropriate for the hospital in Fann. But there was still an old pavilion in which that was done. It was horrible. The plug was simply stuck in the socket in the wall and then something broke in the brain" (Niermann 2005: 114). If the front of the story of the early years of Fann—the part that is commonly told and celebrated—is about the demedicalization of psychiatry and the establishment of culturally specific forms of therapy within the clinic, this is the back story, often concealed from view.

There is another "back story" as well. A few years after the Fann clinic was established, a closed psychiatric hospital was built in a suburb of Dakar called Thiaroye. Thiaroye was not like Fann. Progressive stories of openness and care did not abound there. The facility was designated for patients who were deemed incurable, patients who were committed under court order, patients who presented a danger to themselves or others (Storper-Perez 1974). It was distant from Fann and, as such, hidden from everyday view. Yet the facility was also crucial to what Fann itself would become and the reputation it would garner, because the sickest and most difficult to treat patients ended up there. In Collomb's 1965 article on *bouffées délirantes*, at the end of a section in which he describes the excellent recovery rate of Fann patients thus afflicted, he asks the question: "What is the future of those patients that are not cured?" Some, he explains, are taken home and cared for by their families, and are seen regularly on an outpatient basis. Others, he writes, "(those who are rejected by their family or isolated) are transferred to a psychiatric service for chronic cases *(service des chroniques* [Thiaroye]*)* where therapeutic activity (other than the administration of neuroleptics) is somewhat limited" (1965b: 212). Collomb and the Fann School took pride in their ability to distance themselves from the carceral colonial regime and conventional psychiatric practices that had come before them, but in reality, they were still entangled in them.

Collomb's Politics

Fann *was* a product of the late colonial regime, and Collomb *was* a French military doctor who had assumed his position in Dakar before Senegal's independence. Nevertheless, Collomb would come to define the Fann project as a radical departure from colonial psychiatric practices in sub-Saharan Africa. Colonial psychiatry, he insisted, had been *at the service of* colonial regimes of power. Collomb distanced himself—and the Fann School—from this tradition. In 1975, for instance, he reflected that

> [t]he colonizer . . . had but one attitude: superiority, which necessarily led to a false vision of the other, the colonized. The other was not only different but was denied his values, his culture, and his skills. The colonizer's gaze did not see him as an equal . . . but as an inferior being who had a long road to travel to attain the level of the white man; even his capacity to travel the road was contested. This racial dogmatism shaped attitudes, behaviors, and observational biases and elaborated baseless rationalizations. . . . The doctors who accompanied the colonizers had a similar attitude, though perhaps tempered by the ethics of their profession. (1975: 93)

Here Collomb denounces the colonial project, distancing himself from both its politics and its psychiatric practices and marking himself as an independence-era (even anticolonial) innovator. He follows this with a statement that speaks volumes about the philosophical approach undergirding his clinical practice. He states that in the postcolonial era, "racial dogmatism" has come to be replaced by "a doctrine that is less destructive from the point of view of human relations, but almost as dangerous from a scientific perspective: the dogmatism of equivalence (*le dogmatisme égalitaire)*" (93). The rightful assertion that all people are equal, he says, is often twisted into an assumption and expectation that all people are—or should be—the same. In the interest of equality, *difference* somehow becomes unspeakable. But, Collomb seems to be asking here, can there not be both difference *and* equality? Contemporary readers may indeed cringe at such an idea—many are surely reminded of the "separate but equal" doctrine that underpinned Jim Crow–era segregation in the United States—but questions related to how difference gets recognized, acknowledged, neutralized, and assimilated, especially in multicultural liberal democracies, have been at the forefront of debate in recent years (Coulthard 2007, 2014; Fassin 1999; Fassin and Rechtman 2005; Giordano 2014, 2015; Povinelli 2002; Taylor 1994). In that conventional Western psychiatry assumes itself to be universal and based upon the belief that all people experience mental illness and respond to treatment in the same way, it fails to recognize alternative ontologies and epistemologies of health, illness, and healing. Is this not, Collomb seems to be asking, an act of violence in and of itself?

Of course, the end of colonial rule in Senegal was a *fait accompli* by the time Collomb penned these words, and it is important to note that Collomb was not nearly as trenchant in his critique of colonialism earlier on in his career. Like Rainaut before him, it might be more appropriate to call Collomb a colonial liberal than an anticolonial radical. In chapter 4, I shall say more about the parallels and points of contrast between Collomb's work and that of Frantz Fanon; here I shall say only that while both men were critical of the universalizing tendencies of Western psychiatry, Collomb did not overtly frame his work at Fann within a larger political project. He was not a political figure. In an article that stands as the only sustained comparison between the work of Collomb and Fanon, Alice Bullard (2005a: 241) similarly remarks that "Collomb largely segregated his psychiatry from political events." This is not to say, however, that Collomb's work existed in a political vacuum, or that it was not influenced by the politics of the day and, in turn, put to political use. As the Fann group came to understand conventional Western psychiatric models to be limited in their ability to address and treat mental illness in Senegal, they entered their practice into conversation with—and allowed it to be modified by—local exegeses of madness and therapy, and by "culture" itself. This was a key point at which Collomb's project at Fann intersected with Senghor's vision for Senegal, and it was for this reason that the Fann School earned the president's praise.

SENGHOR'S VISION FOR SENEGAL

When Leopold Sédar Senghor (1906–2001) became the first president of independent Senegal in 1960, he envisioned for the new nation a distinctly

Senegalese style of modernity. During his nearly five terms and twenty years in office, he worked to create modern citizens and to define Senegalese national identity by molding political subjectivities and aesthetic sensibilities alike. According to Markowitz (1969: 12), Senghor desired to "stimulate in all people of Senegal a new awareness, sense of commitment and moral awakening in order to achieve unity and economic development." He did so by promoting educational initiatives, cultural enrichment programs, and the arts. It has been estimated that while he was president, Senghor channeled nearly 25 percent of Senegal's national budget into the Ministry of Culture (Harney 2004: 15).

But upon what was Senghor's vision for Senegal based, and why exactly did Senghor take special interest in Collomb's project at Fann? In this final section of the chapter, I discuss how Senghor's ideas about Negritude not only informed his political philosophy as president, but also became the national style and symbol of the nascent Senegalese state. I suggest that Fann was hailed by Senghor as an exemplary institution because it both embodied this national aesthetic and actualized his vision of a new kind of Senegalese modernity.

Negritude as Cultural Movement, National Aesthetic, and State Ideology

Both Senghor's political philosophy and the new Senegalese modernity that he promoted as president were greatly influenced by Negritude, a concept that Senghor himself had played a part in articulating some three decades earlier. While studying in Paris during the 1930s, Senghor had met a number of writers, poets, philosophers, and activists from French West Africa and the Caribbean, including Léon-Gontran Damas and Aimé Césaire. To Senghor, Negritude represented an ontological fact—a condition of black existence and being black in the world (Clifford 1988). His concept of Negritude took a divergent path from that of Césaire, who had coined the term in his 1939 poem, "Cahier d'un retour au pays natal."[18] To Césaire, Negritude was the invocation of a shared experience of racial, cultural, historical, and political subjugation—not a natural or essential characteristic of blackness. He asserted: "My Negritude has a ground. It is a fact that there is a black culture: it is historical, there is nothing biological about it" (Césaire 1976: 60 [trans. Eshleman and Smith 1979: 23], quoted in Arnold 1999: 37). Later, Césaire distinguished his perspective even further, stating that

"Senghor made a kind of metaphysics out of negritude; there we parted company. He tended rather to construct negritude into an essentialism as though there were a black essence, a black soul . . . but I never accepted this point of view" (Césaire [interview] quoted in Attoun 1970: 111–12, translated and quoted in Arnold 1999: 44).

As a reaction against colonial racism, alienation, and the presumed superiority of Western values, the Negritude writers composed poetry and prose celebrating black experience—Senghor would later refer to this as a celebration of "African ontology" (1966: 3). Senghor's Negritude, referred to by Jean-Paul Sartre ([1948] 1976: xl–xli) as a distinctly "anti-racist racism" (*"racisme antiraciste"*), described Africa's children as sharing a fundamental spirit and unity that was different from—and in opposition to—that of "the white man" (Zahar 1974: 63). According to Senghor:

> The African has always and everywhere presented a concept of the world which is diametrically opposed to the traditional philosophy of Europe. The latter is essentially *static, objective, dichotomic*; it is, in fact, dualistic, in that it makes an absolute distinction between body and soul, matter and spirit. It is founded on separation and opposition: on analysis and conflict. The African, on the other hand, conceives the world, beyond the diversity of its forms, as a fundamentally mobile, yet unique, reality that seeks synthesis (Senghor 1966: 4; italics in original).

Senghor's Negritude sought to embrace and elevate the essence of African experience; it was a positive valuation of the history, beliefs, and "values of traditional Africa as they are embedded in the thought systems and social institutions of African societies, and especially as they inform the mentality of the African" (Irele 1990: 73). Viewed by many as a necessary tool in repairing the historical and psychological damage done by colonialism, Senghor's Negritude was also met with harsh criticism—and even condemnation—by scholars and intellectuals across the Diaspora for both essentializing and depoliticizing black experience (see especially Césaire 1976; Fanon 1963; Soyinka 1976; Mphahlele 1962).

"Above all," writes Markowitz (1969: 43), "Negritude was a Paris invention." Although crediting Paris for the movement is perhaps taking things too far, it is worth asking whether Negritude could have germinated elsewhere, or during any other historical period. The young black French-speaking intellectuals who met in Paris during the 1930s had come from different corners of the world; French colonial rule and its policy of assimilation had brought them together. Having mastered French language and culture, they were part of an elite social stratum in their homelands. Many had received scholarships and promotions to continue their studies at Parisian universities. Many were Francophiles, and a good number, including Senghor, were granted full French citizenship.

Years later, Senghor (1966: 2) would write that Negritude had been "developed . . . as a weapon, as an instrument of liberation." For their poetic expression of black experience, however, Negritude writers were particularly well received by the French avant-garde. By the 1920s, modernism and the appeal of *l'art nègre* had ushered in a fashionable interest in Africa (see Archer-Shaw 2000). In addition, ethnological research in Africa and the Diaspora had acquired an important status among the French intelligentsia. Writers such as Leiris, Métraux, Bastide, Griaule, and Pidoux were making major contributions in ethnology during that time, especially in the area of dynamic possession rituals and therapeutic rites. James Clifford (1988) has described the way in which ethnography and surrealism found each other—and even merged into what he has termed "ethnographic surrealism"—in Paris between the wars. In the shattered and fragmented aftermath of the Great War, Clifford explains, surrealism sought new models and other realities. By way of ethnography, Africa offered surrealism the alterity it desired:

> For the Paris avant-garde, Africa . . . provided a reservoir of other forms and other beliefs . . . the other (whether in dreams, fetishes, or Lévy-Bruhl's *mentalité primitive*) was a crucial object of modern research. Unlike the exoticism of the nineteenth century, which departed from a more-or-less confident cultural order in search of a temporary frisson, a circumscribed experience of the bizarre, modern surrealism and ethnography began with a reality deeply in question. Others appeared now as serious human alternatives. (Clifford 1988: 120)

Negritude was born and thrived in this milieu. Senghor established himself as a central figure in the movement between the wars, and after World War II his fame continued to grow.[19] Still dedicated to literary pursuits and more prolific than ever, Senghor became actively involved in politics during the postwar years.[20] With this shift into the world of politics also came a shift in his concept of Negritude: whereas Senghor had once posited Negritude as the rejection of Western values and the elevation of "Africanness," he now asserted that Africa and the West were intertwined and invaluable to each other. Negritude, Senghor would write as the first president of Senegal, "has enriched European civilization and has been enriched by it" (1964: 10). By the mid-1960s, Senghor (1966) was referring to Negritude as a "humanism of the 20th century" that had much to contribute to what he called the "Civilization of the Universal":

> Negritude is . . . the sum of the cultural values of the Black world, as these are expressed in the life, the institutions, and the work of Negroes . . . Our sole preoccupation since 1932–1934 has been to assume this negritude by *living* it and, having lived in, to seek for its deeper meaning, to present it to the world as the cornerstone in the construction of the "Civilization of the Universal" (1964: 12, reproduced in Senghor 1966: 1).

A "Civilization of the Universal," said Senghor (1966: 5), was much needed in the "divided but interdependent world of the 20th century," and Negritude had an important role to play. His new approach "emphasi[zed] . . . the singularity of the black's contribution to civilization" and aspired to demonstrate the value and significance of Negritude to all peoples of the world (Markowitz 1969: 40).

Senghor's concept of Negritude evolved alongside—and in conjunction with—his political career; it had a direct bearing upon both his political philosophy and his vision for newly independent Senegal. As art historian Ima Ebong (1991: 130) suggests: "It was when [Senghor] attained this dual role as culture broker and president that Negritude began to achieve the status of a national aesthetic, transgressing its boundaries as Senghor's own personal philosophy, to inhabit a more public place as the 'cultural constitution' of the nation." Senghor's early nation-building projects celebrated tradition, authenticity, and an African "essence," claiming these to be at the very heart of the modern nation. It is important to note that within his own political discourse and philosophical writings on Negritude and the "Civilization of the Universal," Senghor had little to say about the place and role of Islam in West African tradition and culture (Back 2004). In his view, it was the idea of a shared African spirit that would unite the country, not religion nor religious unity; Negritude values had the capacity to transcend religious difference. The "spiritual socialism" that would become the trademark of the new nation—and was staunchly supported by both the devoutly Catholic Senghor and his Muslim compatriot in statecraft, Senegal's first prime minister Mamadou Dia—was founded on principles of secular governance.[21] It was Negritude that would become the national style and symbol of Senghor's Senegal; in it, what E. V. Daniel (1997: 309) would call the "aestheticizing impulse" of the new nation-state found its form.

L'Ecole de Dakar *and* l'Ecole de Fann

The privileged place of Negritude in Senghor's Senegal inspired the creation of an intellectual and artistic movement during the years following independence. The movement was focused especially around the University of Dakar and *l'Ecole Nationale des Beaux Arts* in Dakar. *L'Ecole de Dakar* (The Dakar School), as the movement was called, sought to embrace Negritude in such diverse fields as literature, philosophy, history, science, and the arts; it also sought to articulate "traditional Africa" in distinctly modern ways. *L'Ecole de Dakar* played an important role in Senghor's vision of modern Senegal, and the movement received both support and accolades from his government for expressing a new kind of Senegalese modernity. In his 1980 work entitled *La poésie de l'action: Conversations avec Mohamed Aziza*, for instance, Senghor asserts that *l'Ecole de Dakar* exemplified modern Senegalese thought. Here he traces the origins of the movement—and the modernization of Senegalese thought itself—back to the "handful of students who founded the Negritude movement" in the 1930s (1980: 180). Further, he explains:

> It is necessary for us Black Africans ... to root ourselves in the values of Negritude, to hold on to our gifts of analogy and of rhythm.... We must not imitate nature, but recreate it by rethinking it, and especially by dreaming it. It remains that, without abandoning the art of our ancestors, we want to enrich ourselves with the fecund contributions that come from abroad.... It is also necessary for us to assimilate the discursive reason of Europe into our own way of thinking. The problem is that all too often, we ... turn our backs to logic.... It is against this laxity—a laxity to which our political writers frequently succumb, not to mention our philosophers—that the Senegalese government has been reacting since independence by prioritizing mathematics on the one hand, and the black imagination on the other. *It is this double effort to reconcile authenticity and modernity that characterizes that which is known as l'Ecole de Dakar* (181; my emphasis).

After independence, Senghor tells us, the will of the government and the creativity of *l'Ecole de Dakar* were aligned in an effort to craft a new Senegalese modernity by merging the traditional and the modern—the "art of our ancestors" with the "discursive reason of Europe."

Although *l'Ecole de Dakar* is best known today as a literary and artistic movement that came out of Senegal during the 1960s and 1970s, Senghor himself actually insisted that it was not in these areas but in medicine—and in the field of psychiatry in particular—that some of "the most positive work was accomplished by *l'Ecole de Dakar*" (1979: 137). The unique theoretical and clinical orientation of the Fann Psychiatric Clinic during the 1960s and 1970s not only attracted Senghor's attention, but earned Fann's brand of psychiatry a prominent position within *l'Ecole de Dakar*. In fact, in an interview that appeared in Senegal's most widely circulated newspaper in 1998, the director of Fann went so far as to boast: "If one speaks of *l'Ecole de Dakar* at all, it is because of psychiatry."[22]

The Fann Psychiatric Clinic, then, became a jewel in Senghor's crown, an emblem of his vision for a new and distinctly Senegalese modernity. But in those early independence years, was Senghor at all uneasy about crediting Collomb and his (mostly French) colleagues with this achievement? The answer, it seems, is no. Senghor's ideas about the "Civilization of the Universal" all but required the blurring and crossing of racial boundaries. To Senghor, some of the most compelling examples of the modern expression of Negritude in art were also of European—and not Senegalese—origin. Early in the twentieth century, Europe's images and ideas of Africa had been central to the development of European modernism. Decades later, Senghor would uphold European modernism as an example of what Negritude—as a new African modernism—could (and perhaps, should) look like. Extolling the work of Picasso, for example, he once declared: "No artist could be more exemplary. He is a model for *l'Ecole de Dakar*, and his closeness to us here is a rich inspiration" (Senghor 1977: 324, translated and cited in Ebong 1991: 131).[23] In a 1966 essay, we see Senghor grappling with his own expectations and anxieties vis-à-vis modern African art:

> Recently M. Lods [a Belgian national who taught at *l'Ecole des Beaux Arts* in Dakar during the 1960s] ... was showing me the pictures his students intend exhibiting at the projected Festival of African Arts. I was immediately struck by the noble and elegant interplay of shape and colour. When I discovered that the pictures were not completely abstract, that they portrayed ladies, princes and noble animals, I was almost disappointed. There was no need for me to be: the very interplay of coloured shapes perfectly expressed that elegant nobility that characterizes the art of the Southern Soudan (1966: 7).

As Senghor explains here, the shapes and colors were right, but there was still something wrong. The fact that the pictures were "not completely abstract"— i.e., that modern African art had not yet been freed of its representational forms and figures, as had European abstract art—had given Senghor a moment of pause. Although he was almost disappointed, it suddenly struck him that this was one of African art's defining characteristics.

Just as Senghor praised Picasso as a model for *l'Ecole de Dakar*, he applauded Collomb and the other doctors at Fann for affirming Negritude ideals and promoting a new model of Senegalese modernity. The two men were, in fact, well acquainted. Senghor not only praised Collomb for being a "Frenchman [who] knew how to kill the most firmly established prejudices" (1979: 139) but even went so far as to credit him for having made himself *nègre avec les nègres,"* or "black among blacks" while working at Fann (138). I heard similar sentiments about how Collomb "made himself black" or "was like an African" during my fieldwork stay in Dakar, especially from the men and women who had worked with Collomb at Fann. Aissatou, who had been a nurse from 1962 until 1992, put it like this:

> Collomb loved Africa, you see. He lived in Africa from the time he was young until he retired from Fann in 1978 and went back to France. He was forced to leave Fann, you know, because he was a military doctor, and because he was French. When he left, he said, "I am leaving, but my heart will stay here." And in France, well, it wasn't very long after he left Dakar that we received news of his death. I think he belonged here. Africa was like his own country (*comme son proper pays*)! He participated in rituals, he knew everything about Africa. In the end, he was like an African.

In Senghor's eyes, Collomb's ability to move across cultural landscapes and blur racial boundaries was absolutely desirable; throughout his life, Senghor proudly and vocally attempted to do the same. In fact, his hopes for achieving a "Civilization of the Universal" were predicated on this very movement. And just as Senghor saw Collomb as a man of the independence era who made a great contribution to the new nation, many of the Senegalese women and men who worked alongside Collomb and his colleagues as nurses, social workers, and translators during the 1960s and early 1970s express similar sentiments. Further, they equate the early years of Fann not only with Senegalese independence but also with the feelings of hope, optimism, and progress that permeated the era.

In the next two chapters, I explore what Bissell (2005: 216) has termed "multiple strands of remembrance" in order to engage with two very different sets of stories that circulate about the early years of Fann. The first set, heavy with nostalgia for Collomb's Fann and bitter about its demise, describes the 1960s as the "golden age" of the clinic. The second takes a much more critical view of this era and explains why it necessarily had to come to an end. As I have already suggested, Fann is a powerful lens through which the postcolonial state was (and continues to be) experienced by those who inhabited it; the way people remember the Fann Psychiatric Clinic has much to say about how they relate to the larger social and political transformations that have taken place in Senegal since the nation's independence in 1960. While these stories unsettle and even disrupt one another, they remain entangled and entwined; neither can be told without the other, but together they remain apart. The content of these stories—as well as the force of their telling—challenges the pastness of the past.

RUPTURE

A Letter Unanswered

THINGS MIGHT HAVE BEEN OTHERWISE. One letter might have changed everything.

In the summer of 1953, Frantz Fanon wrote a letter to Léopold Senghor, who was by then living back in Senegal, in Dakar. The two had moved within the same intellectual circles in France and had both been part of the journal *Présence Africaine*; they were, according to all accounts, still on good terms at the time. Fanon had just successfully completed a battery of intensive examinations; he was now qualified to hold the coveted position of *chef de service*, or director, of a psychiatric hospital in France or one of its colonies. According to Alice Cherki, who would later work with Fanon at Blida-Joinville in Algeria, the place he had wanted to work more than any other was Dakar, not only because of his desire to learn more about Black Africa or his commitment to anticolonial thought and action, but because he thought Dakar a perfect place "to both practice psychiatry and to continue his study of societies in which the modern and the traditional exist side-by-side" (Cherki 2006: 24). Senghor was, at that time, a deputy in the *Assemblée Nationale Française* representing Senegal. Fanon wrote to him hoping that his friend might help him find a job.

I should say this: I have not seen the letter myself. I am not entirely sure it still exists, or that it ever did. I have seen it mentioned in passing in several French and English sources, with the earliest reference coming from Hussein Abdilahi Bulhan's *Frantz Fanon and the Psychology of Oppression* (1985). None of the authors who mention the letter, however, give any indication of having seen it themselves, and none cite the letter directly. This is not to say, of course, that the letter does not exist. It is simply to point out that the letter, which has come to be taken as fact, may not be.

Still, the very possibility of this letter invites us to imagine how many things might have turned out differently. What if Fanon had been hired in Dakar in 1953, in the place of Jean Rainaut, as the *chef de service* of *Cap Manuel*? What if Fanon had been in charge of overseeing the move from *Cap Manuel* to Fann, and what if it had been he and not Collomb who had set the course for the clinic after independence? How would Fanon have shaped Fann as its director? And what would have come of Fanon's presence in Dakar (instead of Algeria) during the late 1950s and the early independence years? Would he have had Senghor's ear, perhaps influenced him? Would Fanon have openly challenged Senghor's Francophilia and his desire to maintain close ties with France after independence? Would "Fanon's Fann" have been anathema to the distinctly Senegalese modernity that Senghor promoted during the nation's early years? And what would have come of Blida-Joinville, of the Algerian War, of Fanon himself?

But perhaps the most poignant question in all of this, for me at least: *Why didn't Senghor respond to Fanon's letter?* Did Senghor already view Fanon as a potential adversary? Were Fanon's politics already incompatible with Senghor's vision of what Senegalese independence could and should look like? Why didn't Senghor simply write back to Fanon and tell him that there was no available position for him in Dakar? Would it have been an uncomfortable letter for Senghor to write—a task that ended up being put off indefinitely? Did Senghor mean to respond, but just never get around to it? On Fanon's end, how did he understand the silence? Did this make him resent Senghor, or lead him to question Senghor's character and ambitions?

THREE

Nostalgic for Modernity
(Or, Looking Back on a Golden Age)

Namm reytil weer.
[*Lit.*: Nostalgia does not kill the moon / month; *Fig.*: Nostalgia does not stop time.]

—WOLOF PROVERB

MARIE-CLAUDE WAS A YOUNG WOMAN WHEN SHE began working as a nurse at Fann in 1961. During our many conversations, she proudly and passionately told me stories about the early years of the clinic. One of the very first things Marie-Claude said to me as we sat down in her living room for the first time, however, was not about Fann per se but rather about the era more generally:

> When I was young, you know, Dakar was known everywhere as the Paris of Africa. That was during the 1950s. You should have seen Dakar back then! It was a beautiful city. It didn't look anything like it does now. It was so green! And clean. The fountains all over the city worked and people would walk by and throw their *sous* in them. And during Senghor's time! Senegal was a very important country back then, and Dakar was a fashionable place. People would dress up and go downtown just to stroll along the boulevards. Yes, Senghor's Senegal was really something. It was so different back then.

On a most basic level, Marie-Claude's words read as a simple narrative of nostalgia—a story of a rich and resplendent "back then" that bears little resemblance to the "here and now." Her reflections also bind the late colonial era to the early independence years in an almost seamless fashion, simultaneously underscoring the continuity of the period and more generally alerting us to the limits of thinking about these and other historical eras as "discrete domain[s] of social relations and politics, of experience and memory" (Stoler and Strassler 2000: 9).

Although Marie-Claude's nostalgic recollections exemplify but one of many disparate and contested "strands of remembrance" (Bissell 2005: 216) that circulate about the early postindependence years, her sentiments are shared by a number of other Senegalese women and men who worked as nurses, social workers, and translators alongside Collomb and *l'Ecole de Fann* during the 1960s and 1970s. These "middle figures" (Hunt 1999) were also part of a growing middle class in independence-era Dakar. They had been deeply invested in the new and distinctly Senegalese style of modernity—rooted in Negritude ideals and actualized in the work of the Dakar School—that Senghor promoted during those years (Ebong 1991). When they speak nostalgically about the early days of the Fann Psychiatric Clinic, their stories reflect—and are embedded within—an even deeper sense of nostalgia for Senghor's Senegal. At the same time, their stories about the "golden age" of both institution and nation hinge upon the very loss of that era. As they underscore the vast disjuncture between then and now, their nostalgia for that other time serves as an indictment of the failures of the present, both within the Fann clinic and of the state more generally.

In this chapter, I explore the nostalgia of these "middle figures" as both a narrative mode and a cultural practice (Bissell 2005; Stewart 1988) that acts as a vehicle for social commentary and political critique. I insist that nostalgic stories of Fann's early years are a salient form of memory work. As such, they cannot and should not simply be dismissed as bad history, or as fantasy spun from dreams of a time or place that never "really" existed; nor should they be approached as points of access to a "true" or "real" past. Instead, these stories highlight memory work as an interpretive, imaginative process and nostalgic remembrance as a mode of speaking about the past that speaks critically to, and about, the present.

I begin, then, by considering anthropology's nostalgic foundations and by questioning both the possibility and limitations of an ethnographic engagement with nostalgia before turning to a more general discussion of the topic. In many ways, my discussion reaffirms and extends current scholarly understandings of what nostalgia *is* and what it *does*. However, my analysis of the nostalgic stories of Fann's "golden age" (and by extension, of Senghor's Senegal) diverges from this literature in one significant detail. It has been said that nostalgia and modernity are two sides of the same coin—that nostalgia is as much a shadow or byproduct of modernity as "tradition" is said to be (Boym 2001; Robertson 1990; Stewart 1988). From this point of view, nostalgia typically takes as its object an unscathed and harmonious past, a time in which everything was simpler, slower, and more "natural." In contrast, the object of nostalgia in stories about Fann's "golden age" and Senghor's Senegal *is modernity itself*, or more precisely, what I refer to as the "phantasm of modernity," meaning not only the lived reality of the era but the future it promised and the progress it seemed to assure. What one encounters in these stories is what Ferguson (1999: 13), in the context of Zambia, has called "modernity through the looking glass, where modernity is the object of nostalgic reverie, and 'backwardness' the anticipated (or dreaded) future." Stories about Fann's "golden age" and Senghor's Senegal, then, summon memories of better times that locate hope itself in the past, as something belonging to an altogether different era.

In the final section of this chapter, I begin to consider Marie-Claude's comments about Dakar's seamless transition from colonial jewel (the "Paris of Africa") to cosmopolitan capital of independent Senegal ("Senghor's Senegal") from a more critical point of view. Nostalgic stories about Fann's "golden age" and Senghor's Senegal do not circulate uncontested; as I discuss in the chapter that follows this one, many who have since been affiliated with the clinic refuse such tales outright. For the Senegalese psychiatrists who inherited the Fann Psychiatric Clinic from their European predecessors in the late 1970s, both Fann and Senghor's Senegal were too closely linked to the colonial regime that had preceded them; the era represented more of a bridge between the colonial and the postcolonial than a departure from the colonial. In their eyes, this bridge had to come down eventually.

NOSTALGIC ENGAGEMENTS

Even as a very green ethnographer, it did not take me long to recognize nostalgia to be a dominant mode of reflection and a shared narrative framework for talking about the past among those who worked alongside Collomb and his colleagues at Fann during the 1960s and 1970s. It has taken me much longer, however, to figure out how to productively engage with this nostalgia. Van Dijk (1998: 155) has suggested that because nostalgia is "primarily relational" and "refers back to relationships with people, spaces, and places," it is often difficult for "the anthropologist . . . to enter this realm of yearning." From the very first life histories I collected from these men and women, however, I found quite the opposite to be true. So captivating were their stories, and so deeply did they resonate with my own (admittedly romanticized) ideas about the brilliant optimism of independence-era Senegal, I sometimes felt overcome by a kind of "armchair nostalgia" (Appadurai 1996: 78) that caused me to long for this past that was not even my own. Although I was absolutely drawn in by stories of Collomb's Fann and Senghor's Senegal, I also felt unsure about how to approach this nostalgia without infusing or conflating it with my own desires—without myself slipping under its spell. This, I think, is a familiar problem within anthropology.

From Marx's idyllic precapitalist societies to Tonnies's *Gemeinschaft* and Durkheim's simple society, and from Boas's salvage anthropology to Levi-Strauss's *Tristes Tropiques*, anthropology and social theory have themselves been highly nostalgic in their depictions of lost ages, disappearing cultures, and faraway places. Likewise, critical discourses surrounding modernity, progress, and globalization have tended to reify the "back then" and the "over there" as viable alternatives to the modern world—alternatives that are, nevertheless, quickly slipping away. Nostalgic longing for the world that modernity is imagined to have replaced is a "distinctive issue of modernity" itself (Robertson 1990:49). This issue has been implicit in the rhetoric of modernity and pervasive in its worldview, despite the fact that nostalgia is often dismissed as fantastical, ahistorical, or even reactionary.[1]

A text that aligns itself well with my own thinking on the subject is Svetlana Boym's *The Future of Nostalgia* (2001). Reflecting on postcommunist nostalgia in Eastern Europe and Russia, Boym distinguishes between two different types: the *restorative* and the *reflective*.[2] Restorative nostalgia attempts to lay claim to the past (or an imagined past) and mobilize it in the present. It is both selective and creative in what it chooses to pluck out of the past; often, it venerates origins and preaches a return to them in the future. People engaged in this kind of nostalgia "do not think of themselves as nostalgic; they believe their project is about truth," writes Boym (2001: 41). And if restorative nostalgia makes claims about truth, then it also makes claims about power and justice. In other words, restorative nostalgia is first and foremost a political endeavor. Van Rijk (1998: 156) suggests that this type of nostalgia might also "be viewed as *politicized cultural memory*, syncretically blending the longing for a past and its evocation within present social reality *to create a* specific route to empowerment" (italics in original). Restorative nostalgia finds affinity with other times and places, which are often imaginary but sometimes not, in an effort to bring those other times and places into the present. We would do well to remember, however, that the act of summoning the past in this way can be fraught with peril. As Marx warns in *The Eighteenth Brumaire of Louis Bonaparte*, the demise of all revolutionary activity comes about when, in moments of "revolutionary crisis" or fear, those involved "anxiously conjure up the spirits of the past to their service and borrow from their names, battle slogans, and costumes in order to present the new scene of world history in this time-honored disguise and this borrowed language" (Marx 1972: 595).

In his description of the French Revolution, Marx states that "the heroes, as well as the parties and the masses . . . performed the task of their time in Roman costume and with Roman phrases" (595). Here Marx asserts that during the critical moment of the revolution, the inability to generate new responses for the challenges of the day led the revolution to invoke the ghosts of the past; calling on the past, claims Marx, paved the road for the establishment of French bourgeois society. To Marx, then, restorative nostalgia would likely have been viewed as distinctly counterrevolutionary.[3]

Boym, like Marx, is suspicious of this use of the past. Restorative nostalgia, she writes, "reconstruct[s] emblems and rituals of home and homeland" (2001: 49) and "characterizes national and nationalist revivals all over the world, which engage in the antimodern myth-making of history by means of a return to national symbols and myths" (41). As a powerful political tool, restorative nostalgia has indeed been at the service of many modern states. In the case of newly independent Senegal, restorative nostalgia was mobilized with a highly stylized twist: Senghor promoted the development of a national aesthetic that would articulate and accentuate elements of "traditional" Africa in the most modern of ways.

In contrast to this restorative nostalgia, says Boym, is reflexive nostalgia. Whereas the former "manifests itself in the total reconstructions of monuments of the past," the latter "lingers on ruins, the patina of time and history, in the dreams of another place and another time" (41). Reflexive nostalgia understands time as irreversible and the past as a faraway place (see also Foster 1988). Marilyn Strathern (1995: 111) similarly describes synthetic nostalgia as that which takes as its object a past that is lost to the present, and thus "mourns for what is missing from the present." From a certain angle, perhaps, this type of nostalgia bears a closer resemblance to melancholia than to mourning, at least as Freud would have it ([1917] 1957). Sealed off from the present, the past is as an altogether "other" time recalled in daydreams and reverie. While "restorative nostalgia evokes a national past and future," writes Boym (2001: 49), reflective nostalgia is "oriented toward an individual narrative that savors details and memorial signs" and is thus "more about individual and cultural memory." In her view, the two are decidedly different in scope and aim, and while they "might overlap in their frames of reference," she writes, "they do not coincide in their narratives and plots of identity" (49). The nostalgia expressed by Marie-Claude and her colleagues both acknowledges and challenges Boym's division between the restorative and the reflexive. Stories of Fann's "golden age" are at once narratives of self, institution, and nation; they are both personal and historical. In this sense, as Bissell (2005: 240) writes, nostalgia is "uniquely capable of . . . crossing boundaries between public and private spheres. In the nostalgic domain, the personal is inherently political and vice versa." Reflecting on that other time, the women and men who worked at the clinic chart their memories and experiences of the early years of Fann upon the *topos* of Senegal's independence era. What is more, in describing a "better" past and its subsequent demise, they offer a powerful critique of the present while at the same time acknowledging the impossibility of return. After all, there is no story of nostalgia that is not also a story of loss, failure, or fall.

MIDDLE FIGURES, LOOKING BACK

Within the past fifteen years or so, scholars of African history have paid increasing attention to the role of "African intermediaries"—interpreters, clerks, functionaries, nurses, teachers, letter writers, and so on—as active agents in the articulation of colonial knowledge and power (Hunt 1999; Lawrance, Osborn, and Roberts 2006). Working at the interface of cultural, political, economic, and therapeutic structures and regimes, these men and women acted not simply as pawns of imperial order but as " 'gate-keepers,' or 'brokers' . . . between subject populations and external sources of power / patronage" (Austen 2011: 22; cf. Austen 2006; Cooper 2002). While these "middle figures" mediated knowledge systems, they also established themselves as knowledge producers and important historical actors in the "dialogical emergence" (Tedlock and Mannheim 1995) of colonial modernity. Occupying this critical juncture at the interstices of different cultural orders, these "emerging évolués or hybrid middle figures . . . helped beget a new creolized lexicon . . . in keeping with the concrete, contradictory modernity they imagined as theirs" (Hunt 1999:12).

Although the colonial era had officially come to an end by the time Marie-Claude and her colleagues began working as nurses, social workers, and translators at Fann, they were in many ways positioned as "middle figures" within the clinic. Far from marginal, these men and women worked as intermediaries between Fann's mostly foreign doctors and local patients, and between psychiatric knowledge and Senegalese culture more generally. They were, in fact, key agents in the articulation of Fann's unique therapeutic economy—an economy in which "culture" was very highly prized. For this reason, they were also model citizens of the distinctly Senegalese style of modernity that was envisioned by Senghor, and they felt deeply connected to his national project through their work at the clinic.

The nostalgic recollections of these "middle figures" are deeply personal and highly individualized; they tend to fix upon common themes, follow familiar plots, and display similar affective orientations and excesses. Above all, they describe the dynamic ambiance that Fann had during that time. Remarking on the sharp contrast between Collomb's Fann and the inadequacies of the present-day clinic, they speak also of the abundant resources that were at the clinic's disposal, and of Collomb's own wealth and generosity. The stories tell of the sense of community and kinship these "middle figures" felt toward the rest of the staff (and some of the patients) during that time. They depict Collomb as a kind, charismatic leader and tireless researcher, insatiably curious about "all things African." Finally, they talk of Collomb and his colleagues' active commitment to understanding local beliefs and practices, and the group's desire to create a truly transcultural psychiatry.

Marie-Claude, whose words opened this chapter, started at Fann in 1961 and worked there until she retired in 1989. "I have seen it all," she laughed, explaining:

> I was working in the *Pavillon des Dames*, you know. It was much different than it is now. We usually had over thirty patients at a time; I bet they don't have half that many today. It was such a lively place; very animated. There were activities going on all the time. We made *attaya* (tea) together often. Theater troupes came regularly to perform for the patients. We had our *pénc* (town hall–style group therapy) sessions each Wednesday, and other divisions held their *pénc* sessions on different days so everyone in the clinic could attend. We never missed a session!

Pénc sessions still take place at Fann today, as I discuss in chapter 6. According to many who worked at Fann during Collomb's time, however, they no longer function as they once did. These days, not many people get involved, and doctors themselves rarely attend. "I think it is a question of motivation," said El Hadj, who worked as Collomb's principal translator during the 1960s and 1970s. He continued:

It is really too bad. The *pénc* sessions used to be very dynamic. They used to help the patients. They helped the patients get up and move around and talk. I remember, patients would wake up on *pénc* days saying, "Today is the *pénc*! Get dressed!" It was something they looked forward to.

According to Marie-Claude, patients were encouraged to participate in *pénc* sessions and other activities; they were given numerous opportunities to socialize as well as express themselves both verbally and artistically. Not only that, she added, but the nurses and doctors often took part in the activities right alongside them. Over the years, as described in chapter 2, diverse forms of therapy and numerous leisure activities were offered to patients, from drawing and painting to doll-making and *batik* dyeing. Every few days, all of the women from the *Pavillon des Dames*—patients, nurses, and social workers alike—would gather in the kitchen to cook large meals for everyone at the clinic, which were then eaten communally. "It was a social activity, a way to pass the time," Marie Claude explained, "but it was also a form of occupational therapy for the women that rehabituated them to daily activities." Many of the women, she said, were somewhat hesitant to participate in art therapy or contribute to the *Pinthioum Fann*; they felt more comfortable performing activities that were familiar to them, like cooking. From time to time, the clinic would have what they called "*les journées portes ouvertes*" (open-door days), during which people from outside the clinic were invited in to share the meal.

Patients were at ease at Fann, Marie-Claude remembered; they got to know each other well. Even when no activities were planned, they would make *attaya* (tea) together on the verandah and talk. The clinic staff also got to know patients well; like Marie-Claude, many spoke in terms of family and kinship when describing the early years of Fann. They, too, talked about how sharing in their daily activities made patients and workers like kin, and suggested that this sense of community helped patients in their recovery. Retired nurse Seynabou also pointed out that doctors and nurses did not wear white coats to set themselves apart from the patients, as they do now. "I think that it helped patients feel more integrated, less isolated," she explained. "We were like a big family. And I think that helped patients get better." Many others also commented on the fact that the clinic staff was like a family unto itself. Aida, who was a social worker at Fann, said of the strong relationships that developed: "We all knew each other very well. Everyone worked hard together. That was the best part for me. Between all of us working together, it was as though we were a family."

Almost all of the women and men who worked at Fann during the 1960s and 1970s mentioned the clinic's whitewashed facades, courtyards, and clean interior spaces. They also talked about how back then, unlike now, the clinic did not lack resources. According to Bintou, who began working as a nurse in the *Pavillon des Dames* in 1971:

> The clinic used to provide everything for the patients. There were fresh linens on the beds. There was good food—three meals a day. You wouldn't believe me, Katie, if I told you. For breakfast, there were *petit pains*, with butter and jam! Coffee and milk, too. Sometimes, at around 10 or 11 in the morning, they would bring the patients a snack, like yogurt or something. Now, you know, the food they give patients is barely edible, if offered at all.

The clinic lacked nothing; patients wanted for nothing. In these men and women's stories of Collomb's Fann, recollections of abundance and plenitude overflow the boundaries of the institution, making reference to the era as an altogether better time. As El Hadj insisted:

> Times were different then, and Fann was different, too. What an ambiance the clinic had! There was money then, and there was no shortage of personnel. Nothing was missing! . . . And the patients—they were spoiled, truly spoiled! Yes, life was much easier then than it is now.

But where exactly did the money come from? Fann was not a private clinic; as a teaching clinic affiliated with the University of Dakar, its funding came mostly from the French and Senegalese governments. According to El Hadj, Collomb and his colleagues often solicited outside sources to supplement the clinic's needs. "Money was easier to come by back then," he told me. "And Collomb was well connected. He knew people all over the world. All he had to do was ask and he got whatever he needed." El Hadj remembers, for example, going to the French Embassy with Collomb on several occasions for financial and material support. In addition to being well connected, Collomb was a man of significant means—he was, after all, equipped with his own private jet—who often paid for a great deal out of his own pocket. As Bintou related:

> He gave a lot to his patients and was very generous. He even put his own money toward celebrations at the clinic. I remember one morning he arrived very early, earlier than usual, and I was there working. It was the morning before *Korité* (the Muslim holiday of Eid al-Fitr). He came in and put 25,000 francs [about $50 USD] in my hand and said, "Here, this is for tomorrow, for the patients."

Many people who were connected to the clinic during the 1960s and 1970s mentioned Senghor's appreciation of both Collomb and Fann, and told me that Collomb could call Senghor for whatever he needed. As El Hadj related:

> President Senghor was proud of Fann! He was very interested in Collomb's projects at the clinic, and they became good friends. Oh yes! Anything that Collomb asked for was his. Easily. Yes, he got whatever he wanted—easily, easily. Senghor knew he was a hard-working kind of man, a man who knew how to do his job and do it right!

When I asked El Hadj if Senghor and Collomb shared the same political views, though, he looked at me as if I had committed a great offense by even asking such a question. "Ah, no! Oh, absolutely not!" he replied emphatically, shaking his head. "Collomb wasn't political at all, and rightly so! He didn't involve himself in politics. He was *apolitical.*"

Along with the strong sense of community and abundant resources at the clinic, many describe their own dedication to—and investment in—both Fann and Collomb's project. They portray Collomb as having been deeply committed to the clinic and almost always present. As Aida recalled, she and the others were motivated by the rigorously collaborative work environment that he encouraged at Fann:

> Collomb was devoted to the clinic, and he was dedicated to his patients. He arrived early in the morning and stayed late, very late, at night. Often, he would work all weekend long. And he expected the same of us, of course! We worked hard, but I did not mind. We had the feeling, back then, of being part of something important. We were all young, you know; most of us were in our twenties or thirties. . . . Everything that went on in each division, day or night, we wrote down in a notebook. Collomb would come in each morning, read through the notebook, greet the patients, say hello to us, and then go and speak with each doctor. He was always moving around and busy, but he was always available.

Perhaps one of the most prominent aspects of Fann's "golden age" described by the Senegalese women and men who worked as nurses, social workers, and translators during the 1960s and 1970s was Collomb and his colleagues' respect for—and desire to collaborate with—traditional healers. This, they say, no longer exists at Fann. Aissatou explained that Collomb's great dream was to create a veritable transcultural psychiatry. He was acquainted with healers from all parts of Senegal, and he often consulted them about specific cases he saw at the clinic. Collomb, Aissatou said, would explain his views about psychiatry, and tell them about the kind of work he was doing at Fann. Many made regular visits to the clinic to see patients or attend special events. To visit those who lived too far from the clinic to make the trip, Collomb would take his private plane. He wanted to get healers and psychiatrists to acknowledge each other's work and to collaborate effectively. Among Collomb's greatest interests, Bintou told me, were spirit possession (*ndëpp*) ceremonies—he went to great lengths to attend these. According to several of the retired nurses, *ndëpp* ceremonies were even held in the court-yard of the clinic from time to time, although as I shall discuss later in this chapter, this assertion is hotly contested today.

Many who worked at Fann during the 1960s and early 1970s remember these years as the best of their lives; the "golden age" of Fann was also *their* "golden age," and with that particular kind of nostalgia the aging often have for their youth, they describe themselves as having once been strong and energetic, happy and healthy. As Marie-Claude leafed through her old photos with me one day, she shook her head and laughed. "There I am! Can you believe I was that young once? Not bad looking, either!" she joked. The pic-ture, which had been taken in 1966, showed a beautiful, smiling young woman standing next to the unmistakable personage of Henri Collomb.

Nostalgic stories of Fann's past are often recounted with dramatic flair; these are wistfully told stories, loaded with emotion, heavy with longing for an irretrievable past, and tinged with anger at its loss. This is not to say, how-ever, that the events described by these men and women did not "really" hap-pen or that their stories are untrue. To be clear, it is not the proximity to (or distance from) "fact" or "truth" that I find most compelling about these sto-ries, or about nostalgia more generally. Rather, it is the affective mode in which the stories are told, and the commentary they convey about the vast disjuncture between then and now. In order to properly engage with nostal-gia, I argue that we might do well to dispense with the idea that it is nothing more than distorted or romanticized history. Instead, as Bissell (2005: 218) has suggested, "we need to engage with [nostalgia] as a social practice that mobilizes various signs of the past . . . in the context of contemporary strug-gles." Bissell's statement is reminiscent of Kathleen Stewart's (1988) assertion that nostalgia is altogether misunderstood when approached in terms of what Susan Stewart (1984: ix) had called a "social disease." Instead, Kathleen Stewart (1988: 227) writes, nostalgia is better understood as a "cultural practice, not a given content; its forms, meanings, and effects shift with the context—it depends on where the speaker stands in the landscape of the present." In my own encounter with stories of Fann's golden age, I find it most fruitful to approach nostalgia as an active and directed way of speaking about both past and present that carries with it an element of institutional and political critique. Viewing nostalgia only in terms of its personal / psychological dimensions (as disposition or affect) or dismissing it as "bad" history may hinder our ability to see the ways in which nostalgia, as a narrative mode, becomes mobilized and performed within these different contexts.

The Senegalese men and women who worked alongside Collomb during the 1960s and 1970s describe themselves as having been entirely committed to Fann's project, just as they were invested in Senghor's vision for a new kind of Senegalese modernity. As described in chapter 2, Collomb's project at Fann and Senghor's Senegal were, in fact, closely bound in the minds of many, including President Senghor himself. The men and women who worked alongside Collomb at Fann, then, not only recall a time when they themselves were young, enthusiastic, and full of hope for the future. They remember a time when they were actively engaged in the national project—and by extension, the very future of Senegal—through their work at Fann. This they contrast with the sense of dispossession and dislocation they have felt vis-a-vis the state since Senghor's departure from office in 1980, which was also around the time that Senegal began to feel the effects of structural adjustment, privatization, and trade liberalization that paved the way, as I discuss in chapters 5 and 6, for Senegal's neoliberal turn.

MODERNITY (AND ITS PROMISES) AS
THE OBJECT OF NOSTALGIA

On one level, these stories describe Collomb's Fann as a radically different institution that was both nested within—and emblematic of—an altogether better era. But there is an added dimension to this nostalgia that makes it all the more salient, for the stories do not only invoke the material reality of what once was (a present of / in the past), but also the promises of the past that never came to fruition (the imagined futures of / in the past). As the women and men who worked alongside Collomb at Fann speak of that other place in time, they allude also to the promises of Senghor's Senegal, and the sense of hope that those years are said to have engendered. "It was an exciting time back then," recalled Seynabou. *"On avait de l'espoir"* (There was hope, one had hope). Others speak of the optimism that filled those years, and of the way they once envisioned the times to come. It is important to note that their stories pose a challenge to Bissell's (2005: 221) assertion that "nostalgia requires an object world to seize on—buildings, fashions, images, and the ephemera of everyday life." Most often, the object of nostalgia in these stories is not an "object" at all, but rather an idea, a hope, or a dream for the future that was never allowed to materialize.

As with nostalgia, "hope . . . is itself embedded within historically and culturally specific understanding" (Crapanzano 2003: 15); it too may be approached as a narrative mode that serves as a vehicle for social commentary and political critique. Reflecting on hope and desire alike, Crapanzano reminds us that "neither . . . can be removed from social engagement and implication" despite the fact that we often tend to "place them insistently in the individual" (25). It is certainly not rare to hear people throughout Senegal and across the Diaspora reflect upon the hope and optimism that permeated the independence era. Boubacar Barry, a well-known Senegalese historian, expressed a similar sentiment several years ago, at a Columbia University brown-bag seminar, when he talked about the great promise people had back then for the future, for the newly independent nation, for Africa, for black culture, politics, philosophy, and art. During the lecture, he also described what he called a "space for dreaming" that existed during the 1960s—an inspired space that fostered hope for the days ahead. After the talk, when asked to comment upon his hopes for the future of Senegal, he responded: "Back then, there was a space for dreaming. But now? That is a difficult question. To have hope for the future, one must first have a space for dreaming. It is difficult to dream again."

Like those who speak nostalgically about Fann's "golden age" and Senghor's Senegal, Barry makes reference not just to the independence era itself, but to what Reinhart Koselleck (1985) might call the expanded "horizon of expectation" that existed during that time but has since receded. Koselleck describes the "horizon of expectation" as a future imaginary, a space into which all possibilities for the future are inserted—and brought to bear upon—the present. I suggest that the distinctly Senegalese style of modernity promoted by Senghor during the years following independence laid claim to the certainty of an ever-expanding "horizon of expectation." Against this backdrop, Marie-Claude's memories of dressing up to stroll along the boulevards of Dakar depict an emerging modernity that was at once cosmopolitan, fashionable, and self-conscious. It was also optimistic about its future and, above all, confident of its own progress and advancement. For the men and women who worked alongside Collomb and his colleagues, the object of their nostalgia is this very modernity, or more precisely, the "phantasm of modernity," meaning not only the lived reality of the era but also the hope it inspired, the future it promised, and the progress it assured. In other words, the "phantasm of modernity" at the root of this nostalgia is the ever-expanding "horizon of expectation" that Senghor's brand of modernity guaranteed, and the sense of loss conveyed by stories of that "other place in time" stems from their tellers' experience of—and investment in—the emerging Senegalese modernity that was disavowed and abandoned before it was ever truly achieved. Their "horizon of expectation" was foreshortened right before their eyes.

What distinguishes nostalgia for Fann's "golden age" (and by extension, Senghor's Senegal) from the nostalgia described in much of the literature on the subject is that it does not lament the loss of an "authentic" past or long for a mythical time in which everything was (or is imagined to have been) simpler, slower, and more "natural." These stories, I argue, complicate and add dimension to the idea that nostalgia, as the longing for a lost past, is a byproduct of modernity. In these stories, modernity itself is the object of nostalgia rather than simply a condition of its possibility.

Although James Ferguson's *Expectations of Modernity* (1999) does not engage with the topic of nostalgia per se, there is a great deal of resonance between a facet of his project and this facet of my own. During his fieldwork stay in the Zambian Copperbelt town of Kitwe during the late 1980s, Ferguson was confronted by an overwhelming sense of despair about the nation's decline. Zambia's industrial and economic boom of 1960s went bust during the 1970s, ushering in a severe economic crisis that impacted people's lives in a multitude of ways. Ferguson (1999: 12) explains that his book does not seek to write a history of the crisis but rather to

> trace . . . its effects on the people's modes of conduct and ways of understanding their lives. For the circumstances of economic decline have affected not only national income figures and infant mortality rates but also urban cultural forms, modes of social interaction, configurations of identity and solidarity, and even the very meaning people are able to give to their own lives and fortunes.

Rather than concentrating on the nostalgic aspect of people's stories about a better time, Ferguson approaches Zambia's state of decline as an economic and social *fact*, which allowed him to "concentrate on the social experience of 'decline' itself" (15). In so doing, he interrogates and attempts to deconstruct what he calls the "modernization myth" as it operates in three distinct but interrelated spheres: in academia (specifically in anthropology and the other social sciences); in modernization and development discourses; and "real life," as it has shaped and structured urban Zambian's expectations of their futures.

Certainly the men and women whose nostalgic stories form the backbone of this chapter would argue that the overwhelming sense of "decline" plaguing Senegal since the late 1970s should be approached as *fact*. There has indeed been widespread criticism within Senegal regarding the nation's economic, political, and even moral decay over the past four decades. However, many refuse this nostalgic mode outright and instead take a critical view of both Collomb's Fann and Senghor's Senegal, insisting that Collomb and Senghor were actually part of the problem. Although I cannot speak about Zambia, I can say with certainty that in Senegal, there are other ways of speaking about the "golden age" that portray it differently; there are other voices occupying other positions, with other interests in mind. In this light, I take to heart Bissell's (2005: 216) comment:

> Nostalgic discourses . . . circulate in a social terrain in which diverse forms of memory are at play. A truly ethnographic engagement with nostalgia requires that we acknowledge and seek to account for multiple strands of remembrance, seeing how they coexist, combine, and / or conflict.

Nostalgia, as Boym (2001: xvi) has suggested, might just as well be directed at—or rooted in—the "unrealized dreams of the past and visions of the future that became obsolete" as it is in "ancient regime[s] or fallen empire[s]." But what does it mean to locate hope for the future *in the past*—when hope itself becomes an object of nostalgia? When nostalgia (directed toward the past) takes hope (directed toward the future) as its object and loops back on itself, it indexes a present that was lost before it ever came into being. The temporalities of hope and nostalgia become entangled in this discursive movement, producing what Jacques Derrida (1994: xx) might well have called a spectral moment or a "moment that no longer belongs to time." Here, stories about the "golden age" of Fann—and the hope-filled years that followed independence—haunt the present with specters not only of a lost and irretrievable past, but of an *other* present that never came into being. And in the movement between pasts of the present and futures of the past, linear or progressive time is destabilized and thrown into question. The present, for

the men and women who worked alongside Collomb and his colleagues, is
not what they imagined it would be.

NOSTALGIA SPEAKS OF THE PRESENT

Predicated on—and constantly reaffirming—the vast disjuncture between
then and *now*, stories about Fann's "golden age" undoubtedly say as much
about the present as they do about the past. Many of the men and women who
worked at Fann during the 1960s and 1970s say that they are deeply saddened
to see the clinic as it is today, as it has come to be—a shell, they say, of what it
once was. According to Aissatou, the Fann of the past and the Fann of today
are not even comparable; they are two completely different places. The clinic
lacks the resources it once had, she and others say, but that does not explain
all of the changes that have taken place there. They insist that the clinic began
its decline when Collomb and his European colleagues left in the late 1970s
and Senegalese psychiatrists took over. "Since Collomb's departure," Bintou
told me, "psychiatry at Fann has fallen into banality (*tomber dans la banal-
ité*)." Further, many explicitly compare Collomb's departure and the subsequent decline of Fann with Senghor's departure from office in 1980 and the
social and economic crises that hit Senegal around that same time.

If the nostalgic recollections of Fann's "middle figures" appear to share a
common narrative framework and produce a seemingly inexhaustible supply
of stories about Collomb's Fann, their depictions of the 1980s and early 1990s
are, in comparison, sparse and unelaborated. Stoler and Strassler (2000)
describe encountering a similar phenomenon when they interviewed
Indonesian women and men who had worked in Dutch colonial homes as
domestics, groundskeepers, and nursemaids in colonial Netherlands Indies.
"In contrast to the elaborated, oft-repeated stories of the Japanese occupation,"
Stoler and Strassler explain, their interlocutors' memories of the domestic
work they carried out during the late colonial era "seemed uncrafted, rough-
hewn and apparently unrehearsed," leading Stoler and Strassler to suggest that
"[p]eople seemed unused to talking about, and perhaps even recollecting,
these experiences" (14). Marie-Claude and her colleagues had much to say
about the present-day clinic, however. When I asked them to describe the
differences between the past and present-day institution, they told me that
the doctors currently working at Fann no longer care about culture or tradition. "They believe only in Western medicine (*les traitements occidentaux*),"

Marie-Claude intimated. Seynabou responded similarly, explaining that "Collomb thought that to treat madness, one had to take culture into account." She thought for a minute and continued, "Senghor thought the same about developing Senegal. It was part of the era, I think. After Collomb and Senghor, things changed." Bintou insisted that while the European doctors had respected traditional therapies and were driven to learn more about them, the Senegalese doctors rejected traditional therapies in favor of conventional Western psychiatry. Likewise, Aissatou opined:

> The doctors working there today, they don't accept tradition. They don't want collaboration [with local healers]. Collomb accepted it! He collaborated—truly collaborated—with healers! While he was at Fann, healers came through the clinic all the time. But after he left, they were no longer welcomed there. They eventually stopped coming.

Aissatou's assertion that the doctors at Fann did not accept tradition has two meanings. On the one hand, she says, they are refusing to consider traditional beliefs; on the other, they are denying the history of Fann itself. The latter assessment was echoed by Seynabou, who told me that the present-day Fann operates as though it has no memory of its own past; as if it had no history. As I discuss in greater detail in the chapters that follow, the Senegalese psychiatrists who replaced Collomb and his colleagues view their relationship with both history and tradition in a very different light.

Perhaps the most contested memory that Seynabou, Aissatou, and the others shared with me about the early years of Fann had to do with whether or not *ndëpp* ceremonies were ever organized at the clinic. According to them, Collomb's desire to collaborate with local healers led him far beyond mere observation or dialogue. They insist that Collomb not only attended *ndëpp* ceremonies outside of the clinic, but that he actually organized, funded, and participated in them at Fann. As Aissatou told me:

> We held *ndëpp* sessions at Fann back then, in the courtyard. The one I remember best took place behind the *Pavillon des Dames*, and it lasted for several days. It was held for a young woman by the name of Fama Diop, and the attending healer's name was Fatou Mbaye. It was remarkable! And the young woman seemed to get better after it was over.

Aissatou explained that while *ndëpp* ceremonies were not performed regularly at Fann, they were indeed organized there from time to time. The men and women currently working at the clinic, however, deny that *ndëpp* ceremonies ever took place in Fann's courtyard. Dr. Mamadou, a psychiatrist working at Fann in 2002, suggested to me that time or fantasy had perhaps distorted people's memories. Several other doctors have likewise scoffed at the idea that *ndëpp* ceremonies had been held in the courtyard, and laughed while dismissing such claims as make-believe. They insisted that such stories grossly misrepresent Fann; while Collomb and his colleagues were curious about—and even had a "scientific interest" in—local healers and their techniques, their idea of collaboration never went so far as to carry out *ndëpp* ceremonies at Fann. "There are *limits*," Dr. Mamadou told me, smiling. "Collomb was a *doctor*, after all."

Although the doctors currently working at Fann accept Collomb and his colleagues as innovators and express some degree of indebtedness to them, they also agree that a modern psychiatric clinic is no place for healers or traditional therapies, let alone *ndëpp* ceremonies. As Fann's previous director explained to me over and over again, patients do not come to Fann to consult traditional healers; they come to receive the kind of treatment that a psychiatric clinic has to offer. "If patients wish to consult healers," he said, "they can, and many do—outside of the hospital. But it is not Fann's place to facilitate these relationships."

Those who worked at the clinic during the 1960s and 1970s, however, applaud Collomb for having accepted tradition. Like Senghor, they praise Fann for having once been a place where traditional African therapies and Western models of mental health care entered into dialogue with one another to create a new—and uniquely Senegalese—style of psychiatry. They resent the fact that traditional beliefs are no longer important at Fann; that the European doctors thought more about tradition than the Senegalese doctors do now. The doctors who work at Fann today, they say, do not want to remember; they refuse tradition, they refuse history, and they refuse to inherit the past. I shall look more closely at these accusations—and also the way the current Fann doctors respond to them—in chapter 5.

THE "PARIS OF AFRICA," SENGHOR'S SENEGAL

As a social practice and a form of memory work, nostalgia cannot be properly interrogated without considering both the context in which it is mobilized and the various subject positions of its speakers. Above all, the way the "middle figures" described in this chapter remember Fann has much to say about how they relate to—and make sense of—larger social and political transformations that have taken place in Senegal since the nation's independence in 1960.

Marie-Claude and her colleagues embraced Senghor's vision for a new Senegalese modernity, which celebrated Negritude as the cornerstone of a "Civilization of the Universal" and strongly affirmed close French-Senegalese ties. Her reference to Dakar as both colonial jewel (the "Paris of Africa") and cosmopolitan capital of independent Senegal ("Senghor's Senegal") did not simply imply a seamless transition between the two eras; in her view, the "Paris of Africa" and "Senghor's Senegal" were one and the same. Although the early independence era was exciting and full of promise, Marie-Claude did not experience it as a time of great change from what had come before.

Marie-Claude had just turned 18 years old when Senegal gained its independence; she was 20 years old when she began working at Fann. She described herself as a "naturally curious child," and because she "wished to be as clever as her older brother," she excelled as a student at the local missionary school. Marie-Claude simply loved learning, and geography was her favorite subject. Like other Senegalese children enrolled in French schools, she too had learned that her ancestors were *les Gauls*, although she laughs about it now. Her father was one of a handful of Senegalese men who had risen up through the ranks of the French military, and her mother, like Senghor himself, was Sereer and had come from a "good Catholic family." Her family was far from rich, Marie-Claude told me, but they were very well respected in the community.

Marie-Claude's family, and Marie-Claude herself, were not only committed to *la Francophonie,* they were invested in—and dedicated to—the path of modernity that the French colonial encounter had offered and Senghor's Senegal had extended. As part of a rising middle class in urban Dakar,[4] they were educated, modern, and well represented by President Senghor, who favored continued cooperation and collaboration with France after independence. Indeed, Senghor drew the bulk of his support from this growing middle class.

Senghor's vision, however, was not promised equally to—or shared by—all, nor was his desire for continued collaboration with France. Thus, Marie-Claude's nostalgic reflections about Dakar's seamless transition from colonial jewel (the "Paris of Africa") to cosmopolitan capital of newly independent Senegal ("Senghor's Senegal") was met with strong criticism by those who felt Senghor's Senegal to be too close to the colonial regime that had preceded it.

Likewise, for the first generation of Senegalese psychiatrists who would eventually replace Collomb and his European colleagues at Fann in the late 1970s, Collomb's continued directorship at the clinic represented an ongoing and stifling link to the colonial world.

From this "landscape of the present" (Stewart 1988: 227)—a landscape in which Marie-Claude and her colleagues feel utterly dispirited and displaced—recollections of both Collomb's Fann and Senghor's Senegal give rise to memories of better and more hopeful times. Their nostalgic stories recall an innovative experiment in cross-cultural psychiatry as well as the realization of a distinctly Senegalese style of modernity. Above all, their reflections reaffirm a shared sense of bitterness that this present is not what the past imagined it would be. Nostalgia, this active conjuring of an "other" time, necessarily troubles and inhabits the present.

A Terrible Cry from the Past

UN CRI TERRIBLE DU PASSÉ IS A POEM WRITTEN BY Demba (Magatte Ndiaye). It appeared in the patient-run publication *Pinthioum Fann* in January 1986.

Un cri terrible du passé

Un cri lugubre à travers les avis touche mon SANG
Quel est ce frisson, qui me pénètre
Quand hier, depuis . . .
J'ai admiré la lance de mon pere?
Si l'Afrique me baigne d'Effroi!
Qu'est ce qu'elle cache
Ces rimes qui gravitent sa tombe?
Afrique!
Non ce n'est qu'un souvenir qui affirme
Quand les humbles touchent le Soleil et s'exhilent[1]
Tout pousse et nous repousse à être indulgent
l'Afrique!
Non plus la colère
Qui enseigne le malheur à nos fils
Car l'Occident semble se ressaisir
Il m'a appris à danser
Sur le coudes de ses melodies

A terrible cry from the past

Through the announcements a somber cry touches my BLOOD
What is this shiver that penetrates me

When yesterday, since . . .
I admired my father's spear?
If Africa bathes me in Dread
What is she hiding
These rhymes gravitating toward her gravestone?
Africa!
No, it is only a memory that avows
When the humble ones touch the sun and turn to exile
Everything pushes us towards and away from indulgence
Africa!
No longer the anger
that teaches our sons sorrow
For the Occident seems to recover
He taught me how to dance
On the bends of his melodies

FOUR

The Ink That Marked History

THERE ARE OTHER STORIES THAT circulate about collomb's Fann as well, other "strands of remembrance" about that era that stand in stark contrast with—and remain unassimilable to—the nostalgic recollections of Fann's middle figures. For although the clinic continued to flourish during his late 1960s and 1970s, the first generation of Senegalese psychiatrists who were being trained by and working under Collomb and his European colleagues remember the period as one characterized by *friction*. As this new generation came into its own and began to seek legitimation in its own right, it also began to put distance between Collomb's "culture" project and its own orientation, which assumed—as its point of departure—the universality of the human psyche as well as the universal applicability of psychiatric medicine. By the 1970s, Senegalese psychiatrists working at Fann were distancing themselves from the brand of psychiatry that had been established as Fann's trademark. This group, which would eventually replace Collomb and his European colleagues and "Senegalize" (*sénégalisé*) the clinic, was as wary of Collomb's collaboration with local healers and healing traditions as it was reluctant to engage with or report on the cross-cultural research that had been initiated by the Fann School. And although the head of this group, Babakar Diop, was himself psychoanalytically trained and oriented, his troubled tenure as the first Senegalese *chef de service* (director) of Fann from 1978–98 also corresponded with a weakening of the clinic's psychodynamic approach and a growing reliance on pharmaceutical care.

In this chapter, I reflect upon the "Senegalization" of the clinic and ask why this new generation found it necessary to put distance between their approach and the brand of cultural psychiatry that had been promoted by

Collomb and the Fann School. The irony of this story, of course, is that while the European doctors had wanted to "Africanize" psychiatry by letting local beliefs and healing practices inform conventional psychiatric methods, the "Senegalization" of the Fann moved the clinic in the opposite direction, away from these very questions of culture.

As I build upon this new generation's recollections of the transitional period of the 1970s, I frame my discussion around a story that has come to figure prominently in the moral and historical imagination of the clinic— that of the untimely passing of Dr. Moussa Diop, a promising young psychiatrist who was expected to take Collomb's place and become the first Senegalese director of Fann. Diop's death, which occurred in 1967, was a harsh blow to the clinic; to this day, many people associated with Fann's past still whisper that he fell victim to invisible (occult) forces, namely witchcraft. In the wake of Diop's death, Collomb ended up staying on as the director of Fann for eleven years longer than intended, during which time he faced growing opposition from the Senegalese psychiatrists who were eager to take his place.

Moussa Diop's death came up quite frequently in conversations I had with people about the dissolution of Collomb's Fann, not only because it was a tragic event that had befallen the clinic, but because it was an event that many understood to have radically altered the course of the Fann's history. Some thirty-five years and more after Diop's passing, the story of his death was still affectively loaded, and still a source of inexhaustible speculation and intrigue for my interlocutors. I came to understand its invocation as a form of memory work that allowed tellers to situate themselves in relation to a kind of moral imagination of Fann's past. There were two divergent modes in which the story was told. The first described Diop's death in terms of what it ruined or destroyed. As detailed in chapter 3, the men and women who nostalgically remember the 1960s as Fann's "golden age" expressed certainty that Moussa Diop would have continued Collomb's project and carried on his legacy; in their retrospective view, his death prefigured the decline of the institution. In contrast, the second mode in which the story of Moussa Diop's death was told seemed to cast the tragic event in terms of the limits—even the impossibility—of Collomb's project of transcultural psychiatry and the lessons it provided for the future of the clinic. This particular framing of Diop's death, I suggest, also recalled the failures and limitations of Senghor's ability to build a distinctly Senegalese modernity—a modernity predicated upon both the politicization of Negritude and the notion of a "Civilization of the Universal." From this perspective, Moussa Diop's death is understood to mark the beginning of the end of the era of collaboration and cooperation in which Collomb's Fann and Senghor's vision for Senegal flourished.

A prominent Senegalese psychiatrist who served as director of Fann from 1998 until his retirement in 2012, and who first came to the clinic as a medical student in the early 1970s, once told me that the death of Moussa Diop "*a fait couler beaucoup de l'encre.*" In literal terms, this expression means that his death "made a lot of ink run or flow," or in other words, much was written about the event (presumably in ink). Idiomatically, the expression means that the death attracted a good deal of attention or has generated a good deal of commentary. As a nonnative French speaker, though, I am captivated by the image and idea of this ink—ink flowing from a pen, ink used in a printing press, ink that runs, trickles, marks, and blots. I take this ink not only as a reference to writing, textuality, and legibility, but to flows of ink that may both inform and menace memory and identity, and to the writing of history itself. It is with this ink in mind, then, that I proceed.

THE END OF AN ERA

In a photo in Senegal's daily (generally, pro-government) newspaper, *Le Soleil,* dated July 19, 1978, Collomb stands in the foreground like a proud soldier, chest thrust forward and arms pressed stiffly into his sides, as a crowd looks on. Another man stands facing him with a medallion in his hand—a National Medal of Honor, to be exact. His eyes are focused on Collomb's lapel, as if he is calculating where and how to affix the honor. "Professor Henri Collomb," I imagine the man saying, "in the name of the President of the Republic of Senegal, and by the power thus invested in me, I hereby name you '*Grand officier de l'Ordre national du Lion.*'"

I have looked at this photo many times, wondering what Collomb was thinking that day, and how he felt about his long tenure at Fann coming to an end. He had, after all, occupied the post since 1959, the year before Senegal's independence. So much time had passed, in fact, that many around Fann had begun to wonder whether he would ever relinquish his position. "I remember," said El Hadj, who had worked as Collomb's principal translator,

> we were going somewhere one day, I'm not sure where, and I asked him, "But why do you want to go back to France and quit your job here?" He said, "I have to leave, because Senegal wants to Senegalize *(Sénégalisé)* the clinic. That's why I have to go, not because I want to. Otherwise I would stay." So I

asked him, "But where will you go? You have been here almost twenty years!" He told me that he would be working at a hospital in Nice.

Collomb had not planned to stay at Fann as long as he had. He often told people that he had intended to leave as soon as the young Senegalese psychiatrist, Moussa Diop, had been awarded the title of *professeur agrégé* by the University of Dakar. The title *professeur agrégé* confers the highest academic rank in the French university system; in order to receive this nomination, one must pass the highly competitive *agrégation* examination. Since Fann serves as a teaching clinic for Université Cheikh Anta Diop, the director is required to hold this title. Dr. Moussa Diop—Collomb's apprentice, confidant, friend, and peer—was to be the first Senegalese *professeur agrégé* in psychiatry, and the first Senegalese heir to Collomb's post at the clinic.

Fann would have flourished under Diop's direction, Collomb later told people. Moussa Diop would have built upon Fann's already well-established reputation as an innovative, experimental, and highly unconventional psychiatric clinic. He would have continued the project that, under the direction of Collomb, had become Fann's claim to international renown and debate— the project of building a distinctly Senegalese psychiatry that entered into dialogue with local exegeses of madness and its cure. This was the project to which *l'Ecole de Fann* had dedicated its research, writing, and clinical practice for many years.

That Moussa Diop was to take Collomb's place was no secret. Marie-Claude told me that Moussa Diop's passion for psychiatry had led him straight to Collomb; that on the day of their meeting the two men embarked upon an extraordinary relationship. Collomb, referred to by some as "the father of Fann" (*le père de Fann*), was said to have found a son the day the two met.[1] Indeed, Moussa was (and still is) referred to as *le fils spirituel*—the spiritual son—of Collomb. As the two men worked side by side for several years, their bonds of fictive kinship grew strong. "Moussa *was* Collomb," El Hadj insisted, projecting their closeness into a somewhat mystical realm of resemblances: doubles, echoes, twins, reflections, magical correspondences. El Hadj spent a great deal of time with both men and knew them both well. "Yes," he repeated, "Moussa *was* Collomb!" With that, El Hadj covered his mouth with his hand and shook his head. "The day Moussa died . . . I saw Collomb cry that day, oh how he cried. To think of it now! Shaaa-dut-dut-dut . . ." Tears welled up in his eyes, and still shaking his head, he grabbed his mirrored aviator sunglasses off the table and put them back on.

Alphonse, who first came to the clinic as a medical student in the mid-1970s, told me that Collomb often talked about Moussa Diop and made references to the fact that his untimely death was what kept Collomb working at Fann for so long:

> Honestly, I think that when Collomb came to Fann as a *coopérant*, he thought it was going to be a relatively short stay. His job was to instruct Senegalese medical students in psychiatry and to train someone who could take his place [as the director of the clinic]. Then he was to leave, and go back to France. That is the role of a *coopérant*, after all! But in Collomb's case, the person he trained to fill his shoes died before he was able to take over. So he stayed around. He submitted a request to the government, asking to keep his position. The government accepted. He stayed. And he often explained his extended stay by saying, simply, "I have been here as long as I have because the person who was to take my place died, and there was no other."

Here is the story—a condensed version of the many tellings I encountered during my time at Fann. The year was 1967. Moussa Diop, who had completed his medical studies several years earlier, was practicing psychiatry at Fann and working toward the distinguished title of *professeur agrégé* that would make him eligible to act as director of Fann. Moussa Diop was in his early forties; he was charismatic and well liked by many, and great things were expected of him. Quite suddenly, however, he fell ill. "It all seemed to happen in a matter of days," remembers Aissatou. "One day he was perfectly healthy, but then all of a sudden, he was sick, so sick! He had an X-ray taken and some tests were run. I remember the day when he went into the office of one of the other doctors and they looked at the results together—he knew he had cancer, and he knew then that it wasn't going to be OK." As it turned out, the official diagnosis was liver cancer. Nothing could be done to stop the disease, which proved to be aggressive and resistant to treatment. Moussa Diop passed away shortly thereafter, after having been transferred to the Fann clinic, as per his request. He was just 43 years old. In an obituary penned by Collomb (1967: 182), he is described thus:

> Moussa Diop lived two cultures. He had the rare privilege of being profoundly African, and of remaining completely so despite long experience of acculturation in Europe. Not only was he perfectly able to manipulate Western language, logic and technique, he was also able to perceive and experience it as a Westerner. He had made the journey from his culture to ours, and he asked us to follow the same path from our culture towards his own.

According to many who worked at Fann during the 1960s and 1970s, Collomb never recovered from Diop's death. As Aissatou confided, "He [Collomb] even kept Moussa Diop's picture—several pictures—in his office, long after he passed away. One day when I went in there for something, I saw the pictures and said, '*Professeur*! All of these photos here, you are holding on to pictures of the dead!' And he said, 'But Aissatou, these photos are all that is left.'"

. . .

Several months into my dissertation fieldwork stay at Fann, after I had already heard numerous stories about Moussa Diop and his untimely passing, I sat with the then-director of Fann, whom I shall refer to here simply as the Professor. The Professor and I had come up with an arrangement that seemed to be working well for both of us. I would spend several hours each week helping him with his English and, in return, he would answer any questions I had about Fann, past and present, and put me in contact with people I wanted to talk to about my project. Engrossed in this collaborative endeavor, we spent several mornings each week together in his office. As if engaged in important official business, he would tell his secretary that he was not to be disturbed. This day, we had begun working through *The Autobiography of Malcolm X*. The Professor read aloud to improve his pronunciation, stopping periodically to ask about words he did not recognize and jot them down.

After his English lesson, it was my turn to ask questions. "Today I would like to learn a bit more about Moussa Diop," I said to him. "I would especially like to know more about how his death affected the clinic. What happened at Fann after Moussa Diop died?"

With his hands folded on the desk in front of him, the Professor leaned forward to close the gap between us. He knew I had heard the story before. He sighed. "You know, the death of Moussa Diop *a fait couler beaucoup de l'encre*." He tilted his head forward and shot me a meaningful look over the top of his eyeglasses to be sure I understood. And as with most of the other times he had given me that look, I was not at all sure what he meant. I waited for him to say more.

"His death scared away a lot of people who almost specialized—who had wanted to specialize—in neurology and psychiatry." He paused again for a moment, and then continued:

People understood Moussa Diop's death as an unnatural death. Because, well, they thought that it happened because he worked in the field of psychiatry. It is a dangerous field; some people think that there are evil forces that will attack those who try to intervene. Because . . . if a person treats someone who is thought to have been attacked by evil forces, it is as though that person is stepping between him and those evil forces. Therefore, well, people thought that he was a victim of witchcraft (*dëmm, sorcellerie-anthropophagie*).[2]

By making reference to the power of invisible forces in the visible world—forces that are thought to be especially augmented in and around Fann—and even alluding to the fact that people understood Moussa Diop to have been a victim of these evil forces, the Professor brought forth a number of images and associations regarding the unexpected loss of Moussa Diop, the outcomes of that loss, and the possible meanings that have become attached to it. At the same time, by bracketing his comments within "some people think," the Professor distanced himself from being implicated in such occult forces. "The tracery of suppositions through which conjectures of responsibility for evil can be surmised," Adam Ashforth (2005: 15) reminds us, "is made from the skeins of gossip and speculation—oft-repeated, half-remembered—that are the living history of a community." As is often true with stories that invoke invisible forces and spirit worlds, the mention of Moussa Diop's death suggests and circulates the possibility of danger, and implies (among other things) the need for vigilance, prudence, and protection. But what kind of danger is being referenced here? From what—or from whom—must one protect oneself? The story of Moussa Diop's death resists being condensed into any singular, comprehensive meaning. Perhaps it could be said that its very power lay in the multiplicity of meanings that it communicates.

Especially important to my way of thinking about the stories of invisible (occult) forces that circulate about Moussa Diop's death is the work of what is commonly referred to as the "modernity of witchcraft" school (Comaroff and Comaroff 1993; Geschiere 1997; Moore and Sanders 2001). What is compelling to me about this approach is that it insists on taking witchcraft stories not as atavistic remnants of a "traditional" way of thinking, but as particular ways of understanding events that occur in complex—and undeniably modern—sociopolitical environments and institutions. According to Comaroff and Comaroff (1993: xxviii–xxix), "witchcraft is a finely calibrated gauge of the impact of global cultural and economic forces on local relations, on perceptions of money and markets, and on the abstraction and alienation of 'indigenous' values and meanings. *Witches are modernity's prototypical malcontents"* (my emphasis). Far from "stamping out" witchcraft beliefs and accusations, modernity and its effects have done just the opposite. Indeed, if stories of occult forces circle about excessive accumulation and fame just as they hover around unexpected tragedy or failure, then modernity has provided ample space and opportunity for witchcraft to flourish.[3] As discussed in chapter 2, the early Fann clinic was celebrated by Senghor as an exemplary institution of the newly independent state and hailed as a model of a distinctly Senegalese brand of modernity built upon Negritude ideals. Fann was indeed a modern site, but with a twist: in lieu of banishing spirits and healers from its premises, the institution sought to invite them in, observe them, and even tame them. For at least some people working at Fann, however, Moussa Diop's death marked an early blow to the certainty and optimism of Collomb's project. In the end, the clinic generated a witchcraft story of its own.

I should note here, in case it is not already clear, that I am much less concerned with assessing or debunking the "real" or "true" role played by occult forces in the death of Moussa Diop than I am with understanding how stories of occult forces are mobilized by speakers and made to carry meanings that extend far beyond the person or event being spoken about (see White 2000). What interests me is thinking through the discursive and imaginative effects this witchcraft story may generate. For those who inherited the clinic from Collomb and many of the doctors currently working at Fann, a crucial point was to be made—and lesson to be learned—through this story of Moussa Diop's untimely death. From their point of view, the story stands as a first whisper of the limits of the clinic as a site of collaboration between Western medicine and local models of health, illness, and therapy. In reflecting upon the possibility of multiple transgressions that may arise in such a collaborative endeavor, the story of Moussa Diop's death was mobilized in this way to both highlight the limitations of Collomb's project of transcultural psychiatry and to affirm the validity of Fann's philosophy vis-à-vis treatment and therapy *since* the era of Collomb.

DANGEROUS SPACES AND PERILOUS FIELDS

The Fann Psychiatric Clinic was just over ten years old at the time of Moussa Diop's passing. The institution's reputation was at its zenith; its whitewashed façades still glowed brightly under the midday sun. Everyone in Dakar, it seemed, knew of the place. "Back then," Aissatou told me, "working at Fann was really something. We were part of something important. The clinic was famous then, you know!" By the mid-1960s, both Collomb and Fann had not only secured a spot in the city's popular imagination, they had also caught the attention of mental health care specialists around the world. As discussed in the previous chapter, many who worked alongside Collomb and his team during the 1960s—especially nurses, social workers, and translators—still talk about how the feelings of hope and optimism that marked the era were reflected in the institution. No matter how visible and self-assured Fann had become, however, and no matter how solid it appeared to be, Moussa Diop's death would recall the instability at its very foundation.

As the Professor intimated, many people associated Moussa Diop's mysterious death with his involvement in the field of psychiatry, and with the Fann Psychiatric Clinic in particular. It seems that his fate served to remind people that psychiatry in Senegal—especially the distinct brand of psychiatry for which Fann had become well known—was dangerous endeavor. But why was psychiatry in Senegal (and the Fann project in particular) perceived to be so dangerous? In this section, I look to those who inherited the clinic from Collomb and his colleagues—namely, the first generation of Senegalese psychiatrists, those who were said to have "Senegalized" the clinic—to offer insight into this question.

At the time of Moussa Diop's death in 1967, only three other Senegalese medical students had completed their training and established themselves as psychiatrists. All were younger than Moussa Diop. None was yet in a position to take over Collomb's post, for each would have to wait years before he could sit for the examination required for him to earn the title of *professeur agrégé*. The most senior of these three men was Babakar Diop, who was working at a hospital in Bordeaux during the early and mid-1960s and was thus unconnected to the early years of Fann.[4] After Moussa Diop's death, Babakar returned to Dakar at Collomb's request and began working at Fann. The two men were on amicable terms at the start, but their approaches and orientations would diverge in the years that followed. After Collomb's departure in 1978, Babakar Diop would become the first Senegalese *chef de service* of Fann.[5]

Shortly after returning to Dakar, Babakar Diop attended a Colloquium of African Psychiatrists during which he gave a paper entitled *"Sur la formation des psychiatres négro-africains en France"* ("On the training of black African psychiatrists in France"). In this paper, Diop (1968: 169–70) made a curious reference to the potential dangers of psychiatry in Senegal, noting that these dangers are especially serious for African psychiatrists:

> Encountering the other (the patient) has ... serious consequences for the African who is trained in French schools. He commits a transgression in penetrating the domain of mental illness, a domain that is traditionally reserved for healers who are invested with the power to heal.[6]

The passage, so eloquently written, nevertheless raises more questions than it answers and compels us to take a closer look. Diop notes that an act of transgression takes place when an "African," who has been trained to be a psychiatrist in "French schools," offers psychiatric care to African patients. The transgression is, in effect, the result of not one but two boundaries being crossed. The first boundary is that which divides Africa from the West, or in this case Senegal from France. This boundary, constructed and continuously reconfigured over centuries of conquest, colonization, and contestation, is not an impassable wall but, rather, a border zone within which meaning and identity are both generated and undermined. What is implied perhaps in Babakar Diop's statement is that to be trained in French schools necessarily engenders a turning away—or even an abandonment—of one's past.

And it is here that a second boundary is crossed. The "domain of mental illness" in Africa, Babakar Diop suggests, is a sacred dominion reserved only for healers with special knowledge and power. The psychiatrist is not and can never be a healer, thus his or her appearance within this sacred domain is a breach of its very integrity. Babakar Diop signals that this transgression has "serious consequences" for the African psychiatrist who has committed it.

But just what sorts of consequences might the psychiatrist face? Are these consequences thought to be intellectual, moral, social, physical, psychological? Recall the Professor's statement:

> [Psychiatry] is a dangerous field; some people think that there are evil forces that will attack those who try to intervene. Because ... if a person treats someone who is thought to have been attacked by evil forces, it is as though that person is stepping between him and those evil forces.

The Professor here describes psychiatry as a domain occupied by aggressive, invisible enemies or forces—a domain in which anyone attempting to intervene becomes vulnerable and risks "attack." Here nobody is impervious; everybody is at risk. The sources and origins of these hazards are many. As previously discussed, Wolof and Lébou healers in the Senegambia region commonly acknowledge that a diverse band of invisible beings, including *rab, tuur, djinné*, may be at the source of mental distress, including *rab, tuur, djinné*, and many others. Other invisible forces might also be the cause of mental disturbance and behavior changes, including *liggeey / maraboutage* (spell casting; sorcery) and *dëmm* (witchcraft, or *sorcellerie-anthropophagie*). Healers hold specialized knowledge about these forces, and are thus sought for their ability to quell them. They have at their disposal certain measures of protection that others do not normally have—psychiatrists included. According to the Professor, the psychiatrist is at risk because he puts himself in harm's way when he intervenes or "steps between" the patient and the forces that are persecuting him. By entering this space, the psychiatrist thus becomes a target for harm.

Here an important question begs consideration. Babakar Diop was referring specifically to the "serious consequences" an African psychiatrist might face for meddling in the domain of mental illness. But would the risks not be comparable for psychiatrists from Europe or other parts of the world? If psychiatry is indeed a domain occupied by invisible forces, why would African psychiatrists be more susceptible to those forces than their European counterparts? People at Fann (and, in fact, around Dakar) had vastly different opinions to share about this. For instance, a young Senegalese psychiatrist currently working at Fann scoffed at the very question, explaining to me: "Yes, *rab* and *tuur* are an undeniable part of Senegalese culture, but we see this as a kind of description or expression of what is going on for the patient, not the cause of the patient's troubles. No psychiatrist—African or otherwise—has to fear these things." I shall say more about this perspective, and others like it, in the next chapter. The Professor, on the other hand, resorted to a kind of relativism. "Belief is everything," he told me. "The Western psychiatrists are impervious to evil forces because they are protected by their nonbelief (*l'incroyance*). The best that most African psychiatrists can hope for is disbelief (*l'incrédulité*) which, you know, still assumes an underlying belief (*la croyance*). Believing in invisible beings makes you vulnerable to them." The Professor's statement seems to be a variation and (rational) extension of the widely held belief that invisible forces will attack those whom they know best.

Others told me that, in fact, Western psychiatrists *are* equally at risk, but they may either (1) suffer in ways less visible than their African counterparts or (2) be naïve with respect to the "true" source(s) of their suffering. Perhaps the most unexpected and captivating responses, however, came from three nurses who worked at Fann during the 1960s and 1970s. According to these women, Collomb and his European colleagues would have been just as vulnerable to invisible forces as their African counterparts. "[Collomb] was like an African," Aissatou told me. "In a way, he was even more African than many Africans!"[7] The reason no harm came to Collomb and his colleagues, the women told me, was not because they were white. It was because they were protected from invisible forces *by* invisible forces. As Aissatou explained, "Collomb had *rab* (spirits) that protected him here, and they protected Fann."

· · ·

If, as Babakar Diop asserted, the field of psychiatry in Senegal occupies a kind of border zone and the psychiatrist necessarily commits an act of transgression, then the Fann Psychiatric Clinic might have been viewed as especially dangerous. Fann *was* a border zone of sorts—a place of contact and encounter, experimentation and openness. Collomb worked alongside healers and even welcomed them into the clinic; l'*Ecole de Fann* occupied itself with studies of *rab* and *tuur, dëmm* and *liggeey,* not to recast them in psychoanalytic terms, or relegate them to the inner workings of the psyche, or translate them into the language of medical psychiatry as symptoms of psychopathology, but to enter into dialogue with and remain open to them, and to hold them in tension. Collomb and l'*Ecole de Fann* resolutely insisted on taking these forces as a point of departure for understanding mental illness in Senegal.[8] Likewise, they stressed that coming to terms with these forces was key to an effective therapeutic process. It was Fann's very openness, however, that would come to be recognized as its greatest vulnerability. Following Moussa Diop's death, Fann was also perceived as a place of instability and anxiety, limitations and unpredictability. But this is only part of the story.

According to several of the Senegalese psychiatrists who inherited Fann, Collomb and his colleagues seemed to take questions of invisible forces both too seriously and not seriously enough. There was a kind of playfulness in Collomb's dabbling, the psychiatrist Abdou told me. He continued:

> The white doctors, you know, they were in ecstasy over all things African. The Senegalese doctors ... were not interested in these things in the same way. They found these questions to be banal, irrelevant. They didn't claim to be healers and they didn't want to be; in fact, they wanted to distinguish themselves from them.

According to Abdou, Collomb's preoccupation with invisible forces was at once naïvely childlike and exceedingly arrogant. It was naïve because it assigned such importance to local exegeses of mental illness. (Psychiatry, Abdou insisted, functions much better without this.) And it was arrogant because it assumed that such topics could be studied and "understood" in the first place. Senegalese psychiatrists, he explained, insist on distinguishing the role of the doctor from that of the healer. Collomb and his colleagues blurred these worlds; they flaunted their imperviousness from the "serious consequences" that Babakar Diop would later warn about. They invited invisible forces into Fann with the assumption that these could be tamed or even harnessed; they assumed that psychiatry would somehow maintain the upper hand.

Moussa Diop's death, however, caused the first major crack in the veneer of Collomb's project. It reminded people that psychiatry in Senegal was an unstable and hazardous endeavor; it brought to the surface many of the anxieties that already occupied the field. Further, the event was taken by many to be a sign of the project's ultimate inability to control the invisible forces that were present at Fann. For if Collomb and his colleagues were vulnerable to these forces, what sort of assurance would they be able to offer to Fann's patients? Moussa Diop's death, then, threw into question the very possibility that Fann could succeed as a site of collaboration between Western psychiatric medicine and local models of health, illness, and therapy. This doubt, in turn, obliquely reflected back on Senghor's national project, which was facing increasing scrutiny and opposition as the 1960s wore on.

THE VICISSITUDES OF SENGHOR'S SENEGAL

In a critical analysis of contemporary art in Senegal, Ima Ebong (1991: 129) describes an artistic assemblage she once saw in Dakar: "A simple construction hanging from a tree: a mask bound by a rope, like an unsevered umbilical cord, to a flagpole that bears a weathered Senegalese flag." The mask, here standing as a generic symbol of African tradition and authenticity, represents Negritude. Tethered to the Senegalese flag with a "rope, like an unsevered umbilical cord," it suggests the extent to which Negritude was at the service of—and dependent upon—the newborn state's nation-building projects. To Ebong, the assemblage was not only reminiscent of the aesthetic formula that dominated political, cultural, and artistic movements—and typified *l'Ecole de Dakar*—during the 1960s; the assemblage also hinted at the limitations of this aesthetic and foreshadowed its eventual abandonment.

Building a new Senegalese modernity upon the foundations of Negritude was a fragile process. In an attempt to consolidate a homogeneous national identity, Senghor's government—like many other postindependence governments in sub-Saharan Africa—privileged the idea of a shared African essence, and disregarded the ethnic and religious differences within Senegal's borders. This shared African essence, however, had to be recognizably modern. It was above all self-conscious and highly stylized, appealing mostly to the growing urban middle class in Dakar. Mbembe (2001: 12) has written more generally that in postindependence Africa: "[any] discussion of the possibility of an African modernity was reduced to an endless interrogation of the possibility ... of achieving a balance between his / her total identification with 'traditional' (in philosophies of authenticity) African life, and his / her merging with ... modernity." This, according to Mbembe, was primarily due to "the tension inherent in the twin project of emancipation and assimilation" (12).

Perhaps no one was more caught up in this duality than Senghor himself, who was the steward of Senegalese independence, but also favored a close political relationship with France—he remained deeply committed to French language and culture—throughout his life. Although Senghor spoke passionately about the fundamental injustice of colonialism, he did so without putting distance between himself and the Metropole. Senghor never rejected the idea that colonized peoples had gained something important from their colonizers. In a 1963 essay that appeared in the journal *Présence africaine*, Senghor praised cultural exchange that fostered the creation of the "Civilization of the Universal," and even credited colonialism for being the first step toward bringing the races close together:

> Since the beginning of the century, the gap between people and nations has been narrowed progressively as a result of three factors: the extension of European colonization, the intensification of intercontinental relationships, and the independence of former colonies. The cumulative action of these three factors has thrown the races closer together, showing them their brothers in a new light, and the complementary values of their different civilization. It is in this contest that we must study negritude. (13)

For those who were to inherit Fann from Collomb and his colleagues and thereby "Senegalize" Fann, Senghor's discourse of closeness and continued collaboration would prove to be troubling at best. But it was not solely because of his national aesthetic that Senghor faced growing scrutiny, nor was it simply due to his desire to maintain a close political relationship with France. Both Senghor's aesthetic vision and his ideological position were called into question with increasing frequency as he became enmeshed in political battles and was confronted with opposition. Already in 1962, Senghor had taken drastic measures in order to keep his presidency intact; he accused his prime minister and longtime companion, Mamadou Dia, of conspiring to plot a coup against him. Senghor had Dia arrested for treason and imprisoned for life, although he was pardoned and released in 1974, some twelve years later (Le Vine 2004). In 1967, the year of Moussa Diop's untimely and mysterious death, an attempt was made on Senghor's life. The would-be assassin, Moustapha Lô, was sentenced to death for treason and executed by a firing squad. Senghor was publicly criticized for his unwillingness to grant the man clemency (Benoist and Kane 1998). Less than a year after the assassination attempt, massive riots broke out at university when students and workers not only demonstrated in favor of education reform, but also voiced their dissatisfaction with Senghor's consolidation of power. These protests were answered by a heavy-handed military presence and French intervention; Senghor was again harshly criticized (Hanna 1975). Despite growing opposition to his policies and practices, however, Senghor would remain in office until he resigned in 1980. His protégé, Abdou Diouf, went on to serve as Senegal's second president from 1981–2000.

It was against this backdrop, then, of Senghor's own compromised and crumbling vision that both Moussa Diop's death and Collomb's extended tenure at Fann took place. For the first generation of Senegalese psychiatrists eager to replace Collomb and his colleagues, a new direction was as desirable as it was necessary.

KILLING THE FATHER

The Senegalese psychiatrists who inherited the clinic remember Moussa Diop's death as a turning point of sorts. On the one hand, as discussed above, it marked the impossibility—even the failure—of transcultural psychiatry. On the other, it marked the very beginning of a new way of doing things at Fann. Even though Collomb remained at Fann some eleven years after

Moussa Diop's death and his vision was not disavowed overnight, the event significantly altered both the ethos and the future direction of the clinic. Put simply, no other Senegalese psychiatrist wanted to take up the mantle of Collomb's project or continue down the path he had paved. By the mid-1970s, Senegalese psychiatrists at Fann (along with those who had come from other parts of sub-Saharan Africa) began to distance themselves from the brand of psychiatry that had been championed by Collomb and *l'Ecole de Fann*, looking instead to a practice that assumed—as its point of departure—the universality of both the human psyche and psychiatric medicine. In a discussion of psychiatry and psychotherapy in postcolonial Morocco, Stefania Pandolfo (2000) has described a similar process of turning away from relativism. She notes that it was as if relativistic approaches, which treated local healing practices as a "culturally specific form of healing, and an effective one, ha[d] the risk of replicating the colonial operation of circumscribing an indigenous mentality and pathology as something specific to a dominated race, in this case, 'one's own'" (130). If colonial psychiatry had at once been "locked into a discourse of difference" and "unable to contain any notion of difference that was not directly tied to the question of inferiority and the necessity of subordination" (Vaughan 1991: 115), then from the point of view of this new generation of Senegalese psychiatrists, the Fann School's fixation on cultural difference signaled that it had not fully broken free of this past.

All of this is not to say that the changes that took place at Fann were precipitated solely by Moussa Diop's death or by rumors of invisible forces that occupied Fann. As Abdou told me quite frankly, the new generation of Senegalese psychiatrists that Collomb had trained was becoming restless. He continued:

> When I arrived as a student in 1974, some doctors were already complaining about the fact that [Collomb] hadn't yet left. They wanted him to leave; it was my impression that he prevented them from expressing themselves a bit. . . . The service was divided. There was a team of Europeans led by Collomb, and another team of Africans that assembled around Babakar Diop.

While many psychiatrists who had been present at Fann during the 1970s were uncomfortable with Collomb's extended presence at the clinic, some asserted their opposition in more emphatic terms. Alphonse, for instance, went so far as to say that even though Senegal had gained its independence in 1960, the doctors at Fann did not really receive *their* independence until 1978:

Until 1978, there was an uncontested master (*un maître qui était incontesté*) at Fann. Collomb was everyone's master; he had trained everyone. Well, when this master went away, the doctors he had trained finally got to have their independence.

In all of my interviews and conversations at Fann, this was as close as anyone ever came to explicitly labeling Collomb a colonial "master." It was also as close as anyone came to describing Fann as a colonized or occupied territory. In Alphonse's eyes, the colonial era (at Fann, at least) came to an end only with Collomb's departure, nearly two decades after Senegal officially gained its independence.

Throughout much of sub-Saharan Africa, the "process of professionalisation [was] part of decolonization; it coincided with the Africanization of staff and curriculum" (Last and Chavunduka: 1986: 10). In Nigeria, for example, "[t]he process of decolonization of medical services was . . . connected with the emergence of the independent nation-state and with the process of modernization and development upon which independent nation-states embarked" (Heaton 2013: 19). During the 1950s and 1960s, Nigerian-born psychiatrist T. Adeoye Lambo and his colleagues working at the Aro Psychiatric Hospital in Abeokuta championed an innovative approach to psychiatry that was closely linked to larger assertions of political autonomy and, eventually, the birth of a new kind of postcolonial modernity in Nigeria. In Senegal, however, the Africanization of posts did not happen as quickly. Frantz Fanon would end up a vocal critic of Senghor for precisely this reason, and he had sharp words for Senghor's regime in *Wretched of the Earth*: "We know the fierce words of the Senegalese patriots, referring to the maneuvers of their president, Senghor: 'We have demanded that the higher posts should be given to Africans; and now Senghor is Africanizing the Europeans'" (1963: 45). Fanon does not name the Fann clinic specifically, but we need only recall the fact that Senghor credited Collomb for having made himself *"nègre avec les nègres,"* or "black amongst blacks" while working at Fann (Senghor 1979: 138) to see what Fanon might have meant.

Collomb's status as a colonial agent was, for Alphonse at least, not forfeited at the time of independence. And despite the fact that Collomb described the Fann project of the mid-1960s as a radical departure from colonial psychiatric practices in Africa, the extent to which Collomb and *l'Ecole de Fann* considered the social, political, and economic consequences of colonialism on mental health during the early years of Fann is less clear.[9] As Bullard (2005a: 227) reminds us, "Even psychiatrists overtly critical of racism or colonialism were caught within broader political and social structures that exploited the colonized.... Medical complicity with ... imperialism could arise even in situations where the conscious intentions of the doctors were otherwise." It would be erroneous, then, to conflate Collomb's position—or his work at Fann—with that of Frantz Fanon, despite the fact that both were staunch critics of the "universalist aspirations of Western psychiatry" (226). Fanon, who was born in Martinique and received his medical degree in Paris, worked as a psychiatrist in Algeria and spoke out about the effects of colonialism on the mental health of colonized and oppressed peoples. His experiences as a psychiatrist, he emphasized, could not be separated from his politics, which led him to become an outspoken critic of colonialism. As Philippe, a Senegalese neurologist[10] who began as an intern at Fann in 1970, explained to me, Collomb's project was vastly different from that of Fanon:

> Did Collomb and *l'Ecole de Fann* make a break from colonialism? I think it is important to distinguish politics from medicine in this case. Yes, of course, some psychiatrists were influenced by Frantz Fanon ... but Collomb, well, I think his brand of psychiatry was much more a mutation than a revolution, if you know what I mean.... Yes, Collomb's merit was to have been a good mutant *[Oui, le mérite de Collomb, c'est d'avoir été un bon mutant]*.

Here, Philippe mentions Fanon only to contrast him with Collomb. In his view, Fann's project did not imply a radical political consciousness on the part of Collomb; it was far from revolutionary. It did, however, signal a transformation within Western psychiatry, especially as practiced in Africa. Philippe's astute comment demonstrates a certain ambivalence toward Collomb and *l'Ecole de Fann*—an ambivalence he shares with many of the other Senegalese doctors and psychiatrists who were trained by Collomb and *l'Ecole de Fann* during the 1970s.

To Alphonse at least, Collomb was a remnant or carryover from the colonial era whose time at Fann was up. Much more common in my interviews, however, were demonstrations of ambivalence regarding Collomb; these included many references to Collomb as a father figure. "[Collomb] was, in effect, the father (*le père*) of Fann," explained Abdulaye, who worked as an intern at Fann during the 1970s. All of the psychiatrists at Fann are well versed in the Oedipal conflict; the intended meaning of such a statement is as complicated and multilayered as one might expect. On the one hand, Collomb trained the first generation of Senegalese psychiatrists; it was he who built the reputation of the clinic and put Fann on the map. His students were thus deeply indebted to him. As the head of the clinic, he was benevolent but demanding. On the other hand, his "children" were grown. They too wanted to assert themselves. Ibrahim, who was trained by Collomb and then went on to practice psychiatry in Mauritania, summed up the divisions he perceived at Fann during the 1970s:

> There were little rivalries, there was some bad blood (*des mésententes*), if you will. That was how I saw things, anyway. There were some difficulties in getting along—it was the attitude of the occidental who refuses the father, who is always in conflict with the father, who never accepts him but who is nevertheless indispensable to him because everything he does refers back to him.

Bertrand, a French psychiatrist who had worked alongside Collomb for several years, went so far as to describe the factions and divisions at Fann during the 1970s as hostile: "Babakar and his group, they wanted nothing more than to kill the father."

By the mid-1970s, the new generation of Senegalese psychiatrists, led by Babakar Diop, felt themselves ready to take control of Fann—to "Senegalize" the clinic. However, their approach to mental illness and psychiatric practice would turn out to be quite different from that of Collomb and his colleagues. Although Babakar Diop was well versed in psychoanalytic theory and had, in fact, been analyzed by Lacan himself (Guèye 1998: 5), the clinic would eventually turn away from psychoanalytic and psychodynamic interventions and analysis. While this was in part due to the growing financial constraints of the clinic during that period, it may have likewise been driven by another important factor. Just as Lambo and the first generation of Nigerian psychiatrists working at the Aro Psychiatric Hospital in Abeokuta during the 1950s and 1960s had championed the "medicalization of the mind"—in other words, the paradigm of biomedical psychiatry—because it "allowed for [the] depathologization" of the African psyche and brought Africans "into a universal medical framework that treated them as psychological equals" (Heaton 2013: 12), so too did the new generation of Senegalese psychiatrists at Fann, but starting in the 1970s.[11]

Along with this declining interest in psychoanalytic and psychodynamic intervention at Fann also came the abandonment of the Fann School's culture project. After Collomb's departure, healers were no long welcomed into the clinic. Research into local exegeses of mental illness was halted. The idea of Fann as a site of collaboration between Western psychiatric medicine and local models of health, illness, and therapy was abandoned. If the openness of Collomb's Fann had served to usher in invisible forces that could not be controlled, the clinic's doors would be closed. As Abdou explained above, the Senegalese doctors "didn't claim to be healers and didn't want to be . . . they wanted to distinguish themselves from them." Alphonse reflected on the changes at Fann in this way:

> The originality of *l'Ecole de Fann* was its emphasis on culture, and the fact that it took into consideration the differences between peoples [*l'homme dans sa diversité*]. But everything evolves, and in general, everything evolves for the better [*Toute chose évolue, et évolue en general en bien*]. That is the way of things. Modern psychiatry is much more effective and much more efficient than it used to be.

Alphonse stresses here that advances in modern psychiatry, based primarily on biomedical and psychopharmacological models, have made it quite efficacious. In his view, interrogating culture or seeking out alternative therapies no longer makes sense. Alphonse both credits and disavows Collomb's project—Collomb and *l'Ecole de Fann* were innovative in their time, he says, but their time necessarily had to come to an end. Things changed, and in his view, changed for the better.

THE CHANGING OF THE GUARD AS AN ABSENT PRESENCE

Babakar Diop took over as the director of Fann in 1978, shortly after Collomb's departure. This much-anticipated "Senegalization" of the clinic, however, brought with it a number of unexpected hardships. Shortly after Babakar assumed his position as Fann's *chef de service*, he was struck with a mysterious illness that worsened with time, incapacitating him for the rest of his life. There was, and still is, a great deal of speculation surrounding his illness—one psychiatrist currently working at Fann told me that it was most likely multiple sclerosis, while others suggested fibromyalgia or a degenerative muscular disease. Although Babakar Diop was quite ill, he did not relinquish his position as director of Fann right away. Rather, he became something of an "absent presence" at the clinic, making appearances when he could, and appearing to be in great pain when he did, but otherwise staying away most of the time. In the end, Babakar Diop did not officially step down until 1998, twenty years after he replaced Collomb. He passed away only two months after his retirement.

In a touching obituary that appeared in the journal *Psychopathologie afri-caine* a short time after Babakar Diop's death, the succeeding director of the clinic (the Professor) describes the impact of Babakar Diop's illness on Fann, explaining that the high expectations that had been placed upon Diop's shoulders resulted in broken dreams. Consequently, he writes, this led to a "profound and agonizing interrogation of modern psychiatry as it is prac-ticed in Africa by Africans trained in Western medicine" [*"un questionne-ment profond et angoissant quant à la pratique en Afrique de la psychiatrie moderne par des Africains formés a la médecine occidentale"*] (Guèye 1998: 4). The parallels between the untimely death of Moussa Diop and Babakar Diop's extended illness are hard to miss, and they are often paired in people's minds. Both events were open to the interpretation that mysterious—or out of the ordinary—forces had a hand in causing them. And both events proved to be junctures in the life of the institution. From the perspective of the men and women who had worked alongside Collomb and *l'Ecole de Fann* during the 1960s, however, Babakar Diop's illness was not only a horrible tragedy; it was connected to Moussa Diop's death in that it served as an indictment for the dismantling of Collomb's project. As Aissatou explained:

> The clinic changed after [Collomb] left. Babakar Diop fell ill right away. After a couple of years, he could no longer walk without assistance. He could barely write. And when he spoke, he spoke so softly! He saw many doctors, oh yes, and he even went to hospitals in France, but nobody could do anything for him. It was a mystery. He was sick for such a long time—almost 20 years! Everybody told him he should consult a healer, but Babakar didn't accept this for himself. He was like a European, you know. What I want to say is this: Collomb had *rab* (spirits) that protected him here, and they protected Fann, and Babakar did not acknowledge them or make offerings to them. That is why he got sick.

For Fatou and her colleagues, there was an important lesson to be learned from Babakar Diop's illness. In Fatou's opinion at least, Babakar Diop had strayed too far from Collomb's project. Diop's colleagues, of course, did not see things in a similar manner, for they were occupied with maintaining the clinic in his absence and were concerned about the future. Without Babakar Diop's active leadership, what would happen to Fann? What would happen to psychiatry in Senegal? As Guèye wrote, Babakar Diop's illness inspired "compassionate sentiments from everyone around him" while at the very same time "creating an ill-defined state of fear" (Guèye 1998: 4). Fann was once again seen to be a dangerous place, and psychiatry a perilous field, but for different reasons than before. Whereas Moussa Diop's death had been understood by the first generation of Senegalese psychiatrists as both a symbol of the limits of Collomb's project and an invitation to rethink psychiatry in Senegal, Babakar Diop's extended illness offered no such interpretation. Caught in limbo, the newly "Senegalized" institution was forced to operate without an effective leader or a coherent sense of direction for two decades. What is more, the period of Babakar Diop's directorship at Fann, which spanned roughly the same period as the tenure of Senegal's second president, Abdou Diouf (1978–98 to 1981–2000, respectively), was also a period during which Senegal's economy went through IMF and World Bank–inspired transformations that had rippling effects on the social sector (Kelly et al. 1995; Easterly 2005). This, in turn, meant dramatic budget cuts at the CHNU *de Fann*; these cuts had a profound effect on the resources and day-to-day functioning of the psychiatric clinic. I examine these changes in greater detail in the next chapter.

Stories surrounding the dissolution of Collomb's Fann often mark Moussa Diop's death as a turning point of sorts. For the men and women who worked alongside Collomb and his colleagues, his death was the first great tragedy to befall the clinic. It was also the unfortunate beginning of the end of an era that had been filled with optimism, confidence, and the certainty of progress—Senghor's Senegal. For those who were to inherit Fann from Collomb and his European colleagues and "Senegalize" the institution, however, the event was demonstrative of the failure of Collomb's project—and by extension, Senghor's Senegal. The event provided them with the justification they needed to move Fann in a new direction.

The Professor's statement that Moussa Diop's death made a great deal of ink flow can thus be read in several different ways. On the one hand, his death led to the eventual ruination of Collomb's project; it blotted out and made unintelligible a certain track of history. From this perspective, the ink spill destroyed the project that Collomb had started. This was articulated as a great tragedy by some people; for others, it represented an opportunity anew. In that Moussa Diop's death recalled not just the limitations of Collomb's project but the dangers of psychiatry in Senegal as a whole, however, new starts were not impervious to the spilled ink. Moussa Diop's death marked the field of psychiatry in Senegal with fear, self-doubt, and a suspicion that would never quite be allayed. In fact, it would only be intensified by the illness of Babakar Diop. As one of the first Senegalese psychiatrists to be trained at Fann once told me:

> Yes, well, after all, I chose a career in politics, you see. I was one of the first [Senegalese] students trained in psychiatry, but I only did clinical work for a short time. I liked it very much, but other opportunities presented themselves. I can't say that I left psychiatry because I was scared, no, but I think there was—and still is—a lot of fear around psychiatry here. I mean, look at the case of Moussa Diop! Look at what has become of so many of them! No wonder people think it isn't safe!

For the men and women working as psychiatrists at Fann circa 2000, coming to terms with this legacy at Fann—and attempting to place themselves within the institution's lineage—was a difficult and complicated process. In chapter 5, I consider how the doctors working at Fann during the late 1990s and early 2000s positioned themselves in relation to these various "strands of remembrance" of the institution's layered past.

Each in His Corner

"I WAS NOT COLLOMB'S STUDENT, I WAS HIS FRIEND," Demba said to me one day. "I did not come here as a *dof* (Wolof, meaning crazy person). That is to say, there was something—a supernatural power (*un pouvior sur-naturel*) that led to my coming here. I inherited it from my family but it also existed at Fann. Collomb, he also had powers. There is no such thing as coincidence.

"Sometimes Collomb would say, 'Walk with me.' And we would walk and walk, around the compound grounds, over back by the kitchen, here and there. There were lots of stray cats—twenty or so—around these parts. And he would ask me, 'How are the cats? Are they getting enough to eat?' I found this somewhat strange, you know. He took them very seriously. Why was he always asking about the cats? Why did he care about them? In the mornings, too, he'd ask me: 'Did you sleep well? Did you take care of my cats?' Then I realized: He knew something, and he was doing research. It wasn't every cat that he was concerned with, only a few amongst them. They were something, or someone, to him. He would tell me: 'Not all of the cats here are Senegalese.' The colonists brought trees and animals with them from Europe. I also have encounters with these cats. For example, the other day—and this happens a lot—one of the cats came into my room. There's one in particular who visits me like that lately. I'll be sleeping, and then all of a sudden, I wake with a start because I feel someone next to me. And it's the cat. It's like my wife the way it stays next to me! Yes, Collomb had a certain affinity for these cats. You too, when I look at you, I see that you are like a cat!"

Demba was growing more agitated by the second. I sat next to him on the bench, awkwardly, quietly. I wasn't sure how to respond to this story of Collomb and the cats, and these nightly visits. And I was trying to figure out what he meant by drawing me into the story the way he did. The silence dragged on. This was one of the times I was recording our conversation. When I go back and listen to it, the silence still seems to last forever.

Demba shifted; now he was angry. "The doctors here now [in 2003]—everyone is shut away in their office. Before, there were *pénc* sessions, communal meals—things were happening! Now, well, there's a kind of incapacity that's beginning to set in around here. They don't take care of patients anymore. They're working for something else, but not the patients. They are only interested in their documents and their meetings. The clinic doesn't belong to the patients anymore."

"How could they make it better? What would have to happen?" I asked.

"They have to integrate us again! They have to SEE us!" Demba shouted. "They should be retracing the steps of Collomb! Collomb, he wanted to discover everything. He was open. He had time. He would say: 'Come sit and talk with me. I am here.' In the past, it was never a question of dossiers. It was about trying to get at why a person was suffering. It was about getting to know about the person's lineage. They would ask: 'What is the source of this person's illness? Why did his family bring him in? Is his family against him? What does his illness mean in the family? Is he married or not? What is his story?' Now, everybody has his car, his office. They keep the doors shut. Each person is in his own corner. There is no longer an African style around here. Nobody ever asks: 'Why are you suffering? What are your aspirations, your dreams?'

"Collomb, when he was here, he never stopped helping me. Now they do nothing. I come back and they tell me they can give me an injection that will calm me. Those injections do calm me, but they also bring on bad side effects. They make me slow and stupid. So why don't they support me in other ways? Why don't they give me a scholarship (*une bourse*) to work in art therapy, or to do writing? I'm just wasting my time here. Why does nobody help me? Everyone here is against me now."

FIVE

Strategic Ambivalence

BIRAGO AND I OFTEN CROSSED PATHS and exchanged short greetings during my fieldwork stays at the Fann Psychiatric Clinic in 1999 and again from 2001 to 2003. A stocky, slightly unkempt man in his sixties whose usual attire included an oversized T-shirt and cropped pants, he was almost always in a hurry, rushing around on what appeared to be important hospital business. Nurses and secretaries were often looking for him to relay a message or perform some task for them, and I frequently noticed him ducking into doctors' offices. He was clearly not a doctor, nurse, or social worker, nor was he a member of the maintenance staff, but it was obvious that his presence was important to many in the clinic.

One day I asked the Professor about Birago's official title. "Ah, well, Birago. His is an interesting story," the Professor said. He continued:

> He used to work here as a nurses' aide and earn a salary from the hospital, but he reached retirement age about four years ago. So, yes, he has been retired for three or four years now! He collects a small social security check every few months, but it is not enough for him to live on. He lives around here—not far from the clinic—in a one-room place. He's been living in that same place for a long time, more than twenty years at least. It's the kind of arrangement a man might have before he is married, but Birago is married, and he has many kids. It's just that he has never been able to move into anything bigger. He lives there with his whole family, all in that one room.

> Birago's position is very difficult. Even though he's retired, he still comes to work every morning. I can't tell him not to come, you know, and he can't just stay home. There is nowhere for him to go! If you visit these houses in the SICAPs during the day, you will never find anyone at home.[1] Sometimes there are sixteen people who live in two rooms, and they can't just stay around there all the time. They have foam mats (*matelas*) that they sleep on, and they

roll them up and put them away every morning. So I cannot tell him not to come! He doesn't officially work here, but he still finds odd jobs to do and is able to make a little money that way. Madame Dieng in the document center, for instance, is very happy to have someone like Birago around. She can send him downtown or ask him to go to the post office. And the doctors have him run blood samples to the laboratory.

I benefit from him being here, too. Sometimes I have errands for him to run, and I pay him what I can out of my own pocket. This morning I came in and I had a check that needed to be deposited at the bank. He went and came back, and I give him a little something. And sometimes I give him and his family a sheep for *Tabaski* (Eid al-Adha). Lots of people have him run personal errands for them, like paying the electricity and such. I mean, what can I do? He's retired, but he has worked here for years. I cannot tell him not to come anymore. He's not hurting anybody by being here. On the contrary! He helps everyone.

For many people I met while living in Dakar during the late 1990s and early 2000s, making ends meet required an ever-increasing amount of creative problem solving, entrepreneurialism, and flexibility. It also meant drawing on existing moral economies and fashioning new—and oftentimes contingent—social relationships. Times were tough. In the years since 1980, Senegal had received twenty-one loans from the IMF alone (Easterly 2005), but as with all IMF and World Bank loans, there were strings attached: in order to receive the loans, Senegal was required to restructure its domestic economy and implement dramatic reforms that turned out to have far-reaching consequences for millions of its citizens. These Structural Adjustment Programs, or SAPs, privileged "productive" spending while at the same time spurring significant budget cuts in the social sector—the domains of education and health care were particularly hard-hit (Diop 2002; Kelly et al. 1995; Easterly 2005). The impact of these reforms—and of the pushes toward privatization and trade liberalization that are so characteristic of neoliberal restructuring (Harvey 2005)—had rippling effects on every facet of life in Senegal.[2] Prices of everyday items skyrocketed in 1994, for example, when the currency (fcfa) went through a devaluation of 50 percent and controls and subsidies were removed in order to encourage a boom in foreign investment (Diop 2002; Dembele 2005; Kelly et al. 1995).

During my first stay as a university exchange student in Senegal from 1995–96, talk of the everyday difficulties people were facing in the wake of *la dévaluation* was ubiquitous, and nearly every person I met spoke of going abroad (or sending their children abroad) to find work and make money.

Students at the university had experienced an *année blanche* (a canceled school year) in 1988–89, and an *année invalide* (invalidated school year) in 1993–94; even for students lucky enough to secure a coveted place at the university, the dysfunctional educational system meant that it was exceedingly difficult to make progress toward a diploma.[3] I watched as many of my new friends and acquaintances, young and old alike, devised short-term money-making strategies and concocted plans they hoped might provide them with some measure of longer-term financial security. In these affairs, my own role often went far beyond that of a simple observer or collector of stories: from accompanying friends to the U.S. Embassy for visa appointments, to giving English lessons and helping people find short-term research assistantships, to assisting students in their navigation of North American university applications, to lending small and large sums of money, I was frequently (sometimes willfully, but other times reluctantly or even unknowingly) woven into the schemes and dreams of friends, interlocutors, and acquaintances.

An unlikely folk hero, known for his ability to muddle through even the most difficult of situations, emerged as a veritable cultural icon in Senegal during this same period. Goorgoorlou,[4] as he was called, was the main character of a popular comic strip that shared his name. The comic had first appeared in 1989, as a regular feature in the weekly Senegalese satirical newspaper, *Le Cafard Libéré*.[5] Penned by cartoonist T. T. Fons (Alphonse Mendy), *Goorgoorlou* quickly became so popular that the weekly comics were brought together and published as collected volumes. In 2001, the well-loved comic strip was adapted into a television series on RTS (*Radiodiffusion Télévision Sénégalaise*, Senegal's national television network). The series, which featured actors Habib Diop and Seune Sène, began to appear five nights each week, in five-minute sketches of tribulation and sheer hilarity, right before the 8:30 p. m. news program. The segments opened each evening with a scene featuring percussive *sabar* music and dancing, with Goorgoorlou right there in the middle. This music was something of the "theme song" of the show, and woven into it was a Wolof proverb frequently heard on the streets during that era: "*Yàlla, Yàlla, bey sa tool,*" which literally means "pray to God, cultivate your field" but was commonly invoked to mean anything from "God helps those who help themselves" to "prayer alone won't get the job done."

How to describe this Goorgoorlou? He was a rather unremarkable—but infinitely relatable—middle-aged man of limited means and few employment prospects living in Yarakh, one of Dakar's *quartiers populaires* with his wife,

Diek, his son, Modou, and his daughter, Aida. "STF" (*sans travail fixe*, or without steady work) and living in the wake of heavy-handed structural adjustment and economic reform, Goorgoorlou had to rely on pure ingenuity, the help of his social network, and a good dose of luck to scrape together the money he needed to get through each day. Locked in a constant struggle to secure his D. Q. (*dépense quotidienne*, or daily expenditure) and provide for his family, Goorgoorlou regularly devised (or was lured into) big schemes that often became quite messy, and rarely amounted to anything more than trouble.

Goorgoorlou, or Goor (Wolof *goór*: man) for short, had broad appeal and a huge fan base during the 1990s and early 2000s precisely because he was so identifiable as an "everyman." Readers and viewers saw themselves reflected in this character of Goorgoorlou—in his struggles and his ceaseless scrambling, but also in his tenacity and resilience, as well as in the absurd and impossible situations in which he was often caught. Against the backdrop of structural adjustment, devaluation, and governmental incompetence—and against the odds—Goorgoorlou somehow always managed to get by, though sometimes just barely. In so doing, he provided an oblique (and oftentimes not-so-oblique) social and political commentary on the failings of the post-colonial state, and on the problems faced by ordinary people on a daily basis. The brilliance of comic strips like *Goorgoorlou*, explained Massimo Repetti (2007: 24), is that they "juxtapose 'how we are' (daily life) with 'how we try, yet fail to be' (due to the irreversible absence of a civil life, revealed by the authors' criticism of corruption and inequality in the postcolonial state)." As such, comics may be viewed as "acts of moral protest which, by putting popular indignation down on paper, show the impossibility of a different way of life" (24–25). In one poignant and memorable scene, for example, Goorgoorlou hears of the government's plans to devalue the CFA franc; he grabs a shovel and begins digging a hole in his own courtyard, with feigned resignation. Diek is there with him, and she too is concerned. How on earth would they make their way? "We've already had to deal with the structural adjustment and austerity programs," Goorgoorlou says, partially to himself and partially to Diek. "Now comes devaluation. I may as well just bury myself alive!" (Fons 1999: 24). Goorgoorlou the man, and *Goorgoorlou* the comic, offered potent social and political commentary and a hearty laugh, all at the same time. His struggles were emblematic of the struggles of millions of ordinary people in Senegal and throughout sub-Saharan Africa who, with unrelenting humor and an extraordinary capacity for bricolage, creatively navigated the precarious social, economic, and political conditions that shaped their daily lives (cf. Mbembe 1992, 2001; Hecht and Simone 1994; Simone 2004, 2010).

Goorgoorlou was as much a master signifier and battle cry at the Fann clinic during the late 1990s and 2000s as it was throughout the rest of Dakar. Fann and the larger CHNU had certainly suffered the dramatic social sector reforms and curtailed public health care budgets that were implemented as a result of the SAPs of the 1980s and 1990s. People working within the clinic were trying to get by within a "vitiated state" (Wendland 2012) and health system. At the time of my first fieldwork stay at Fann in 1999, the clinic was severely underresourced and operating at a limited capacity, with one of its five divisions closed down completely. Doctors and staff alike were quick to make reference to the infrastructural and material inadequacies that existed at every level, and that made it difficult for them to do their jobs. The bathrooms were filthy; toilets barely flushed and overflowed regularly. Patients' rooms often lacked furniture; many of them did not have locks and a few were missing doors altogether. Patients refused to stay or to keep their belongings in such rooms because they were afraid someone would steal from them if they left. They were also afraid of being harmed by the other patients, a fear that, according to Dr. Yacine, was not unfounded. "There is only one nurse on duty for the entire clinic at night—for all four divisions," she explained to me. "There are both women and men in here, you know; anything could happen. Sexual assaults, violence, anything." The doctors all noted that they struggled constantly to keep up with the day-to-day demands of the place, and sometimes their frustration got the best of them. There were simply not enough doctors and support staff working at Fann to get the job done.

It was within these gaps created by personnel shortages and material insufficiencies at Fann that a flourishing informal economy had emerged in the clinic. In their ongoing search to make ends meet, many people like Birago saw an opening—informal and unstable, but work nevertheless—at Fann and established themselves in the clinic's moral, therapeutic, and political economy. Fann staff were grateful for these unofficial workers, and they felt a degree of indebtedness—even obligation—toward them, oftentimes compensating them with small sums of money or gifts. It is not an exaggeration to say that doctors, nurses, and social workers depended on this informal support staff to a large degree in order to do their jobs. As Melly (2011: 365) has noted, Dakar's "so-called informal economy employ[s] a large percentage of the able-bodied workforce . . . these seemingly 'marginal' activities are, in fact, central to household, urban, and national economies." From this angle, both Birago's refusal to retire and the Professor's justification for not sending him away represented creative strategies for getting by in a time of economic austerity, and in a place where state support had been dramatically curtailed.

The spirit of Goorgoorlou was apparent at all levels within the clinic. "Goorgoorlou rek!" (Wolof *rek*: only; the phrase thus means something like "the scrambling never ends!" or "nose to the grindstone, like always!"), one of the psychiatrists once said to me, half-smiling and shaking his head as he hastily made his way toward a patient's room. One of the most startling ways that Fann doctors were forced to "make do" with the limitations they faced involved the drug treatment strategies they devised—and constantly had to amend and improvise—for their patients. By the 1990s, in the absence of sustained psychodynamic therapies and interventions, psychopharmaceuticals had become the backbone of psychiatric treatment at Fann, mirroring trends in the United States, Europe, and many other places throughout the world (Lakoff 2005; Luhrmann 2000; Petryna, Lakoff, and Kleinman 2006). Despite the centrality of medication to the therapeutic regimes at Fann, however, many of the drugs were hard to come by, and when they were available, they were prohibitively expensive. In 2003, only a few of the newer medications being used in Europe and the United States were available in Senegal, and most were well beyond the financial means of Fann's patients. The cost of Lexipro, for example, was around 40,000 fcfa ($80) per box in 2003— more than many patients (or their family members) might typically make in a month. The clinic depended on samples and donations—from pharmaceutical companies, NGOs, or international agencies—and often provided short-term supplies of these medications for free to inpatients who could not afford to buy the drugs on their own, but the flows were unpredictable and uneven. As Dr. Yacine explained and as I witnessed several times over, doctors often started patients on the newer, more expensive medications in order to "get their problem under control," at which point they would step the patient down to a cheaper and more widely available neuroleptic and antipsychotic medication, like Haldol (haloperidol), Largactil (U. S.: Thorazine; generic: chlorpromazine), or Mellaril (thioridazine).[6] "This is far from desirable, of course," said Dr. Yacine. "It's hard to practice medicine like that." But, she explained, sometimes the medications ran out and the doctors just had to make do.

The "blunt instrument" antipsychotics listed above, many of which have since been discontinued by pharmaceutical manufacturers because of their serious or even fatal side effects, were still very commonly used at the clinic during the late 1990s and early 2000s. With little background or training in psychopharmacology before beginning my research at Fann, I took some time to understand that much of the "abnormal" behavior I witnessed in the clinic was not symptomatic of patients' psychiatric conditions per se; it was related to the medications being used to treat them. It seems naïve to me now, but I did not immediately recognize the heavy sedation, the jerky, repetitive movements, the shuffling feet, pacing, restlessness, and aphasia for what they were: common side effects of the medications that played a central role in psychiatric treatment at Fann. And yet, even these medications ran low at times: In early June 1999, for example, a shortage of Mellaril meant that many patients had to be switched to other medications in a moment's notice. Fatima was one of those patients.

Fatima, a sturdy 44-year-old headmistress from Dakar, had been treated as an impatient at Fann on two separate occasions before her stay in 1999. Although her condition sometimes improved for short periods of time, her sister Salimata told me, the troubles returned, and always got worse. Fatima's family started to notice changes in her behavior some five years earlier; she became antisocial and aggressive, often acting out in the family and accusing people of trying to harm her. Fatima had always been calm, sociable, and predictable, Salimata explained, but her behavior became erratic and explosive. She started spending money left and right, buying things she did not need and could not justify (*les dépenses non-justifiée*): "She began taking taxis all over Dakar. But then, when she got out, she'd refuse to pay. She'd start screaming at the driver and making a scene. One time, the police even got involved." Fatima's words started to not make sense. During her first six-week stay at Fann, she was treated with the benzamide antipsychotic Tiapridal (tiapride) and released with a prescription, but she stopped taking the medication after consulting a *marabout* in Burkina Faso who told her it was making her problems worse—a point I return to later in this chapter. Shortly after that, in early 1998, Fatima again fell ill. She had just experienced two back-to-back miscarriages and was convinced that her husband was trying to kill her because he no longer loved her. Her sister brought Fatima back to Fann, where she was again prescribed Tiapridal and her condition again improved.

After being released from this second stay at Fann, however, Fatima's problems dramatically worsened. She stopped eating and secluded herself. Salimata suspected that Fatima had either mixed up her dosages or stopped taking her medication altogether during that period; she started to experience hallucinations and extreme paranoia. Claiming that her husband was looking for a second wife and had tried to poison her, Fatima fled back to her childhood home in eastern Senegal. Fatima's parents did not much like Fatima's husband, Salimata told me; he was too reserved, often absent, and never helped the family. "But everyone could see that her problems were bigger than a bad marriage." Salimata brought Fatima back to Dakar to take care of her. It was difficult work, Salimata said, but Fatima accepted her care for a time. That is, until one morning in May 1999, when Fatima's sister woke her up to take her medication and Fatima flew into a fit of rage. "You slept with my husband," Fatima screamed, cursing and flailing her arms at Salimata. "I am going to kill you, right here, right now!" Fatima attacked her sister, hitting her and throwing everything in reach. No one could calm her down. That same evening, Fatima was brought back to Fann for the third time and was immediately prescribed Mellaril. The intake notes described her as paranoid and delusional, with a history of experiencing brief psychotic episodes.

When I first met the sisters, Fatima seemed groggy but restless. She spent a good deal of her day pacing the halls, her expression dazed. Fatima had not spoken for several days, so her sister did all of the talking. I could not compare Fatima's behavior to any previous state, of course, and it was not possible for me to assess the extent to which her comportment had been altered by the Mellaril, but Salimata told me that she had noted an improvement from the constant agitation and explosive anger Fatima had exhibited before being brought back to Fann. I did, however, notice a significant change in Fatima's behavior two weeks later, in the wake of a shortage of Mellaril in the clinic. Fatima was switched to Valium when the Mellaril became unavailable, and she began to talk again, but only to address the doctors and nurses with loud demands and insults, and only in stern French. She refused to speak or respond to Wolof. "They wanted to strangle me," she yelled fiercely in the hall one day, "but I am a doctor (French: *une doctoresse*) to the whole world." During a *pénc* meeting in the same period, Fatima came out of her room down the hall, walked over to the group, and disruptively pushed her way into the middle of a mat around which patients, staff members, and guests sat. In a loud, accusing voice, she demanded to know what everyone was doing there, her level of aggression clearly escalating. A nurse intervened to escort Fatima back to her room, and Salimata, who had been attending the *pénc* meeting, walked back with her. The next time I read Fatima's dossier, I saw that her medication had again been changed, this time to a more potent antipsychotic combination of Haldol and Largactil; each time I stopped by her room to see her, she appeared heavily sedated. I wondered at the time whether doctors would have shifted her to this intensive new medication regime if they had not been forced to switch her from Melleril to Valium in the first place.

Psychiatrists regularly choose to alter the medications they prescribe to their patients, of course, usually because they are not responding positively or they are experiencing undesirable (or dangerous) side effects. At Fann, however, changes were also made to patients' medications because of shortages, or because doctors firmly believed that prescribing cheaper medication to patients who were being discharged and monitored as outpatients was a better way to ensure compliance. Dr. Yacine explained to me that it is never a good idea to prescribe drugs that are impossible to find in the local pharmacies, or that are beyond the financial means of patients. "They are less likely to continue taking the medication if we do." Many of Fann's doctors adopted this practice of medication switching as a creative strategy to promote drug adherence. And while Dr. Yacine noted that it was difficult to practice medicine under such conditions, it was certainly all the more problematic for the patients who were subjected to these altered drug treatments and substitution strategies. Psycho-pharmaceuticals affect both the body and mind; they unquestionably transform both experience and subjectivity. Further, as Petryna and Kleinman (2006: 8) remind us, "drugs and treatment strategies also go beyond the body, affecting and potentially reshaping interpersonal, family, and community domains."

Alongside the structural and material inadequacies that existed at Fann during the late 1990s and early 2000s, doctors and nurses had to contend with personnel shortages at the clinic. "I am doing the job of three people," Dr. Mamadou told me, "and getting paid a fraction of what I would be paid in France or elsewhere!" In addition to making regular patient visits, the doctors were expected to teach and monitor students' progress, and attend (and sometimes lead) weekly case presentations. Dr. Yacine explained that each of the doctors spent at least one morning each week (and for some doctors, multiple mornings a week) doing outpatient consultations or checking in with patients who had recently been released. Doctors were also expected to publish and to attend conferences, of course, even though few had the time or the resources to do so, and there were virtually no opportunities for the doctors to be reimbursed for their travels. On top of all this, many of Fann's doctors made themselves available for consultations and even regular rounds at private clinics in order to supplement their paltry incomes. On several occasions, I accompanied one of Fann's doctors to Dakar's upscale *Clinique des Mamelles*, which does not specialize solely in mental health or psychiatric services, but does accommodate psychiatric patients from time to time.

It should come as no surprise, then, to hear that morale at Fann was low. As Dr. Isseu, a psychiatrist who headed one of Fann's four functioning divisions in 2002, lamented, "it seems that every person around here works for himself; everyone is just trying to get by and get through each day." In this sense, the demands of the clinic precluded the possibility of contemplating or expounding upon Fann's therapeutic philosophy, much less making designs on the future; the doctors simply did not have time for such frivolities. Dr. Mamadou's critique was perhaps a bit harsher: "People are motivated by self-interest and that is all. There is really no collaboration here—there is no working as a team. The responsibilities are not shared or equally divided. That creates lots of tension, and makes it quite disagreeable around here sometimes."

Tensions arose not just between doctors, but also among doctors, nurses, and support staff, many of whom blamed each other for making their work more difficult than it needed to be. For example, after walking into the nurses' station of her division one day to find nearly every nurse on duty huddled around a pile of new handbags and shoes, excitedly handling them and haggling with a nurse who had devised the strategy of supplementing her salary by selling goods at work, Dr. Isseu expressed her ongoing frustration about a few of the nurses who, according to her, were part of the problem. "They sit around all day gossiping; they do their *petits commerces*. I've even caught them selling things to patients and their family members. Can you imagine? And if we need them to do things for us, we have to run after them. They administer medication, and that's it. They just aren't invested." From the point of view of many nurses, however, it was the doctors who were not invested. "We do everything. We keep this place running. We know the patients and see them every day. The doctors, sure, they do their rounds. But often, they're just not here."

The question of whether to continue working at Fann or go elsewhere— namely abroad to Europe or the United States—was certainly one that preoccupied psychiatrists and medical students alike during that era. For many, the desire to leave was quite strong; they frequently asked themselves what was keeping them from going. "Really," Dr. Isseu told me, "many times I have asked myself, 'Will I stay or go?' I cannot say for sure." Many people trained in psychiatry at UCAD do, in fact, end up leaving. One day in 2003, the Professor helped me chart out all of the medical students who had specialized in psychiatry since he had first stepped up as interim director of Fann. As we listed names and talked about the career path of each, we realized that of the thirty or so medical students who had specialized in psychiatry under his tutelage, more than half were then living and working in France, and several more were in the United States or elsewhere. "Many went to France for just six months, to do internships. But now they are French citizens! They just never came back! But what can I do? Their lives are better there; they get paid more and they don't have to work as hard." The transnational emigration of so many young psychiatrists trained at Fann has itself been a kind of institutional "brain drain" that has disrupted historical transmission and troubled group solidarity among those who work at the clinic.

RETHINKING TRADITION, REVISING HISTORY

Central to the critique by Senegalese women and men who worked as "middle figures" at the Fann clinic during the 1960s and early 1970s were two important points. First, they insisted that the doctors and staff working at Fann no longer accepted *tradition*; i.e., they no longer wanted to collaborate with traditional healers or seemed interested in taking traditional exegeses of mental disturbance into consideration, as did Collomb and *l'Ecole de Fann*. Second, they avowed that the institution had forgotten its own *history*. By this they meant that the doctors at Fann had chosen not to remember—let alone honor—Collomb, *l'Ecole de Fann*, or the unique style of psychiatry the group had worked to establish during the 1960s and early 1970s.

In this section, I turn to consider these accusations from the perspective of the doctors who were working at Fann between 1999 and 2003. With the exception of the director of the clinic, none of them had ever met—let alone worked with—Collomb, and they denied having disavowed their cultural traditions or having forgotten the institution's rich history. If anything, they insisted, the "disavowal of tradition" and "forgetting of history" had already taken place by the time they arrived on the scene. And while they were to varying degrees aware of Collomb's contribution to the field of psychiatry, many also displayed what I call "strategic ambivalence" toward both Collomb and the early years of Fann. Oscillating between romanticization, distant praise, dismissal, indifference, and outright rejection, they refused the notion of a lost "golden age" and sought legitimation in their own right as they struggled against the everyday shortages and inadequacies of their clinic.

Ultimately, the way these doctors oriented themselves toward and used the past may best be understood in light of the very *Goorgoorlouisme* that characterized those years. In this sense, both Collomb's name and the clinic's renowned history, as symbolic capital, could be drawn upon as potential resources (or likewise, could be dismissed, ignored, or rejected) for the benefit of the clinic. I begin, then, with a discussion of how these doctors imagined their work as psychiatrists, asking in particular how they situated themselves vis-à-vis these questions of both *tradition* and *history*.

In a 2000 article entitled "L'Ethnopsychiatrie à Fann Aujourd-hui" ("Ethnopsychiatry at Fann Today"), authors Ndoye, Devos, and Guèye (2000: 270) insisted that, "given the plurality of therapeutic options (traditional procedures on the one hand, and biomedical treatment on the other), psychiatrists appear to be ill at ease." Based on open-ended interviews carried out by Anne Devos, a Belgian psychology student who did an internship at Fann during a four-month period in early 2000, the twelve-page article evaluated the state of the clinic and assessed the way in which psychiatrists negotiated both "traditional logic" and what they somewhat vaguely referred to as "cultural elements." It also questioned Collomb's legacy in the present-day institution. I take this article—and especially the polemic assertion mentioned above—as an invitation to discuss the ways in which psychiatrists at Fann came to imagine their role as psychiatrists and to situate themselves in relation to both "traditional" and "modern / biomedical" ideas (an operational distinction that they themselves use) of mental illness and treatment. While their article offered a compelling discussion of issues that are central to my own questioning of the institution, my research elicited several distinct points of contrast.

Was it true that the psychiatrists working at Fann between 1999 and 2003 felt a certain uneasiness about their position vis-à-vis traditional versus biomedical treatment models? If so, what exactly did they find unsettling and how did they express their discomfort? Based on my own conversations with the doctors, it would not be obvious to presume that they were "ill at ease." On the contrary, many exuded an air of confidence in their ability to negotiate traditional exegeses of mental illness in light of a more conventional biomedical approach. Listening to how each of the doctors described his or her practice, it became clear to me that most imagined their role as something akin to that of translator. Fluent in both a "local" and a "universal" language of mental illness and therapy, they understood their job as one of rephrasing and reframing patients' symptoms in terms of the diagnostic criteria offered by a more conventional Western psychiatry, and making these legible to patients in a different way.[7] Their translation work, however, was always uni-directional. Above all, the doctors operated according to a firm belief in the universal basis of mental illness, and they saw culture as that which shapes its experience and expression. Psychiatric knowledge was privileged as true and real, representative of a higher order reality. Patients' stories of *rab* and *tuur* were understood as cultural idioms—a local language of affliction that had to be translated into the universal language of psychiatry before it could be properly treated and cured.

These views bear a strong resemblance to the pathogenic / pathoplastic model described and criticized by Kleinman. According to this model, "biology is presumed to 'determine' the cause and structure of . . . mental disease, while culture and social factors at most 'shape' or 'influence' the 'content' of disorder" (1988: 24). It was not that the doctors ignored or rejected their patients' explanations about the origins of their illness and suffering; in fact, they insisted that it was important to get to know the traditional elements of illness as experienced and understood by the patient. "This," said Dr. Yacine, "helps us to better understand the pathology." From a certain perspective, it could be said that Dr. Yacine and others looked through their patients' stories of invisible forces in order to apprehend the "real" medical conditions at their source; they were sensitive to questions of culture not so that they might identify culture-specific disorders, but precisely so they could peel culture away. Patients' stories were taken seriously by the doctors because they represented the patients' lived and experienced reality, the explanations patients gave were, at the very same time, cast as being subordinate to a higher (rational and knowable) medico-scientific truth. This translating and reframing was especially visible in the monthly case presentations made by medical students, where a presentation was deemed successful when it coherently decoded and recoded patients' symptoms and stories to offer a cogent diagnosis, justify specific drug regimens, and chart patient responses to medication.

Although it may seem like a contradiction, the fact that psychiatrists worked to translate local idioms of mental distress into the language of psychiatry did not necessarily mean that they denied the efficacy or importance of healers, traditional therapies, or *ndëpp* ceremonies. In fact, two of the doctors confided that they had recently visited healers, at the request of their families. They were quick to stress the fact that many healers are no better than charlatans, but then, there are charlatans in every profession. "In any case," said one of the doctors, "it [the healer's craft] is not something that can be entirely rejected." Nevertheless, the doctors were, in their own practice, entirely committed to scientific reason and evidence-based medicine. In their daily practice, they appeared most concerned with evaluating and relieving their patients' symptoms in order to establish baseline mental health; they were not searching for the origins or meaning of these symptoms. In their view, the healers' craft simply had no place in the Fann clinic.

According to Dr. Malick, the psychiatrist must first and foremost approach the patient with the tools of modern medicine, for "that is what the patient will expect." Claiming that his clinical practice was basically culture-free, Dr. Mamadou insisted that "culture plays little to no role" in the way he interacts with his patients, "and besides," he added candidly, "I did not study for over ten years to become a *fajkat* [Wolof: healer]!" In any case, he explained, even when patients came to the clinic with a traditional explanation in mind, the very fact that they sought treatment in a *hospital* (or were brought by family) demonstrated their willingness to think about illness in a new way. Doctors, he said, should respect this fact, and take it as an invitation to do what they do best. "Why play at being a healer? That is not my role," stressed Dr. Alioune. He and the other psychiatrists at Fann went to great lengths to distance and differentiate themselves from local *fajkats* and *marabouts*. In contrast, Dr. Mamadou explained, Collomb and his colleagues "tended to blur those lines." According to Dr. Alioune, "medicine itself has evolved, as has society in general." Patients, he explained, have also changed; what people look for and expect from a psychiatric clinic is different than it was forty years ago. "Because Collomb was French," Dr. Alioune told me,

> he had to go to great lengths to make psychiatry more palatable for people. What he did at Fann was, in a way, just artifice to make [psychiatry] more palatable [French: *faire passer la pilule*; literally "to make pass the pill"] at the moment that [it] was first introduced. This is no longer necessary. More and more patients come to the clinic first, before consulting local healers. More people have faith in what the clinic does.

Dr. Alione's comments demonstrate a degree of ambivalence toward the early Fann clinic's emphasis on culture—the "artifice" of Collomb's orientation, he said, was necessary back then, although always something of a ruse. And such artifice is wholly superfluous today.

I was never able to verify whether an increasing number of patients in fact sought treatment at Fann before consulting local healers; historically, this question was not always asked of patients (or was not always recorded). I was, therefore, unable to gather the data from archived patients' files. My notes from 1999 and 2001–03, however, reveal that almost every patient I spoke with during that time had visited a healer before seeking treatment at Fann, and many continued to see a healer even during their stay at the clinic. Preferring to stay "neutral," as they called it, doctors neither recommended nor discouraged patients from consulting with healers, but they did sometimes give patients permission to leave the clinic for short periods of time in order to do so. "We'd prefer it if they would wait until after they were discharged, but if a patient really wants to go, we cannot forbid it, and we have no reason to do so. And even if we were to try, they would go anyway," Dr. Isseu told me. "We ask only that they refrain from ingesting herbal medications (Wolof: *garab*, which also means 'tree'; this word may also be used for prescription medication) offered by the healers, and that they continue with the medication regimen we have prescribed for them." Still, admitted Dr. Alioune, when a patient asks him for permission to leave in order to consult a healer, "it is difficult to know how to react so that [the patient] will feel understood, not alienated or judged."

Ndoye, Devos, and Guèye (2000) suggested that the Fann doctors generally exhibited tolerance toward local healing traditions, and while I found this to be more or less true, there were hints, perhaps, of annoyance with such practices. Dr. Alioune struggled to remain neutral on the subject with his patients, he said, because in his opinion, patients' visits to healers were sometimes disruptive—even counterproductive—to their treatment at Fann. Such was the case for Fatima, described above, who had traveled all the way to Burkina Faso to visit the reputable *marabout* who had successfully treated her cousin's chronic pain several years earlier. In consultation, the healer had counseled Fatima to stop taking her prescribed medications at once because they were only making her sicker. In the eyes of her doctor at Fann, Fatima's relapse and subsequent descent into even more severe symptoms was precipitated by the *marabout*'s advice. Dr. Alioune was resigned to the fact that most of his patients visited healers before, during, or after their stays at Fann, and I never once heard him talk to patients about their interactions with *fajkats* or *marabouts* in any greater depth beyond simply asking them if they had consulted a healer. Ndoye, Devos, and Guèye (2000: 273) remark that "[a]t Fann ... modern medicine and traditional medicine run parallel to one another, without ever meeting." While this is true in the sense that healers and their therapies were decidedly outside the frame of the clinic, it was certainly not the case for patients and their families, who regularly navigated, negotiated, and made sense of the different therapeutic systems available to them.

In reflecting upon the extent to which the history of the Fann clinic was incorporated in psychiatric practice at Fann circa 2000, Ndoye, Devos, and Guèye (2000: 268) suggest that "all of the doctors are more or less informed by the same central ideas that guided Collomb's team." On the one hand, it was true that Collomb and *l'Ecole de Fann* came up often in conversation, especially between doctors (or staff) and researchers from outside the clinic. Collomb's name commanded respect; it even served as an important currency for a clinic that was stretched well beyond its means. On the other hand, the idea that the doctors were informed by—let alone operated according to—the same sets of ideas or assumptions that guided Collomb and *l'Ecole de Fann* was certainly debatable. In fact, two Fann psychiatrists more or less directly challenged this assertion. Dr. Isseu, for example, told me that her training at the University of Dakar had not included any formal study of the institution's history. Before she started working at Fann, she was familiar with Collomb and *l'Ecole de Fann* only by name.

> Everyone around here assumes that everyone else knows all about Collomb, that they have read his writings and have studied his research. Really, I don't think many have. Most of us have a general idea of what Fann was like back then, but things are very different now. Sure it would be worthwhile to learn more, but look at the current state of the clinic! Our energies are spent on other things. Nobody has time to reflect on such questions!

Several of the elements put into place by Collomb were still in place in 2002 and continue to function today, including the weekly *pénc* meetings and the *accompagnant* policy, although as I discuss in the next chapter, each of these has changed significantly over the years. And while the doctors I spoke to generally extolled the virtues of these activities at their inception and did not hesitate to credit Collomb and his colleagues for their innovative approach to psychiatry, they were also quick to note that the practices Collomb instituted no longer function as they once did. This is not because they are without merit, they say; rather, the practices are both less feasible, due to a lack of resources and personnel, and less relevant to the clinic's approach than they once were. Dr. Mamadou, in fact, confided that he thought the spirit behind these practices had been all but lost; they functioned as little more than empty shells of what they once were. "When it comes down to it, the *pénc* meetings are a waste of time. They are no longer necessary. And besides, there are more important things for us to be doing," he explained. The doctors also expressed mixed feelings about the *accompagnant* policy, but the clinic is so understaffed that they are nevertheless grateful for the extra hands. Dr. Mamadou told me that he often asks himself why the practices are kept in place, seeing that "no one is really committed to them" and "they have lost their therapeutic value." Although Dr. Isseu and Dr. Yacine generally take a less critical stance toward the practices that have remained intact at Fann since Collomb's era, they both also insist that the clinic must evolve at the same speed as the world around it. Practices like the *pénc* and the *accompagnant*, they say, surely need to be reevaluated and updated. "This does not mean turning one's back on the past," Dr. Yacine told me, "but modifying it to better fit the present." Interestingly, Dr. Mamadou suggested one day that perhaps the doctors and staff at Fann were still "going through the motions" because they were afraid to offend Collomb's legacy. Historically, these were the practices that made Fann unique, that put it on the map. What would Fann's international profile be without them? In any case, Dr. Isseu explained, "the quality of the relationship between the patient and the doctor is a much greater factor in the patient's recovery than *pénc* meetings or the role of the *accompagnant*."

Things *were* different at Fann than they had been during Collomb's era. But while the "middle figures" who worked at Fann during the 1960s and early 1970s lament the loss of that special ethos of what they say no longer exists, the doctors working at Fann during the late 1990s and early 2000s were too concerned with the practical problems that confronted them each day to spend their time longing for a past they never knew. This pragmatism was mirrored in their adherence to pharmaceutical treatment strategies as well as in their tolerance of healers, and it was also acted out by way of the "strategic ambivalence" they exhibited toward Fann's past. Here both Collomb's name and the renowned early years of institution operate as symbolic capital. As potential resources, they were put to use when they could meet a need; alternately they were dismissed, ignored, or concealed.

THE FIRST PAN-AFRICAN CONFERENCE ON MENTAL HEALTH

Although the doctors' "strategic ambivalence" toward Collomb's Fann was made apparent to me during our conversations, nowhere was it more clearly demonstrated than at the *Premier Congrès Panafricain de Santé Mentale* (First Pan-African Conference on Mental Health), which took place in Dakar in March 2002. The conference was organized and hosted by Fann in collaboration with *l'Association l'AMI* (*Accompagnement Psychologique et Médiation Interculturelle*), a Bordeaux-based organization associated with the University of Bordeaux that specializes in providing counseling and cross-cultural mediation services for immigrants in France. The event, with its announced theme of "Psychiatry, Psychoanalysis, and Culture," brought together over a hundred African and European mental health care professionals and social scientists to discuss topics ranging from how "culture" can and should (or should not) enter the clinical or therapeutic encounter, to questions related specifically to the diagnosis and treatment of mental health issues among immigrants, to the possibility of integrating "traditional" healers and their techniques into clinical or psychotherapeutic practice.

My involvement in the conference was primarily as an anthropologist and audience member, but because the Fann clinic had served as headquarters for the planning and organizing of the event, I had also gotten swept up in the preparations. When I arrived at Fann to begin my dissertation research in December 2001, countless hours had already been funneled into the conference. The official chair of the event was a clinical psychologist who worked at Fann but drew his salary from IREP (*l'Institut de Recherche et d'Enseignement de Psychopathologie,* or the Institute for the Research and Teaching of Psychopathology), which was under the auspices of the Faculty of Medicine and Pharmacy at the university. In 2002, the chair was—and still remains today—the person at Fann who was most invested in the idea of collaboration between psychiatry and local healing practices, such as the *ndëpp* ceremonies, and most vocal about putting Fann (back) on the map for such initiatives. In some ways, he ambitiously positioned himself as the inheritor of Fann's legacy. At the same time, however, he also expressed a high degree of ambivalence toward Collomb and the Fann School.[8] He frequently traveled to the United States, France, and other parts of Europe to give talks and attend conferences, often promoting ethnopsychiatry and "traditional healing" practices and encouraging their integration into non-Western clinical settings and into clinical work among immigrant populations. Because he was often on-the-go (several of my conversations with him, in fact, took place in his car) and frequently absent from Fann, he only infrequently met with patients at the clinic and did not maintain a steady consultation practice during my research stay.

Almost every doctor and staff member at the clinic—along with many other enlisted volunteers from outside the hospital—was involved in conference preparations in some way, and many were consumed by the roles, obligations, and tasks asked of them. Wanting to make myself useful, and wanting also to integrate myself into the daily goings-on at the clinic, I happily agreed to translate abstracts and manage communications with English-speaking participants, in the chair's name. At the end of my first week, I was formally asked to take part in the conference's "Scientific Committee" and review abstracts and proposals for presentation, and many people commented on how lucky I was to be a part of such an exciting and historic event.

From the chair's point of view, as well as that of many doctors working at the Fann clinic in 2002, the conference provided more than just a forum for evaluating and assessing the state of mental health care in Africa (and among immigrants of African descent in Europe) or proposing new strategies for the future. It was also an opportunity for Fann to put forth a coherent image of itself in the present and for the future—an image that could finally untether itself from and advance beyond the reputation of Henri Collomb and the early years of the clinic. Despite the fact that the conference theme of "Psychiatry, Psychoanalysis, and Culture" could not have been a better provocation to reflect upon the history of the clinic, I quickly came to understand that the conference was decidedly *not* meant to be a celebration or homage to the past, but rather an affirmation of the present. In outlining the event's objectives, for example, the announcement asked participants to consider, "What has been done since Henri Collomb (Dakar) and other pioneers (Lambo in Nigeria)?"—*since* being the operative word. On the one hand, the conference planners attempted to harness the power and prestige of Collomb's name (and Fann's associated past) to draw participants from around the world—indeed, for many international attendees of the conference, the fact that the event had been organized by Fann was significant precisely because of the institution's innovative and illustrious past, and they were thrilled to have the opportunity to tour the place that Henri Collomb had effectively put on the map.[9] On the other hand, however, the Fann conference organizers also desired to show themselves as unique, forward-thinking innovators in their own right, independent of the institution's history. To this end, Collomb's name and a few carefully curated elements of Fann's past were emphasized and elaborated upon, but most of the rest of the clinic's history was downplayed or ignored. The pragmatic attempt to render a highly circumscribed past useful and "usable" (cf. Anagnostou 2009; Blake 1999; Brooks [1918] 1993; Rosaldo 1980) in this way, however, was strongly contested by the few conference participants who had been connected to the clinic during Collomb's era. This included two French psychiatrists who had worked alongside Collomb during the 1960s and early 1970s and were very vocal about the conference's willful omission of Fann's past. They criticized the conference organizers for not having invited Collomb's daughter, Agnès, or the rest of the nurses, doctors, and support staff from that era to participate in the conference. "They surely have an important contribution to make on these topics; their memories must be worth something!," one of the doctors vented to me. In their view, the conference was an active attempt to disavow—even erase—Fann's past.

Perhaps a signal of the conference's relationship to history and memory is evident in the conference's very name: the *Premier Congrès Panafricain de Santé Mentale* was not the first of its kind, not by a long shot. Many conferences with similar names and themes (such as the famous First Pan-African Psychiatric Conference, which was organized by Lambo and his colleagues and held in Abeokuta, Nigeria in November 1961, and which Collomb attended) had taken place all over the continent in decades prior to the event, and many had also been called firsts (cf. Collignon 2004). As a rhetorical device, claiming the conference to be a "first" effectively erased that which had come before it while marking the conference as bold and groundbreaking; the claim signaled a clear desire to start time and history anew. Fann's attempt to build a coherent identity for itself in this manner, however, met with some challenges during the conference itself.

The Contentious Keynote

"No doubt, there are some people here who wish I hadn't been invited," Tobie Nathan said to me as we stood talking at the bar of a small, crowded restaurant during an evening conference reception. In the wake of a highly charged debate about the place of ethnopsychiatry in the modern French state and beyond, Nathan was a contentious choice for keynote speaker at the *Premier Congrès Panafricain de Santé Mentale*. Both the idiosyncratic (and somewhat marginalized) brand of ethnopsychiatry Nathan had pioneered and promoted by way of his clinical work with immigrants in Paris and his charismatic persona had been topics of ongoing debate in France, not just in academic or political circles, but in the larger public sphere. In the context of the conference, Nathan was perceived as something of an unstable signifier—some conference attendees saw him as too controversial, too provocative, and too divisive to unite the group under the common theme of Psychiatry, Psychoanalysis, and Culture.

If we view the conference as a production of the contemporary Fann Psychiatric Clinic, and even more specifically as an attempt by the clinic to consolidate and put forth a coherent identity in the present and for the future, we see also Nathan's participation in the conference served not to clarify but rather to complicate this project. Put simply, the brand of ethnopsychiatry that Nathan espoused was not representative of the kind of psychiatry that was being practiced at or aspired to at Fann around the year 2000. I turn now to Nathan's approach and the debates in which he was enmeshed during the late 1990s to illustrate this point.

Tobie Nathan, a French psychologist and psychoanalyst of Jewish Egyptian heritage, was trained by Georges Devereux and worked closely with him during the early part of his career. In the late 1970s, alongside psychoanalyst Serge Lebovici in Avicenne Hospital's Department of Child and Adolescent Psychiatry, he put into place the first ethnopsychiatric consultation program in France. In 1993, he established the Centre Georges Devereux (CGD), a psychological consultation center geared specifically toward the provision of specialized services related to the mental health care needs of immigrants and their families in France. The center, which was not affiliated with a hospital or a university medical school (Nathan was not a medical doctor) but rather lodged within the Department of Psychology at the Université Paris VIII in the Parisian *banlieue* of Saint-Denis, was the first of its kind.

At the heart of Nathan's ethnopsychiatric practice was the insistence that what he calls non-Western or "traditional peoples" (French: *les peuples traditionnels*) "have their own forms of psychopathology" as well as their own methods of care, and that ethnopsychiatrists "have as much to learn as we have to teach." Ethnopsychiatry, he stressed, "is based on exchange. . . . We engage in learning from other psychiatric traditions that issue from other worlds."[10] To Nathan, the universalist frameworks upheld within both psychoanalytic theory and biomedical psychiatry are little more than an illusion when it comes to offering mental health care to immigrant populations or in non-Western settings, such approaches are ineffective at best and alienating at worst.

At first glance, Nathan's position appears reminiscent of the culturalist orientation espoused by Collomb and his colleagues during the 1960s and 1970s; Nathan's presence at the conference thus seems to recall the institution's past. In actuality, however, Nathan's idea of culture is much more rigid and his position more extreme than the position that had been adopted by the Fann School, and his clinical practice was light years away from the more universalist approach of their successors. Describing culture as an enclosure (*clôture*) that envelops the individual and determines the expression of his or her suffering (Nathan 1986, 1994), Nathan viewed culture and psyche as homologous systems (Nathan 1994, cf. Corin 1997; Streit 1997). In his clinical practice, he insisted upon putting "traditional" etiologies for suffering—and the languages and worldviews that sustain them—at the center of his ethnopsychiatric approach.

First at Avicenne and continuing at the CGD, Nathan and his colleagues assembled therapeutic teams around each patient; these included psychoanalysts, psychologists, cultural mediators, students, family members and caretakers of the patient, as well as "ethnoclinicians" who could speak to the therapeutic traditions found in the patient's country of origin. Each consultation was constructed as a collaborative and heteroglossic cross-cultural encounter, and it was common for such meetings to last upwards of three hours. Following Corin (1997), Giordano (2011: 244) has noted that the impetus for these large consultations was to establish a " 'space of mediation' in which to negotiate a common therapeutic frame" between patient and therapist. Ideally, this space facilitated the speech of patients by enabling them to articulate their suffering in their own language and in light of a larger cultural context. At the same time, it offered the attending therapists enormous insight, not just into the culturally shaped explanatory models for suffering brought forth by the patient, but into the different paths for healing and recovery that might be taken. Nathan's therapeutic interventions were very emphatically not about translating "local" or "traditional" symptoms into a universal language of psychiatry; diagnosis and interpretation were to remain necessarily ambiguous and polysemic (Nathan 1988). Although he was trained in and heavily informed by psychoanalytic theory, Nathan became increasingly ambivalent toward psychoanalysis as his career progressed (Corin 1997), and more apt to subject it to creative adaptation. In a 2006 interview (see note 10), in fact, he reflected on his evolving relationship with psychoanalysis, noting that, "[i]n the process of devoting myself to ethnopsychiatry, I came to understand psychoanalysis as a good method for asking questions, but it is not a therapy."

Nathan had a dedicated group of followers and was enormously popular as a teacher, and his ethnopsychiatric approach was well received outside of France, particularly in Quebec and Italy (Giordano 2014). Within France, however, both Nathan and his approach met with harsh criticism. On one level, he was derided for upholding an antiquated view of both culture and tradition as static, monolithic, and timeless. This view was certainly at odds with anthropological understandings of the terms (Corin 1997), and critics have highlighted the fact that anthropologists and ethnologists were conspicuously missing from the consultation teams that Nathan put together at the Centre Georges Devereux (Andoche 2001; Fassin 1999; Larchanché 2010).[11] It was not just Nathan's reification of a static culture concept that critics found troubling, however, but also its practical application. In Didier Fassin's (2005: 361) view, Nathan's "reification of [immigrants'] cultural otherness" served to naturalize cultural difference at a moment when the marginalization of France's growing immigrant population was more visibly entrenched and more in demand of intervention than ever (Fassin 1999, 2000). For Nathan, ethnopsychiatry and its emphasis on cultural otherness was a clear remedy to this marginalization—a way to restore dignity. Nathan (1994: 190) provocatively insisted that "[i]n societies with large immigrant populations, we must encourage ghettos, yes. Let me say loudly and clearly that we must never force a family to abandon its cultural system." To Fassin, however, Nathan's approach perpetuated discrimination. Nathan located the source of immigrant suffering not in France's exclusionary immigration policies and practices, nor in the failure of the French state to supply adequate, accessible social support services to its immigrant population, but in an irreducible cultural *difference* of immigrants that, he insisted, was overlooked by the presumed universalism of French republicanism, and by the universalism of conventional psychiatry and psychoanalysis. "I think the left has made a grave mistake in forgetting to think about difference," Nathan said in a 1996 interview.[12] To Fassin (2005: 360) and others, though, Nathan's culturalist approach amounted to little more than an "apolitical cultural essentialism."[13]

Nathan came under attack for other reasons during this time as well. Without question, he was a man of great charisma. Outspoken and provocative, he attracted a great deal of media attention during the late 1990s and early 2000s and engaged readily in public debates. In the media, he became known as an expert in all things related to immigration and culture, much to the chagrin of the anthropologists who took issue with his views. Nathan's critics also accused him of cultivating a larger-than-life professional persona. He was chided for the cult of personality he built around himself, which many viewed as anathema to an effective mental health care practice and as overstepping the ethical boundaries of his profession. In addition, by the mid-1990s, Nathan was "increasingly situat[ing] himself on the side of traditional healers or as a kind of meta-healer, able to use basic effective operational elements of traditional techniques" (Corin 1997: 355). For this he was criticized for playing at being a healer, for taking things too far.[14]

To invite Nathan as a keynote speaker at the *Premier Congrès Panafricain de Santé Mentale*, then, was to invite all of these contentious exchanges and opinions to the conference itself. Most every participant knew of Nathan by name and reputation, and attendees from France who specialized in immigrant mental health had followed the debates surrounding Nathan particularly closely. Several participants knew Nathan or had worked with him in the past, including Mary Rose Moro, who had been a student and colleague of Nathan's at Avicenne, but had since broken from his brand of cultural essentialism and distanced herself from the most extreme elements of his practice (Larchanché 2010; Moro, De la Noé, and Mouchenik 2006). The audience received Nathan's address with a wide range of reactions, from sympathy and enthusiasm to skepticism and even outright dismissal.

Inasmuch as the *Premier Congrès Panafricain de Santé Mentale* represented an opportunity for the Fann clinic of 2002 to consolidate a coherent identity that was independent of the institution's past, Nathan's participation in the conference seemed to trouble the whole enterprise. Nathan invoked and praised the pioneering work of Collomb and *l'Ecole de Fann* in his keynote address, but without acknowledging the tension that existed between the past and the present-day clinic. Nathan's own culturalist approach— itself an extreme (even caricatured) version of that which had been embraced by the Fann School—was antithetical to the kind of psychiatry that was being practiced at Fann around the year 2000; his ethnopsychiatric orientation was a far cry from the kind of care that Fann endeavored to provide to its patients. To the then-present Fann doctors, care was less about reaffirming a patient's location within a bounded cultural system than it was about translating their patients' symptoms and suffering into the "universal" language of psychiatry, an approach much more closely aligned with "transcultural psychiatry" than "ethnopsychiatry." This was, however, precisely the approach that Nathan dismissed. "[E]thnopsychiatry," Nathan asserted in an interview several years after the conference had taken place, "is the opposite of transcultural psychiatry, which seeks to globalize the theories of Westerners. When epidemiological studies assess the impact of depression in Botswana and Burkina Faso, the consequence will necessarily be to sell Western drugs to Africans. We could instead emphasize their cultural resources rather than contribute to transforming them into passive consumers."[15]

Healers: Collaboration and Performance

In the opening speech of the conference, Senegalese minister of health and prevention Dr. Awa Marie Coll Seck told conference participants that "[d]uring the next few days, [they would] be discussing the possibility of integrating into [their] practice certain therapeutic techniques that come from different cultural contexts" and that "[they would] likewise be thinking about adaptations to [their] own cultural context." Stressing the need for collaboration between healers and doctors, Dr. Coll Seck reiterated one of the major themes of the World Health Organization's "Health for All" campaign: the need for health care policymakers and biomedical practitioners to approach and collaborate with "traditional" practitioners, validate the role of the "traditional" specialist in the delivery of primary health care, and promote these men and women as key recruits in the ambitious crusade for global health.

According to Dr. Coll Seck, dialogue should be opened between healers and doctors in order to foster an exchange of knowledge and practice because "at least 80 percent of those who seek help in the domain of mental health consult traditional therapists before, during, or after consulting modern health facilities." Although she was quick to point out that traditional beliefs about mental health have at times done more harm than good—this was the case with epilepsy, she said, in that traditional beliefs kept sufferers from seeking simple, effective, and relatively cheap treatment offered by modern health care facilities. She also asserted "that in many cases, traditional practitioners and therapists, in linking treatments with cultural elements, do very significant work." For this reason, Dr. Coll Seck told the audience, "we have made a point to include traditional therapists in your discussions in order to better take into account the cultural dimension of African societies and the reality of the clinic in Africa."

The WHO and its "Health for All" campaign, it should be noted, have their own history of repetition, erasure, and renewal. In 1977, the WHO introduced the slogan, "Health for All by the Year 2000," and the slogan became something of a battle cry at the Alma Ata Conference in Kazakhstan (then the Kazakh Soviet Socialist Republic) the following year.[16] The conference resulted in the drafting of the Declaration of Alma-Ata, a statement of commitment from the WHO and the governments of 134 countries that sought the "attainment by all people of the world by the year 2000 of a level of health that [would] permit them to lead a socially and economically productive life." Especially integral to achieving this goal, stated the

Declaration, would be the accessibility and efficacy of primary health care for all; Section VII of the Declaration described and outlined the meaning of "primary health care" in seven parts, and Section VIII went on to assert that "governments should formulate national policies, strategies, and plans of action to launch and sustain primary health care as part of a comprehensive national health system and in coordination with other sectors."

One of the more popular themes to emerge out of Alma Ata was that governments should recognize and collaborate with "traditional practitioners" for the delivery of primary health care (Section VII, Part 7). This assertion galvanized the already extensive body of research on "traditional healing" and "traditional medicine" that had been accumulating in recent years. In a technical series published in 1978, for example, the World Health Organization reported that the inclusion, promotion, and development of "traditional medicine" was crucial to global health goals, highlighting the necessity of collaborating with "traditional" practitioners, and proposing that (certain scientifically sound) "traditional" health practices and practitioners be integrated and recruited in the battle for a healthful utopia (WHO 1978b).

"Health for All" did not happen by the year 2000, of course; the grand slogan failed to be realized. By the early 1990s, the "Health for All by the Year 2000" mandate was already under review at the WHO. Not only had it been an impossible goal, but health standards were indeed declining in many communities throughout the world. In 1995, then, the World Health Organization launched the "Health for All" renewal process. The initiative promised to review the original "Health for All by the Year 2000" policy, and, after deliberating its strengths, weaknesses, successes, and failures, draft a new declaration to replace it. The document born out of the renewal initiative, which came to be known as the "Health for All in the 21st Century" declaration, was adopted as policy by the Fifty-first World Health Assembly on May 16, 1998. Much of its language stayed the same as the previous declaration.

It was under the auspices of collaboration, integration, and culture, then, that the organizers of the *Premier Congrès Panafricain de Santé Mentale* recruited reputable healers from Senegal and other West African countries to present their technical and practical knowledge at the conference. Remarkable to some attendees, however, was the extent to which the history of the collaborative efforts undertaken at Fann was ignored at, or effaced from, the event. For Soukeyna, a clinical psychologist who was originally from Dakar but had trained in Europe, it was not so much the illusion of newness produced by the conference that bothered her as it was a feeling of injustice, even outrage, toward those who would disregard the past. Soukeyna was affiliated with the CHNU *de Fann* in 2002, but she did not work in the psychiatric clinic (she worked at a different clinic within the compound). Soukeyna harbored some anger at the current state of the clinic for reasons that I will not expound upon, for the sake of confidentiality. She had a long history with Fann; her father was a well-known *marabout* (religious healer) and she knew Collomb when she was young.

One day after the conference, Soukeyna and I sat talking in her office. We had discussed the conference at length in previous meetings, but as the event came up again, I asked her once more what her general impression of it had been. She responded openly, loudly, and unexpectedly. "The conference was a circus! It was a publicity stunt. Psychiatry, Psychoanalysis, Culture! Hmph! Those words already meant something to Fann! But of course they didn't talk about that." The great irony in all of the conference's rhetoric about collaboration and integration was that Henri Collomb and the Fann School *had* cultivated a successful practice of working closely with healers throughout West Africa.

Not only did this history go virtually unmentioned at the conference, but a tragic coincidence occurred on its first day that further underscored this erasure. Daouda Seck, one of the most famous and well-respected healers to have ever worked with Collomb, fell very ill and was hospitalized in the Neurology building of the *CHNU de Fann*, located right next the psychiatric clinic. Two French psychiatrists who had worked alongside Collomb and knew Daouda Seck well took me to his bedside to greet him and to meet his wife, who had been standing vigil next to him. "I'll tell you how serious they are about culture, tradition," one of the French doctors said to me in disgust as we made our way back to the conference after visiting the old healer. "Daouda Seck is there dying alone, right now, right as this farce of a conference is taking place. He's there at Fann, and his family has no money, and he is dying. The man is incredible, do you understand? He is a living library, a national treasure. Not a mention of him at the conference, though. It's as if he never existed. And meanwhile, there they sit, talking about collaboration and traditional therapies." These doctors were outraged by what they regarded as a staggering act of disrespect, and one got up on stage at the conference during the following day to tell the audience of Seck's hospitalization and to pay homage to the man. Daouda Seck—the living library, the national treasure—died within the week.

For some of the local healers who were invited to take part in the conference, too, things did not quite go as planned. There were significant problems with language and translation, for instance. Announcements for the Pan-African conference had said that the event would be accessible to French, English, and Portuguese speakers, but translation of these languages was limited. Of African languages, however, the brochure had made no mention, and nothing was done to accommodate those who spoke neither French nor English nor Portuguese. In that many of the healers in attendance were not fluent in these languages, their exclusion quickly became obvious. A few healers asked attendees who were fluent in both languages to translate for them, on the spot. This was a difficult task, however, and untenable given the speed and specialized language of the presentations.

Several of the healers in attendance also felt that they were not given a proper chance to speak, to be heard, or enter into conversation with other participants. A few weeks after the event, during a visit with a well-known *ndëppkat* (one who performs and commands spirit possession ceremonies) who lives right outside of Dakar, I asked about her impressions of the event, and whether she had felt welcomed and included. "They didn't let us speak!" was her reply. Indeed, instead of fostering exchange and dialogue, the inclusion of healers in the conference at times resembled a spectacle. One such moment took place on the first afternoon of the conference, when a man in a flowing blue *grand bubu* gown was called to the stage to give his fifteen-minute presentation.

The middle-aged man introduced himself to the audience; he had come from eastern Mauritania, where he worked and lived. A healer *de medicine prophetique et traditionelle*, he had been invited, he said, to discuss his practice and share his knowledge and expertise in the domain of mental health. As he spoke, he hovered at a distance from the microphone; his voice cracked and he was barely audible to most of the audience. An audience member sitting in the seats below him called out and gestured for him to move closer.

The healer began his presentation by describing his practice. Most of his patients, he explained, were *victimes de magie* (victims of magic), and it was his work to understand both the type and the source of the magic that made the patient—men, women, and children alike—suffer. People came to him with an array of symptoms, from extreme fatigue, to muddled or disrupted speech, to distraction and, nervousness, to unusual behavior, headaches, and even anorexia. He did not typically charge patients for the first consultation, he told the audience, but treatment usually cost upwards of 7,000 *ouguiyas* (about $35), depending on the patient's ability to pay. The first step in the consultation, the healer noted, was to watch the patient closely and listen to him or her speak. He would then ask a series of questions of both the patient and accompanying family members before making his diagnosis. He explained that the treatments he offered to the patients depended upon many different factors and were tailored to the specificities of each case. He would seek out special herbs or plants for the patient, or recite verses of the Qur'an in her ear; he may give the patient, water that contains verses of the Qur'an or that has had sacred verses spoken into it. And there are special incantations to be recited as well. "It is all in the Qur'an," the healer asserted. And then, for the remainder of his allotted time, he proceeded to recite his more common incantations into the microphone, demonstrating his technique to the audience.

In a 2000 article titled "The Thin Line of Modernity: Some Moroccan Debates on Subjectivity," anthropologist Stephania Pandolfo describes how "traditional therapies" were showcased at a 1992 psychotherapy conference in Casablanca in order to question the extent to which such ontologically dissimilar discourses and therapeutic techniques might be viewed as commensurable, especially in a field of unequal power. Looking back, Pandolfo writes that on her part, she had "believed, at least in an abstract sense, in the ethical possibility of a dialogue between different approaches to subjectivity and alterity. . . . Yet what the [1992] conference urgently made [her] realize was that the historicity of the different subject positionings—[her] own included—could not be bracketed away. Commensurability was not just an epistemological question." To desire commensurability and to speak about "inclusion" is already to occupy a situated position that needs to be interrogated in terms of "decolonization, emancipation, and the characterization of the 'modern' subject" (2000: 130). Not only was such questioning absent from the *Premier Congrès Panafricain de Santé Mentale*, but for many of the audience members who sat before the healer as he demonstrated his techniques, the scene was a spectacle of difference. Some members of the audience looked on in anticipation. Others shifted in their seats, appearing somewhat uncomfortable. Eyes scanned the theater, meeting other eyes. It was hard to discern whether people were glancing about to see how others were responding and to figure out how they themselves should react, or whether they were looking for some sort of commiseration. As a spectacle of difference, the healer's performance seemed to do just the opposite of what it was intended to accomplish; it suggested the limits of collaboration between Western medicine and so-called "traditional" health care practices.

A few weeks after the conference ended, I sat talking with Dr. Mamadou to get a sense for how he thought the event had gone. How, I wondered, would he respond to the critique that Fann's past had been effectively omitted from the conference, even when the conference's central theme of "Psychiatry, Psychoanalysis, Culture" was, to some participants at least, such an obvious allusion to the work of Collomb and *l'Ecole de Fann*? How would he react to the charges that the name of Collomb and the history of the Fann clinic had been used as symbolic capital to advertise the event and draw a large international crowd, but that apart from this purpose, little more had been made of the clinic's past? "Ah," Dr. Mamadou shook his head in frustration. "We are clearly in a difficult position. I mean, how are we supposed to move forward when they insist on living in the past?" To him, the past—and Fann's history in particular—was not some repository of specialized knowledge that contained seeds of possibility for the future, nor was it all that the clinic was and could be. On the contrary, the past was at worst an obstacle—a distraction that drew attention away from the pressing practical issues of the day—and at best a tool or an instrument, helpful only insofar as it could be used in practical terms to service the present.

Dr. Mamadou and others working at Fann circa 2002 appeared less concerned with asserting themselves as heirs to a past legacy than they did with showing themselves to be agents in their own right, creatively trying to manage and respond to the economic and infrastructural constraints of the day. Their "strategic ambivalence" toward the early years of Fann, which oscillated between praise, criticism, indifference, frustration, and outright rejection, was indicative of the kind of bricolage, or cobbling together of resources, that characterized the clinic during that time. This was the very same art of bricolage—popularized by the iconic character of Goorgoorlou—that was employed by people living in Dakar and throughout Senegal to confront the shortcomings of the postcolonial state and make ends meet. Insofar as the Fann doctors were concerned with the clinic's early history at all, then, it was for the practical application of "usable pasts" in the present—history was not an irrefutable inheritance that pressed upon the now, but a tool among others that could be picked up and used at will in an effort to craft a livable life. These doctors were not haunted by the past; to them, there were no ghosts.

A Thing I Could Not See (The Joola*)*

THIS STORY MARKS A GAP. IT SPINS OUT OF MY inability to deal with (let alone represent) a critical event that took place during my dissertation fieldwork stay in Dakar. I will call it a story of ethnographic failure (my own). My intention here is not to seek exoneration through confession, nor am I trying to recuperate this failure and put it toward productive use. Instead, I want to sit with and try to make visible this gap in my work that remains as confusing to me as it is uncomfortable, and that, for a period at least, held me at an impasse.

I am interested in the places and times in which ethnography finds its limits—the events and encounters and experiences we have during fieldwork, but that we intentionally choose not to write about for personal or institutional reasons, or that we sense to be significant, but somehow (for whatever reason) cannot bring ourselves to confront. I am interested also in what we (as ethnographers) won't see; what we can't bring ourselves to witness or experience when we are in the field. What questions can't we ask and where do we choose not to insert ourselves? How do we come to deal with this unseen stuff? It is also about how we sometimes end up writing *away* from the unseen stuff, or even *around* it (where its contours may nevertheless press into our work). Or how the unseen sometimes just brings us to an impasse, whether we see ourselves not seeing, or not. So this interlude is really about *not being present* (or being un-present?) to events in the field, or not being able to write about it, or both.

As I revise this book manuscript, I feel these stories and analyses to be swirling around some sort of dark matter, something that is not visible, but nevertheless *has gravity*. And I'm thinking, well this is just ridiculous and kind of embarrassing, especially given that my entire project is about haunting and memory work, and here this thing is happening in my book, too.

So, what is this absent present event that haunts the rest of my work? This act of rendering the untellable *tellable* is a cheap device, I know. But anyway, here is a quick, and very shaky, attempt. The tone and the words aren't right. But I hope that at least they will give you some idea:

The refrigerated shipping containers arrived first, six of them. That was before anyone knew how many (or how few) bodies there would actually be. Family members and friends of the missing started gathering in the port, too, and within forty-eight hours, the number had swelled to thousands, many of whom had made their way from far away. They were all looking for answers, or maybe for a miracle; at the very least, they wanted to identify and recover their dead. They were frantic and distraught and angry, and it was so hot, and everyone was there, waiting.

Authorities scrambled to set up "crisis centers" to deal with the gathering crowds, and boy scouts distributed water and food to those who had installed themselves near the port. Soon, the notice boards were brought out, then more and more, covered with pictures of bloated bodies and suitcases and personal items that had been pulled from the water near the site of the tragedy. People searching for their missing lined up to pour over the photos in the hope of some sign. Trained health workers were called upon to staff the centers. Fann doctors, nurses, and medical students—everybody went down to the port to provide mental health care and counseling to grieving families, to hand out water, and to be present.

Everybody except me. I stayed at Fann. It was a Saturday morning—September 28, 2002, to be exact—and things were quiet in the clinic, but it wasn't so different from any other Saturday. I spent that day sitting on the verandah with patients and their family members. Although the port seemed far very away, the sinking of the *Joola* was on everybody's mind—all the radio stations were fully devoted to covering the developing story, and conversations at Fann barely strayed from the tragedy. I knew I should be down at the port, but I couldn't bring myself to go. That day and every day afterward, for many days, I thought to myself, "Tomorrow I'll go and offer my help. I'll be present for all the people who have been my friends and interlocutors at Fann over the past three years." Of course it was the right thing to do, and I knew it. But I never went.

The *Joola*, an overloaded ferry, had capsized at sea a few days earlier en route to Dakar from Senegal's southern city of Ziguinchor. The ship was designed to carry about 600 people, including the crew, and it was designed for river travel (it was constructed in Germany to sail the Danube, to be precise). On this particular ocean voyage, which should have taken seventeen hours, there were 1,034 ticketed passengers and hundreds of unticketed passengers on board: as usual, many people had been waved aboard for free, and children under 5 were not required to have tickets.

The rescue effort was slow to start. The *Joola* had capsized at around 11 p.m. on Thursday, September 26, a couple of kilometers off the Gambian coast. The first responders were Gambian fishermen in their wooden pirogues, but they did not start searching until Friday's first light. They recovered a few survivors and many bodies. They saw the overturned boat, which stayed partially afloat and remained visible until 3 p.m. Because of the stifling heat of the interior cabins, most of the passengers had been on the decks when the ferry capsized and had been thrown into the water. But there were also more than 300 people trapped inside the hull. When they pulled a 15-year-old boy from the water at 2 p.m., he reported that he could still hear screams coming from the ship; people were alive inside. But he was the last passenger recovered alive. The heavy-lifting rescue crews and naval boats and divers did not arrive on the scene until the ferry had already taken its place on the sea floor.

Without a passenger manifest, it was impossible to name or even to count the dead. The first number to circulate was 750, then 1,030 people, but the number kept growing and growing. The final death toll was set at 1,863, although some sources estimate that even that was too low. (This would make it the second largest peacetime maritime disaster in history—only the post-collision sinking of the Philippine ferry *Doña Paz* in 1987 was worse; in comparison, the *Titanic* claimed 1,517 lives). There were only 64 survivors. Many, many young children were lost, as well as many teenagers and young college students who had been heading back to Dakar for the start of the new academic year. In the days after the tragedy, Ziguinchor's newspapers reported that a whole generation of its brightest young students had perished when that ferry capsized. There were many sets of siblings on board, and entire families.

In the end, only around 550 bodies were recovered. So many remained at sea, in fact, that lots of people in Dakar and along the coast stopped eating fish altogether in the days and months after the tragedy. (The thought of eating fish that had feasted on the dead was simply too horrible to bear.) Of the 550 bodies that were recovered, fewer than 100 were identified—this was a very low-tech operation (no DNA sampling was done at the scene, for instance, and no international disaster response rushed to the scene). Most bodies were beyond recognition by the time they were recovered and the remains decomposed quickly in the heat. Those who were identified were returned to their families for private burial; the rest were buried in mass graves. In the days and weeks that followed the event, every story that surfaced was even more horrifying than the last. And circulating alongside these stories of unspeakable suffering and loss were the accusations: a corrupt and ineffective government that was not just deemed negligent but responsible for the tragedy; an inexcusably slow response; disorganized rescue and identification procedures; mishandled bodies; few answers; and only a cursory investigation.

So here was this event—a national tragedy of historic proportions—that took place while I was doing my dissertation fieldwork. Local newspapers and radio programs referred to it as "Africa's *Titanic*" and "Senegal's 9 / 11." It deeply affected my interlocutors at Fann as well as my close friends in Dakar for days and weeks and even months after it happened. The government tried to fold the *Joola* tragedy into a narrative of national solidarity through loss and suffering, but this was challenged in meaningful ways with counternarratives of government corruption and impotence. But I just could not face any of it. I could not bring myself to go to the port, and I somehow managed to write my entire dissertation in a way that allowed the event (and the public and professional responses to it) to *just never come up*. No heroic intervention, no compelling account. And the more time that goes by, the more amazing this appears to me.

I don't know why I couldn't face the *Joola* exactly, and I'm not terribly interested in framing my response within the language of trauma. I do know, however, that exactly one year before this, I had been working on a very different project that nevertheless bore many resemblances to this event and its aftermath. I was an ethnographer for an NIH (National Institutes of Health)–funded project that looked at mental health and substance use among firefighters, police officers, and construction workers who were sifting through the rubble of the World Trade Center. I had spent about ten hours a day doing interviews, usually deep into the night, at the edges of "the pit," and in the bars and coffee shops and 24-hour diners that catered to the (mostly) men who were working down there. In this hypermasculine space of guilt, these men worked through their losses by searching long hours for the remains of their firehouse brothers, their police officer friends, and the many others who had just disintegrated when the towers collapsed. (There were hardly any human remains to be found at all, but nobody really understood this, especially at first.) And these men—when they were not on the clock at their jobs, were back at the pit. Some took leave of their jobs altogether in order to search full-time. For many, it was the only place they could be. They couldn't bring themselves to go home. Marriages dissolved.

They couldn't be with their kids. Some slept on cots for a couple of hours here or there, at a makeshift support center nearby, and then woke up and went right back into the pit, because it was the only place that felt right. It was one of the most desperate and self-destructive spaces I had ever encountered, and there was a huge amount of risk-taking going on down there. I was 26 at the time. And these men shared the most intimate details of their lives with me. I worked on this project from September to mid-December 2001, and then I handed all of my interviews over to the project PI as "data". Right after I turned my data over, I left for Dakar to begin my dissertation research.

There was another thing, too. On August 26, 2002, one month before the *Joola* tragedy, I had received a call that one of my closest friends, Jason, had died on the dance floor of a New York club that we had frequented together for many years. After hanging up the phone, I went straight to the airport without a suitcase, flew back to New York, and met our friends, his partner, and his parents and brothers in his apartment, to help plan his funeral. After we had lain him to rest, I got back on another plane and returned to Dakar.

As anthropologists, we often talk about how our own subject positions and life experiences enable us to see and understand certain things in the field that we might not have understood otherwise; this is how we are able to build rapport and be present to certain people and events in the field. And in the history of our discipline, ethnographic accounts of the anthropologist-fieldworker moving from obscurity to clarity—from anthropologist as outsider to "accepted" insider / friend, from chaos to order, from not understanding to AHA! finally understanding!—have been deeply privileged. Anthropologists often describe how they come to "make sense" of those situations, languages, relationships, and worlds of meaning that appeared opaque or wholly mystifying at first glance. At times these accounts have bordered on the trite or the overdramatic or the too-heroic, and at other times they have been profoundly moving. But, it seems that we say a lot less about how our life experiences might inhibit or prevent our understanding of the people and events we encounter in the field, or how these experiences might make it impossible for us to see, or might make us not *want* to see, or may keep us from writing about certain things. That is, of course, unless we are attempting to fold these ethnographic failures into larger stories of clarity, understanding, and being able to finally see what we were not able to see before (think, for example, of Renato Rosaldo's "Grief and the Headhunter's Rage").

Time and distance (and a bit of growing up on my part, maybe) have led me to see more clearly the way I unwittingly wrote the *Joola* tragedy out of my original account, or rather, the way I wrote around it. Privately, I have thought quite a lot about the fact that I never went down to the port to help out. Looking back at my fieldnotes and journal entries, I can see that my attention was stubbornly fixed on other things during that whole period; my fieldnotes reveal that I was overly preoccupied with insignificant infrastructural annoyances at the Fann clinic—haphazard filing systems, the state of the washrooms, the stagnant air, the mildewed everything. My journal takes a wholly different tone. It details the excitement surrounding the birth of a baby boy to my friends Ami and Momar, and describes both the extensive preparations made by the family for the *ngente* (baptism). Interposed with my unfolding account of a larger family drama are entries about the acupuncture treatments I was undergoing for a horrible cough at a new Chinese medical clinic that had recently sprung up near the place I was staying in Dakar. It is all terribly embarrassing to read. In both my fieldnotes and my journal, mention of the *Joola* was minimal. I wrote things like: "It's just horrible. Everybody's talking about it. President Wade announced a national period of mourning. Mass graves have been set up for the unclaimed bodies. People are outraged at the government's handling of the situation." But these were interspersed comments—unelaborated, simple sentences. Even here, in these private writing spaces, I did not dwell or linger on the event and its aftermath.

So while I recognize more than ever the conspicuous absence of the *Joola* from my project, I nevertheless find myself at this impasse. I feel that I can't very well keep the event—and especially my Fann interlocutors' intervention in it—out of my manuscript. At the same time, I can't write it in. I was absent to it; I didn't really register it in the field, and I can't really "make sense" of any of it anyway—not the event itself, nor my own ethnographic failure in not facing it. At this point anyway, the story of the *Joola* stands as little more than a supplement to my manuscript, not as "an inessential extra added to something complete in itself" (Culler 1882: 103) but rather as Jacques Derrida describes the supplement in *Of Grammatology*, as that which is possible and comprehensible (and even *necessary*) precisely because of an originary lack or gap or incompleteness, as that which is essential—but also remains external—to the original story, and as that which draws attention to and reinforces the very gap that it seeks to fill.

SIX

Distinctions of the Present

"YOU SAW THE NEW VIP ROOMS, RIGHT?" Nurse Fatou said to me, waving her hand in the direction of the small buildings that now occupied a corner of the courtyard adjacent to Fann's *Division Sud*. It was 2013. I had just returned to Dakar after a long absence and taken my first walk through the clinic in nearly ten years.

A couple of changes to the built environment of Fann had already surprised me that morning. The façade of the hospital had recently been painted; it glowed a bright white in the March sun. Demba's mural (shown in the introduction) had not been spared. It was gone without a trace, I realized, as I scrutinized its former location. Shrubs had been planted along the walls near the main entrance, and a caretaker with a hose was watering a large patch of grass. Inside the building, plans were being made to reopen *l'Étage Droit*, which had been closed since the 1990s due to disintegrating conditions and budgetary constraints. The clinic had also experienced a major shift in personnel. Some doctors and nurses had retired, while others had taken more lucrative (or promising) jobs elsewhere. After the Professor's retirement in 2012, a doctor who had been working as one of the division heads became the new director of the clinic. Another psychiatrist left Fann to become director of another hospital, and two other psychiatrists had taken jobs with the UN. A similar shift in personnel had taken place among nurses and social workers, where a wave of retirements and job changes led to a flurry of new hires. Those who remembered me from 2003 met me with warm greetings, questions about my family, and chidings for having stayed away for so long.

Now, as I stood there talking with Nurse Fatou, her gesture toward the VIP rooms caused me to shift my focus from the courtyard's newly planted trees to the modest, beige, single-story building. My gaze settled on its line of small windows, then its open door, and finally the empty bench out in front. It was a simple edifice, nothing fancy, but clean and new, and less institutional than the main building. I was puzzled, and curious. When Fatou and others at Fann talked about the clinic's newest class of accommodations, they pronounced the letters V-I-P in measured English ("vee-eye-pee") rather than in French ("vay-ee-pay"). To my ears at least, the acronym stuck out in a jagged, awkward kind of way; I could not help but think of famous NBA players and television personalities, velvet-rope dance clubs, paparazzi, and expensive box seats. What was this new VIP status, I wondered, and who were the *Very Important Persons* staying in these rooms?

In this chapter, I attend to the afterlives and traces of arrangements that were first put into place during Collomb's era, and that are perceptible in the present-day Fann Psychiatric Clinic. As I examine how the physical space of the clinic has been transformed and how practices of care and caretaking have changed at Fann in recent years, I pay special attention to the shifting economies—moral and material, therapeutic and political—that have characterized the clinic over the past two decades, linking these to larger transformations that have taken place within Senegal during the same period. In particular, it is against the backdrop of former president Abdoulaye Wade's neoliberal agenda and in light of his highly contested presidency, which ended with his failed reelection bid in 2012 and the installation of Senegal's fourth president, Macky Sall, that I seek out invocations and modifications of past practices and arrangements at Fann.

Tacking back and forth between the Fann clinic and the city of Dakar more broadly, my discussion centers around four specific features of the clinic that I have seen emerge or evolve since my first research stay at Fann back in 1999. I begin with the recent emergence of the VIP category. As a status closely tied to modes of consumption that draw on media-driven global imaginaries and aspirations, I show that recent infrastructural changes within the clinic and across the city, while allowing their users to make claims about global membership (Ferguson 2006), nevertheless produce new forms of erasure and dispossession—new invisibilities. I then move to discuss the growing acceptance of a new kind of patient attendant at the clinic, the *accompagnant mercenaire*. A dramatic departure from the original *accompagnant* policy that was put into place at Fann in the early 1970s, the *accompagnant mercenaire* is a patient attendant who, by informal arrangement with the patient's family, is paid to do the job. I examine the normalization of this commodified care arrangement against the backdrop of Senegal's neoliberal turn, while also understanding it alongside Fann's current approach to psychiatric care that emphasizes pharmaceutical treatments over psychodynamic investigation or therapy. The third feature I discuss is the transformation of *pénc* meetings at the clinic. Here I suggest that *pénc* meetings, the town hall–style group therapy meetings first introduced at Fann in the 1960s and celebrated both for their leveling effect and their ability to promote liberatory speech, have evolved into surveilled sites of patient responsibilization. I end with a discussion of the once-defunct but now flourishing *Atelier d'Ex-pression*, Fann's art therapy workshop, which has been reanimated with great success thanks to the leadership and vision of the current director of that program. Throughout, I consider how each of these inherited features and practices has been taken up, reworked, modified, or recontextualized to acquire new significance in the contemporary Fann clinic, and in relation to the shifting economies that have characterized the period in Senegal.

VERY IMPORTANT PERSONS

By 2013, Fann offered four different levels of accommodation based on price. The new private VIP rooms were at the top, and they came equipped with televisions, refrigerators, air conditioning, private bathrooms, and specially prepared meals, all for the sum of 20,000 fcfa ($40) per night. One step down, at 8,000 fcfa ($16) per night, were the "1st Category" rooms; located in the main building, these contained two beds each and a private toilet. Below that, at 5,000 fcfa ($10), were the "2nd Category" rooms, which also contained two beds but required patients to use the shared public toilets down the hall. Finally, there were the "3rd Category" rooms, which were shared by four people and also required the use of a shared bathroom off the main hallway, for 2,000 fcfa ($4) per night. Cafeteria meals were included in the cost of the lower three categories, but many patients complained about the low quality of the food and refused it if they had other options—if, for example, they had family or extended relations within Dakar who were able to bring them food, or if the patient's *accompagnant* was able to cook food or to buy it.

As startled as I was to learn about the existence (and high cost) of the new VIP rooms, I was all the more surprised to learn that, despite the fact that their price put them beyond the reach of many in Dakar, they almost never stood vacant. The stepped-up accommodations were in high demand, and they appeared to generate a steady and much-needed source of income for the clinic. Particularly interesting about this is the fact that many of the patients occupying the VIP rooms during my visit in 2013—including two French nationals, a Congolese diplomat's son, and a prominent Senegalese professor at the university—would probably have sought treatment elsewhere (at a private psychiatric facility in Dakar, for example, like *Clinique des Mamelles*) had it not been for the existence of these private, discreet, and comparatively luxurious accommodations. It is not only that people coming to Fann for inpatient care now have the "option" to pay for improved accommodations, but that the existence of the VIP category rooms has allowed the clinic to reach out to a brand-new clientele—a new market and a new kind of health care consumer and global citizen.

While these new VIP rooms at Fann were far from extravagant, they certainly put new forms of social distinction on display like never before at Fann. This is not to say that status distinctions were new to Dakar, or Senegal, or West Africa—far from it. Traditional Wolof, Pulaar, and Serer social organization is caste-based and highly stratified, and power is both gendered and gerontocratic. French colonial occupation of the region tended to capitalize upon these distinctions and superimpose new ones based on education, assimilation, and citizenship. In many ways, the attempts made by Collomb and *l'Ecole de Fann* to minimize social difference within the clinic were contrary to these local realities. What is new about the VIP status, it seems to me, is that it is earned through specifically global forms of consumption and recognition. This VIP is not just a social figure of high status deserving of (or willing to pay for) special treatment. It is an attitude, an image, and an assertion (or aspiration) of affluence that was, above all, a claim of global membership. Here and elsewhere, "VIP" has come to signal not just a certain kind of person, but access to a whole class of elite goods, services, and accommodations that do not simply confirm the high status of their users, but also bestow their own prestige. The VIP status signals global connections, and the ability to cross borders—indeed, to travel freely is an ultimate mark of affluence in today's Senegal.

Outside of Fann and throughout Dakar, the astounding construction boom that had taken place during my absence also appeared to produce dramatic new forms of distinction. Abdoulaye Wade, who was elected president in 2000 under the banner of *Sopi* (Wolof: change), indeed brought many changes to Dakar during his twelve years in office. Above all, Wade's vision for a prosperous Senegal centered around infrastructural development designed to attract foreign investment; his focus was on making Dakar appealing as a global city of trade that could provide its high-profile clients with ample opportunity for leisure and consumption. This translated into massive road, port, as well as airport construction projects (popularly referred to as *les grands travaux*) as well as prestige projects, like the enormous *Monument de la Renaissance*. It also translated into the development of what had once been an open stretch of Dakar's breathtaking coastline (*la Corniche*) into an expanse of luxury hotels, private entertainment and recreation facilities, and Senegal's first "upscale" mall, Sea Plaza, which was unveiled in 2010. With its internationally known luxury brands (Hugo Boss has a store there, as does Apple), restaurants, and bars, Sea Plaza stands as a space of leisure and consumption that is meant to recall—and also join the ranks of—high-end shopping complexes the world over. In the words of Sea Plaza's website:

> Sea Plaza, the ultimate in relaxation and leisure. Sea Plaza is your destination of choice for leisure and relaxation with friends or the whole family. Spend your afternoon bowling or in the arcade, your evenings playing pool or learning to ice skate. Your shopping center offers unique activities in Senegal for all ages.[1]

In a 2013 article for *Jeune Afrique*, journalist Mehdi Ba—a frequent contributor of stories about economic transformation, politics, and daily life in Dakar—draws attention to the "bourgeois-ification" of Dakar (*Dakar s'embourgeoise*), noting what he sees as not only the ascendency of the city's elite class (and the new forms of luxury spending that have accompanied it), but also the ongoing gentrification of Dakar due to high rents and a steady increase in the cost of living. "The Dakar of 4x4 vehicles and sedans," he writes, "has distanced itself from the Dakar of *cars rapides.*"[2] Beyond serving Dakar's own rising elite class, however, Sea Plaza and the grand hotels along the coast aim to provide to an international elite a stay that is at once luxurious, familiar, and pleasing. According to Eric Guèye, the director general of the shopping and entertainment complex, "[o]ur clientele is already familiar with the malls of Paris, Dubai or New York. For them, Sea Plaza will come as no surprise; it is but the normal way of things. Expatriates, members of NGOs and international organizations, all have been waiting for a place like this."[3] Sea Plaza, then, was an attempt to reach beyond the means of even the comparatively well-off middle class in Dakar to an international elite with money to burn.

As I sat talking with my friend Rico shortly after my arrival in Dakar in 2013, I had a barrage of questions for him. I had not yet seen the new

Corniche. "Was everything I had heard and read about Sea Plaza true?," I asked. "Was it really as big and glamorous as people were saying? Was there really a skating rink in there? Who could afford to go there, anyway? Can anybody just walk in, or is it guarded? Would he have any interest in going there with me to see it?" Rico is one of my oldest friends in Dakar; I first met him in 1995, when we were both around 20 years old. For as long as I have known him, he has been scrambling to get by and make ends meet.[4] *"Eh! C'est pas pour moi!"* ("Hey! It's not for me!"), Rico responded sharply, with a slight shake and tilt of his head and a somewhat sarcastic half-smile. His response gave me pause. "What do you mean it's not for you?" I asked. "Not for you, as in: You don't like it? It's not your kind of place? Or not for you, meaning: It's not there for your use; it wasn't built for you?" "Both," he said simply. In the end, I finally convinced him to go with me. We spent a long time watching people as they walked through the sprawling mall. We were catty, the two of us, as we sat together and talked about the people walking by—it was very unanthropological. At one point, he said to me (as best as I can recall):

> There are a few different kinds of people here. There are the people who can afford to shop here—the foreigners, and Senegalese people who get their money from somewhere else. Then there are the people who come here, dress up, walk around, take a few pictures and post them to Facebook—a "look at me living the life" kind of thing—it's all dreaming, all for show, but it's also all completely pretend. Then there are the people who come here and spend everything they have—like 50,000 fcfa ($100) on shoes, and then can't buy food at home.

So dramatic were the transformations that had taken place during my absence from Dakar—not just in terms of changes to the Corniche, but all over the city—that I spent my first few days back feeling utterly disoriented and slightly panicked, trying to get my bearings, getting lost in the very places that I had once known well. Walking around the SICAPS, I had to stop and ask for directions many times over, or I just kept walking in hopes that I would find a building or a road that corresponded to the map I carried in my mind. I stumbled over apologies and gave huge tips to cab drivers after making them drive me around in search of places I could not find. From Dieuppeul and Liberté 5 to the Fann Hospital compound and the Corniche, everything seemed taller, more built up. Construction projects were happening everywhere—home additions and new buildings in various stages of completedness, structures made of bare concrete and wooden support beams and webbed with perilous-looking scaffolding. These "not-yet houses," so eloquently described by Melly (2010), are often built with foreign money, or piece-by-piece by way of remittance payments. Such houses-in-waiting had been present for a long time—I remember being struck by their number even during my first stay from 1995–96 and amazed at how frequently such buildings appeared to fall into ruin before they were ever completed—but in 2013, the projects were even more visible than they had been during my previous stays.

As disoriented as I was by all the new construction taking place in Dakar, and as ostentatious as I found Sea Plaza and the new five-star hotels along the Corniche—one even advertised a Sunday brunch *de luxe* for "only" 25,000 fcfa (around $50)—it was the roads that surprised me the most. New roads, expanded roads, resurfaced roads, redesigned roads, bridges, tunnels, auto-routes—even a toll highway (*péage*) was being built that was designed to turn what was typically a 90 to 120–minute journey from Dakar to Diamnadio (a 40-kilometer journey off the bottlenecked Dakar peninsula) into a joyride that would take less than a quarter of the time.[5] For those who could afford to pay the toll after the autoroute was officially opened in August 2013, the smooth surface of the road and the lightning speed of the trip made the journey so great as to be worthy of its very own YouTube video (there were many). At 1,400 fcfa (approx. $2.85) per car each way, however, many judged this to be too steep a price to pay.[6] "At this price," one car owner was reported as saying to a *Jeune Afrique* journalist, "I do not intend to take the toll road. Fuel is expensive; instead of spending 2,800 fcfa to go to work and back, I'd rather just sit in traffic."[7] The toll payment offers access to a more pleasant and reliable journey for those who can afford to pay; the sensations associated with road travel are themselves a matter of social distinction. Affluence buys speed and the feeling of gliding over the smooth road; it reduces exposure to choking exhaust and stifling heat. Those who cannot afford to pay must continue to take the longer, slower route.

The impetus behind and justification for the autoroute and the many other road construction projects that were undertaken in Dakar was, of course, to alleviate the horrid traffic congestion issues that had been plaguing the city and its suburbs for years, as well as to make it easier for large trucks to transport their goods to and from the port. The projects were promoted for the benefits they would reap for the people: the new roads would save time, boost the economy, and reduce pollution. These infrastructural improvements, however, were not accessible to all, nor were they evenly distributed across the city. Infrastructure, Rodgers and B. O'Neill (2012: 402) remind us, "demarcates both literally and figuratively which points in urban contexts can and should be connected, and which should not, the kinds of people and goods that can and should circulate easily, and which should stay put, and who can and should be integrated within the city, and who should be left outside of it." In the march toward modernization that was imagined by Wade and actualized in the "*grands travaux*," areas of investment and renovation quickly became distinguished from areas of neglect and even dispossession; the latter were frequently among the poorest and most heavily populated quarters of Dakar. Melly (2013: 387) rightfully noted that while the new roads "linked together spaces of governance, global travel, and elite consumption," the rest of Dakar was "left to contend with dilapidated roads unfit for passage, ruptured sewage pipes, frequent power outages, and the seeming lack of state intervention and oversight." Other sections of Dakar and its suburbs were even less lucky. An estimated 30,000 people were displaced between the cities of Keur Massar and Pikine alone in order to build the new Dakar-Diamnadio Toll Highway. Reports stated that residents were given a choice of either (1) being relocated to nearby resettlement village or (2) receiving monetary compensation (from a budget of approximately 31 billion fcfa / $64 million) for their loss of property and livelihood; the choice they were *not* allowed to make, however, was to stay where they were and not move at all.

Above all, the Wade years marked a period of dramatically uneven, mostly foreign-sourced investment (and corresponding divestment and exclusion) around Dakar. Those who benefitted reflected favorably upon the Wade years. Amadou, who is my age and whom I had known since 1995, comes from a highly educated family that has many of its members currently living abroad. He is well employed and travels frequently for work and leisure. He laid it out for me like this:

> When I was going to school [in the 1990s], it was bad then. At *lycée*, we would see people older than us—brilliant, brilliant minds—who had succeeded at every step, who had always been at the top of their class, and they were competing against so many others for so few positions. But now, with the new private enterprises, things are different. For example—if you have a degree and you're not working, really, it's nobody's fault but your own.

According to Amadou, success is possible now like it was not before, and if you are not succeeding, you have only yourself to blame. And yet, there is clearly more to succeeding in present-day Dakar than personal initiative and hard work, and the wealth and opportunity created during the Wade years were by no means equally distributed.

Back at Fann, as I sat talking with the new director on my first day back in 2013, I described my impressions to him about how, to my eyes, things had changed in Dakar. I noted too that there seemed to be more investment in the clinic than there had been in 2003. Was the clinic in a better position financially than it had been back then, I asked. "Not really," he sighed. "It's the state. There's just not enough money. There were big plans to construct a building right here in the central courtyard that would house a library [to expand the documentation center] on the second floor, and a large classroom that could seat a hundred on the first floor. For a long time we've asked for the money but we were not able to secure it. It's been pushed aside for many years now—it's just not a priority." The clinic, according to the director, was still in difficult financial shape. The new VIP rooms had been the only major infrastructural improvements to speak of in the past ten years, he told me. These were working out very well, even better than expected. They were even providing a steady trickle of money where there had been none before.

In 2016, the family of a young patient who had stayed in one VIP room at Fann donated a significant sum of money to the clinic, aimed specifically at the renovation and updating of the VIP rooms. As I sat talking with one of Fann's nurses about this development, she praised the family, but then turned sour:

> But you know what isn't good? In the rest of the [psychiatry] clinic, things are dirty and outdated. Most of the rooms are disgusting. Sometimes when a patient comes here and we show him to his room, he looks at it and says: "This is not good! I can't possibly stay in here!" The rest of the CHNU is relatively well-appointed. It's clean, it's nice. But in here . . . it's like we're not even part of the larger hospital. It really makes me feel bad. And you know: the new CEPIAD (*Centre de Prise en Charge Intégrée de l'Addiction de Dakar,* *or* Dakar Integrated Treatment Center for Persons with Addictions) building. So much is being done for *les UDIs* [les *Usagers de Drogues par Injection*; in English referred to as PWIDs, or *Person Who Inject Drugs*]. They get free screening and testing, free dental care, massage therapy, everything! When I complain about this to people I look like the enemy, I know. But look, on our side of things [the psychiatric clinic], patients have nothing. None of that is free for them! It's not right. The NGOs pay for everything over there! It's a beautiful building and they are so well set up. They have their methadone and their enrichment activities, and it's all free for them. They have so many privileges! Our patients have none of those privileges! It's not right.

CEPIAD, the first clinic aimed solely at the treatment of addiction in West Africa and also the region's first addiction research and training center, had been inaugurated a couple of years before this, and was the result of a partnership between the Global Fund, the Senegalese government, ESTHER (Network for Hospital Therapy Solidarity), the city of Paris, CNLS (National Center to Combat AIDS), and UNODC (United Nations Office on Drugs and Crime). The nurse's reaction highlighted what she perceived to be an uneven investment and distribution of funds across the different units and clinics of the larger CHU complex. In particular, she found it deeply unfair that the psychiatric clinic and its patients received less money and support than the addictions clinic. She phrased her judgments about this in harsh moral terms related to patient innocence and deservingness. Why, she asked, were PWIDs and their recovery being privileged over non-using psychiatric patients? "And to think: those people over there [PWIDs], they've done it to themselves! Yes, I speak my mind about this, but you know, I'm not included in the conversations. My views are not popular."

If the Fann clinic and greater Dakar have indeed been marked over these past twenty years by uneven investment and the uneven distribution of resources and opportunities (as well as new forms of social distinction that have accompanied them), we would do well to recall Ferguson's (2006: 14) assertion: "Africa's participation in globalization . . . has been a matter of highly selective and spatially encapsulated forms of global connection combined with widespread disconnection and exclusion." Economic investment in much of Africa, asserts Ferguson, whether that of multinational corporations or NGOs, has adhered to an enclave model that divides useful and deserving sites, lands, and people from those deemed useless and unworthy; here, "the global" is as much about disconnection as it is about linkage, and the connections made are not within a local, regional or even "a national grid, but in transnational networks that connect economically valued spaces dispersed around the world in a point-to-point fashion" (40). Just as Dakar's new roads, hotels, and spaces of consumption link the city to a transnational elsewhere of global membership, so too do Fann's new VIP rooms, and CEPIAD as well. And while President Wade drew on the language of an "African Renaissance" to describe and justify his *Monument de la Renaissance*, making reference to a shared history of struggle and oppression as well as an emerging, liberated African present, such sentiment has appeared all but absent in other infrastructural investment projects and partnerships. In fact, as Melly (2013: 386) has rightly noted, the "construction of professedly globalized spaces of consumption and circulation" spoke little of "post-colonial ideologies like *négritude* and instead appeared thoroughly detached from histories and shared struggles of past decades." Instead, these spaces seemed resolutely aimed at other consumers and other futures. The Wade-era changes signaled a definitive end to any lingering remnants of Senghor's "spiritual socialism"— not to mention the utter disavowal of any remaining modernist aspirations toward a "Civilization of the Universal." Senghor's vision was replaced by the project of a neoliberal consumption-centered "global" city.

For the large number of Senegalese men and women who were not the direct beneficiaries of Wade's *"grands travaux,"* who could not easily cross borders, and who had not been the targeted recipients of NGO initiatives or multinational corporations, the affluence and evident prosperity of a selected few signaled a "progress" and prosperity that was not their own. As they struggled to make ends meet, the disjuncture between the fortunes of others and the precarity of their own lives was only affirmed by such displays. As an outside observer revisiting Dakar after a long absence, I found quite striking the new signs of wealth, status, transnational mobility, and life *de luxe*—both within the clinic and around the city—that were openly advertised and put on display, as a matter of distinction, in close proximity to the increasingly difficult living conditions faced by many Dakarois. Also striking was the fact that, by 2013 and even more so by 2017, the very same infrastructural changes that had engendered new forms of distinction (and exclusion) throughout Dakar and at Fann had already faded out of view and become the new normal.[8]

THE EMERGENCE (AND NORMALIZATION) OF THE
ACCOMPAGNANT MERCENAIRE

In chapter 5, I described how the gaps created by personnel shortages and material insufficiencies at Fann during the 1980s and 1990s opened a space for the emergence of a bustling informal economy. Perhaps the most remarkable of the informal jobs taken up at Fann during that period was that of *accompagnant mercenaire,* or hired patient attendant. By definition, *accompagnants mercenaires* are not related to the patient, nor are they official employees of the clinic. *Accompagnants mercenaires* (hereafter, AMs) have become increasingly common at Fann in recent years; this arrangement represents a dramatic transformation of the *accompagnant* policy (discussed at length in chapter 2) that was officially put into place at Fann in 1972, while Collomb was the director of the clinic. In its original form, the policy required inpatients to have a family member or close friend—an *accompagnant*—stay onsite with them for the duration of their hospitalization with the expectation that this would greatly improve the patient's quality of care and chance of recovery.

It is especially instructive, I think, to read the transformation of the *accompagnant* policy in terms of the shifting economies within the institution. As an emerging form of commodified care, the AM arrangement should be examined against the backdrop of Senegal's neoliberal turn while also being framed within an understanding of Fann's current approach to psychiatric care that emphasizes pharmaceutical treatment strategies over psychodynamic investigation or therapy. This relationship between neoliberalism and the biomedicalization of health (including mental health and psychiatric care) is an interesting one: along with sharing the basic core concepts of the atomistic and autonomous self, both neoliberalism and biomedicine idealize individual responsibility, rational choice or action, marketization, and productivity. Some scholars working at the interstices of neoliberalism and biomedicine have highlighted the ways in which neoliberal policies and reforms shape research trajectories, thus fostering and favoring the production of certain kinds of knowledge while limiting others (e.g., Valdiya 2010). Others have argued that the rise of biopsychiatry "help[s] to create the social and cultural milieu favoured by neoliberal policies" (Moncrieff 2008: 235), and more pointedly, that biomedicine and its accompanying technologies have been used as a tool of neoliberal expansion (Lock and Nguyen 2010).

Typically, AMs at Fann negotiate the terms of their employment—and also their salary—directly with the patient's family. In 2013 (and still in 2017), their earnings typically ranged from about 2,500–5,000 fcfa ($5–10) per day. The clinic provides no guidelines regarding the hiring of these attendants, nor does it provide a set of standards or best practices regarding patient care. *Accompagnants mercenaires* at Fann receive neither training nor professional support; the care they offer is ad hoc, unsupervised, and highly dependent upon the wills and whims of the AMs themselves. Likewise, these hired attendants receive no job security or protection from the clinic.

Accompagnants mercenaires were not altogether new to Fann when I first visited the clinic in 1999. Earlier versions had, in fact, been noted by Gbikpi and Auguin back in 1978, but they were framed as both an aberration and an object of criticism. By 2013, however, the position had become normalized, although Fann doctors and staff continued to express their disapproval regarding this trend. Without exception, every doctor and staff member I have spoken with over the years has told me that it is always preferable to have a family member stay with the patient. When they speak about AMs in general terms, doctors and staff are quick to note the many ways in which AMs are inferior to conventional *accompagnants* when it comes to the care of the patient. One current psychiatrist at Fann explained to me that because the AM is a stranger to the patient, they cannot provide Fann doctors and staff with any insight about what the patient was like before they fell ill, nor can they easily recognize the progress the patient is making over the course of his treatment. Several nurses related that AMs do not show the same degree of commitment to the patient and their recovery as traditional *accompagnants* do. These paid attendants, they tell me, do not assist with treatment or monitor the patient's day-to-day progress with the same level of attention. Another difference, described to me by a young but well-respected intern currently working in the clinic, is that when family members act as *accompagnants,* the informal "psychoeducation" they receive enables them to assist their patients even after they leave the clinic; they can help the patient with the transition back to normal life and monitor his condition in a way that AMs cannot. In short, Fann doctors and staff describe the services performed by AMs in purely custodial terms; at best, AMs assist the patient with her daily tasks, report worrisome behavior to the nurses, and make sure the patient does not wander away from the CHNU compound unattended.

Based on these statements, one might be led to conclude that Fann doctors and staff are fundamentally opposed to—or at the very least, ambivalent toward—the presence of AMs in the clinic. In everyday practice, however, AMs are readily accepted as key players at Fann, now more than ever. As the Fann's previous director (the Professor) explained to me, "These families now, they all claim to be too busy to send an *accompagnant.* They come in and say to me, 'We are all working or in school; it's not possible for any of us to stay with the patient as an *accompagnant,* but we are ready to pay someone.'" When a family is at a loss about whom they can hire to tend to the patient, the doctors and nurses themselves recommend that the family hire an AM, and even arrange for the parties to meet. Fann staff and AMs know each other well and often work side by side, and when doctors and nurses are asked about specific AMs, they have many kind words to say.

That the AM arrangement is becoming both more common and more readily accepted at Fann, then, points to the needs and desires that have arisen from the intersecting situations of three parties, all of which relate back to the economic shift that has taken place in Senegal in the past three decades. First, wealthier families from abroad, as well as Senegalese families that have been fortunate enough to prosper in Senegal's new economy, may find themselves unable to get away from their jobs to do the work of care that, according to the original *accompagnant* policy, would once have been required of them. They do, however, have money on hand to hire somebody for the job, and they have few reservations about paying for this care. Second, there is a readily available pool of unemployed or underemployed workers— including those who have been excluded from Senegal's recent moves to modernize—who are trying to scrape together a living, and who are willing and able to accept the job of AM. And third, Fann doctors and staff now see AMs in a new and different light than they did in the past—not as obstacles to care but as a class of "helpers" who can both assist the patient and reduce their workload within the clinic.

There is no doubt that the growing acceptance of the AM role by Fann doctors and staff represents a practical strategy for getting by despite the material insufficiencies and personnel shortages faced by the clinic. Alongside all of this, the acceptance of AMs also signals a shift in attitudes regarding psychiatric treatment at Fann more generally. Doctors and staff currently affiliated with the clinic are not as psychodynamically oriented as their 1970s predecessors were. Recall that Gbikpi and Auguin warned of the dangers of rejection (*le rejet*) that were compounded when a paid *accompagnant* was enlisted instead of a family member, noting that the presence of a paid *accompagnant* was both a symptom and an affirmation of the problems that brought patients to Fann in the first place. In contrast, reflecting a more global shift, doctors at the present-day clinic privilege the pharmaceutical treatment of mental illness over a sustained psychodynamic or culturalist approach. When I revisited Fann in 2017, for example, there were three psychotherapists working in the clinic. One saw very few patients because he was involved in so many other professional projects, and another was on extended medical leave. The third was a psychologist from France who was not officially employed by the clinic, but had an arrangement whereby she would offer free sessions to inpatients and charge a small fee to outpatients. According to her, the clinic's psychiatrists rarely referred their patients for psychotherapy, and the work she did with patients often ended up resembling counseling work. It is also important to note that two of the three psychotherapists conduct their sessions in French, as they do not have the language skills necessary to hold sessions in Wolof or any of Senegal's other national languages.

According to the current head of one of Fann's divisions, the patient demand for psychotherapy at the clinic is not great, nor is psychotherapy an obligatory part of patient treatment. Patients expect to receive a prescription (or several) for medication during their stay at Fann, but they are much more reluctant to participate in one-on-one talk therapy sessions, and even less inclined to want to pay for them. In a 2002 interview with Dr. Malick, a psychiatrist working at Fann during that time, he stressed that Fann doctors must "approach the patient with the tools of modern medicine, for that is what the patient will expect." Doctors, he said, should respect this fact. From his perspective, the "tools of modern medicine" are pharmaceuticals.

The growing acceptance of the role of AMs at Fann, then, signals a shift in the clinic's therapeutic orientation as much as it represents a practical strategy for getting by. For the psychodynamically oriented Fann of the 1970s, the presence of the *accompagnant* in the clinic did much more than keep patients connected to their families and ease the workload of the staff. It offered important clues about the relational dynamics that were thought to be at the source of the patient's suffering and allowed doctors to not just observe but to also intervene in these relationships. In contrast, the current doctors and staff at the clinic are much less likely to view family dynamics as the primary source of a patient's suffering (though they do readily admit that familial relationships have a huge impact on the well-being of the patient). From their perspective, mental illness is not a product of relationships; rather, as the biomedical model affirms, it is located in the patient himself. It is not that troubled family dynamics and dysfunctional social relationships are seen as unimportant, but rather that they are understood to be secondary problems that will be ameliorated once the patient has been cured. In fact, in the present-day clinic, relational problems between patients and family members are often read as the very *symptoms* of the patient's illness, and the mending of these problems is taken as a sign of recovery. As Fann's current head nurse explained to me, she can tell a patient is responding well to his medication when she sees him getting along better with his family members. From this perspective, the custodial care offered by an AM, while perhaps less desirable than the care offered by a patient's family member-*accompagnant*, is nevertheless viewed as a passable substitute when there is no other option available.

THE *PÉNC*: COLLECTIVE AFFIRMATION THROUGH
RESPONSIBILIZATION

"It is true what you're saying," one of the clinical psychologist at Fann told me in 2013. "Psychology and psychotherapy are not as important [within Fann's therapeutic repertoire] as medication, and haven't been for quite some time." We were sitting in his office talking about the research I had carried out at Fann from 1999–2003, and I told him of my plans to write this book. The other psychologist working at Fann in 2013, however, was more critical of my line of questioning. Yes, she said, it's true that very few patients at the clinic attended one-on-one therapy sessions, but many do take part in group activities. "And don't forget," she said, "the *pénc is* a form of group psychotherapy!"

When asked what traces of Collomb's Fann still exist in the present-day clinic, Fann doctors and staff are quick to refer to the *pénc* meetings, although they also note that these have changed a great deal since the time of their inception. Some, especially the old-timers, insist that the changes have been far from favorable. Even way back when I first met Demba, for instance, he had adamantly refused to attend the *pénc* meetings, calling them a terrible waste of time because they no longer resembled what they had been when Collomb was present. El Hadj, who had worked as Collomb's principal translator during the 1960s and 1970s, wholeheartedly agreed. "Today the *pénc* is a joke," he told me. "It is theater, and people are just going through the motions. It used to be a form of therapy, but not anymore."

Others, like Dr. Diop, who was head of one the Fann's four functioning divisions in 2013, affirmed that the *pénc* meetings were, in fact, still worthwhile. "The *pénc* is really good for patients, it's not just a performance," she explained. "Each time we do a *pénc*, there are one or two patients who emerge as leaders, who really seem to see themselves and understand their situation. This is an important step for them," she said. It is worth noting here the extent to which the above-stated objective of the *pénc*—the emergence of articulate leaders who are able to narrate their mental suffering in a way that demonstrates self-awareness and an improvement in their condition—departs from the intentions of the *pénc* that were first articulated in the 1970s, when the goal of such town hall–type meetings was to diminish hierarchy, establish community, foster a sense of collective affirmation and validation, and promote liberatory speech among and between participants (Dia 1976, 1977; Dia et al. 1976; Collomb 1975). As discussed in chapter 2, these weekly sessions were first integrated into Fann during the mid-1960s with the goal of creating a village-like sense of community within the clinic. Then, the *pénc* was touted most notably for its leveling capacity; it was a forum in which doctors and nurses came together with patients and their *accompagnants* as fellow community members, and patients were able to share their stories, problems, complaints, and experiences as equals. At *pénc* gatherings, patients were encouraged to speak up and out—at the doctors, about each other, about Fann, or about the world outside. This was a space in which the social principle of healing, which has been described by Petryna and Kleinman (2006: 9) as "based on a consideration of healing as an interactive, social and cultural process that is especially attentive to symbolic and narrative aspects of health and illness," was played out. The special emphasis on dissolving hierarchical power made the *pénc* sessions unique.

Years ago, it was not at all uncommon for each of Fann's weekly *pénc* sessions to attract upwards of fifty or more participants, including doctors, nurses, social workers, patients, *accompagnants*, outside family members, students, and researchers. The meetings were considered a cornerstone and trademark of Fann's early years; they were also points of access through which people from outside the clinic could experience the institution and witness its innovative approach. Local newspapers, such as *Le Soleil* and *Le Quotidien*, regularly featured stories about the *pénc* sessions. The meetings I have witnessed and participated in since 1999, however, have been much less well attended. Often, they are canceled altogether. Doctors complain that nurses are unenthusiastic about getting the patients and their *accompagnants* together for the *pénc* sessions. Nurses, however, see things differently. They insist that the doctors care little about the *pénc* sessions; they always claim to be too busy and rarely find time to attend. Over the years, I myself have noticed that doctors rarely attend (though advanced medical students in residency often do participate). By 2017, at least one of the division heads had abandoned the *pénc* model altogether, instead opting to run weekly group therapy sessions. Like the *pénc*, these are attended by patients and *accompagnants*, division nurses, and medical students, but they are led and moderated by the doctor himself.

During the summer of 1999 and from 2001–03, my participation in *pénc* sessions took place primarily in the *Pavillon des Dames,* while in my subsequent visits I have mostly attended gatherings in other divisions. These experiences have provided me with a picture quite different from that which was described by Dia, Collomb, and their colleagues during the 1970s. In this division, *pénc* sessions usually took place every Wednesday morning. Before the sessions began, nurses would walk through the clinic and invite as many people as possible to take part. Patients and their *accompagnants* were encouraged, but not required, to participate. On average, anywhere from 8–15 people would typically attend, though on several occasions, such as the day that a local newspaper reporter came to Fann to do a story and the day before Tabaski (Eid al-Adha, or "Festival of Sacrifice") 2002, the number was significantly higher.

Around 10:00 a.m., people would begin trickling into the *Pavillon des Dames* and gathering upon the tiled verandah that overlooked a dry, fenced-in courtyard. Participants would seat themselves upon a large plastic mat that had been rolled out especially for the occasion, or they would sit on the wooden benches and chairs that had been brought to encircle the mat. Although in theory all those in attendance were considered to hold equal status and voice without differentiation, in my experience, patients and family members rarely mingled with staff or guests and there was seldom any confusion or ambiguity about who was who. Status markers were clearly legible, as was the deferential behavior of patients and their families toward Fann staff. Staff most often wore their white or colored coats, patients regularly sat on the floor in or near the center, and guests usually sat in the chairs closest to the door.

To begin the session, a nurse or social worker would welcome the group and appoint one of the patients to the job of *jaraaf* (*jaraaf* is the Wolof word for "village leader or chief") for the session. I was told that this was a relatively new practice; it used to be that the *jaraaf* was nominated by those in attendance. Nowadays, one nurse explained to me, the staff simply assigns the role because "it is so much easier that way." The *jaraaf* is chosen based on her ability to speak empathetically and lead discussion effectively. Because of this, the patient selected for the role is usually someone who has been around the clinic for a significant length of time and is judged by the doctors and nurses to have made considerable progress towards recovery. The *jaraaf* performs the role of moderator during the meeting. She might also play the part of peer-support role model to those patients who are less familiar with Fann than she is.

The *jaraaf* normally opens the session by introducing herself and briefly saying a few words about how the *pénc* are run. She then introduces new patients and their *accompagnants,* asking them if they would like to say anything to the group. When Xady, a patient at Fann from June until early August 2002, acted as *jaraaf* in late July, she was first prompted by the attending social worker. She then explained to the other patients:

> It is important for everyone to talk. Each person should say how she is feeling, if she is feeling better, or if she is going to be going home soon. Also, if anyone is having problems with their medication, the staff, the doctors, anything—

they can and should bring it up. Everyone is equal here; everyone should have the chance to say what is on her mind.

While gatherings were originally predicated on the assertion that all people have the right to speak, be heard, and be respected, patients tended to stay quiet, usually speaking up only when prompted. Much more often, *accompagnants* talked about patients, and nurses or social workers gave advice. In this way, rather than troubling institutional power and creating an opening for new forms of sociality and communality, the *pénc* gatherings tended to reinscribe power distinctions and reaffirm the authority of both the staff and the family over the patient.

Of those patients who did speak up, most (like the *jaraaf*) were nearing the end of their hospitalization, and were identified by the staff as being on the road to recovery. They had acquired a certain narrative structure and vocabulary for their illnesses that both guided and framed their comments. One of the most common ways that these patients address the group, for example, is by talking about how much better they have been feeling since their arrival at Fann, thanks to the excellent treatment they have received. Along with this, it is fairly typical for patients to praise and thank the nurses and doctors (sometimes profusely). The illness narratives that are recounted during *pénc* meetings tend to be somewhat formulaic; they often refer to the authority of the institution to organize and make intelligible the stories patients tell about themselves. Patients often begin by talking about what their lives were like *before* they got sick, and then they describe the experience of getting sick as a progressive decline and withdrawal that aroused the concern of those around them. They often note a final event that led their family members or friends to bring them to the clinic, and they often speak of their hospitalization as a period of recovery, reflection, and new insight. In short, typical illness narratives recounted during the *pénc*, which insist upon a very specific kind of self-reflective and self-knowing subject, most often trace the journey from health to illness, and from illness back to the reestablishment of health (Kleinman 1988; Estroff et al. 1991; Good 1994).

As these illness narratives are plotted upon the institutional topography of Fann, the topography itself structures their very expression. Here I take a cue from Jamie A. Saris (1995), who rightly insists that there are factors present, larger than the experiencing self, which mediate and shape the production of a story. He questions the idea that there is a "romantic freedom innate to 'narrative'" and tacitly questions the institutional authority (and basis for knowledge) that shapes illness narratives (65). During the *pénc*, patients refer to their symptoms, diagnoses, medications, and duration at Fann—and also to their interactions with nurses, doctors, and other patients—as a way of ordering their self-presentations. Although the specificities of each patient's case are unique, the structures of the illness narratives shared at the *pénc* are quite similar. To Fann staff (as well as to patients' families) the patient's ability to narrativize her illness in this manner serves as a key indicator of her recovery.

Just as it takes a certain kind of patient to act as *jaraaf*, I argue that only a certain kind of patient has a voice (and gets listened to) within the *pénc*. The idea that these gatherings necessarily foster and support a sense of liberatory speech among patients is questionable, for just as illness narratives appear formulaic and somewhat restricted, group discussions often transform into normative—and normalizing—discourse. Furthermore, although patients are encouraged to participate freely in the *pénc,* and the gatherings are tolerant of outbursts and interruptions, some words and actions are simply marked as unacceptable. Nurses and social workers police the language and behavior of patients in order to gauge their ability to function in a social setting.

During a *pénc* session in January 2002, for example, an important disruption took place. A young woman named Aminata, who was accompanied by her mother, jumped up from the plastic mat where she had been sitting and, standing tall above the others, screamed "WAA SENEGAAL, DAÑU IÑÑAAN!" (Senegalese people, you are all jealous!). Waving her arms, she shrieked and then began to tear at her hair. A social worker and a nurse quickly grabbed Aminata's arms and escorted her back to her room where, I learned later, she was given valium to ease her *comportement agité* (agitated behavior). Aminata was not asked what she meant or why she shouted out like this, nor was her outcry interrogated by the other participants. With her outburst she had been marked as unwell and therefore no longer fit to participate in the *pénc*. Any veneer of equality between participants dissolved at once as the social worker and nurse took her away. The *pénc,* it seems, demands certain standards of self-regulation—indeed, it requires a certain degree of "civility"—for participation.

Dia, Collomb, and others who wrote about *pénc* during the 1970s described the potential for the meetings to create a therapeutic community by allowing patients to speak frankly and openly about their experiences inside and outside the clinic. In turn, they said, this would promote the interrogation of mental illness itself and, by extension, the social worlds that define it. If one were to speculate about the therapeutic philosophy existing behind the *pénc* of today, it would be much more utilitarian and practical. Fann's main priority now, as I have been told many times, is to restore patients to baseline mental health and thereby promote their ability to function normally in their everyday lives. Whereas in the past, patients' self-expression—no matter how shocking or outrageous—was given central importance in the *pénc* and even assumed to hold the key to recovery, patients today must exhibit a certain degree of restraint and self-control during the *pénc* in order to achieve the status of full-fledged member in this therapeutic community. Individual self-expression or "liberatory speech" is monitored and kept within the bounds of the group's expectations; anything perceived as a possible threat to the smooth functioning of the *pénc*—or to the institutional order that supports it—is deemed unacceptable.

Indeed, a patient's ability to act appropriately in the *pénc* has become a diagnostic tool of sorts. Each patient's participation is actively assessed and evaluated by staff and family members as a measure of her illness or health. Thus, the *pénc* has been transformed into an arena in which patients must not only perform their wellness, sociability, and ability to assimilate to the group but also emerge as leaders. In other words, patients must demonstrate that they understand and can manage social expectations appropriately lest they be marked unwell or even escorted back to their rooms. When patients show the staff and attending family members that they are able to comport themselves correctly during the *pénc*, they are considered to be demonstrating their progress toward recovery. This in turn moves patients closer to their release date. Despite having emerged from a communal spirit, the *pénc* appears to have evolved into something more akin to a neoliberal site of responsibilization. Many of the patients, Xady included, seemed to grasp the *pénc*'s responsibilizing and normalizing function quite clearly and know what is at stake in their participation.

ART THERAPY

"This place is different from the rest of the clinic. I feel like I can breathe here." Modou tells me this as we sit down at the large, cluttered table in Fann's *Atelier d'Ex-pressions*, or art therapy workshop. The name of the workshop is a play on words—in French, *les expressions* are expressions, but *les pressions* are pressures; *ex-pressions* also indicates getting rid of pressure or stress. It is February 2017, and Modou has been an inpatient at Fann for two weeks now, having been brought in by his family for what they reported to be *comportement agité* (agitated behavior). The table at which we are sitting, which has enough space for about eight people, is caked with paint and deep with stuff: paper, brushes, and plastic bottles of paint. Around the table, paintings on canvas and paper are stacked and hung, leaning and piled. The small room in the *Rez-de-Chaussée Gauche* is filled to the brim this morning; nine people—seven men and two women—are already squeezed in, with more to come. Alpha Blondy's *Jerusalem* plays on the small CD player, and a man named Djibril sits down at the big blue cooking gas cylinder to make *ataaya* for the group. There are newspaper cones filled with peanuts, too, for sharing. The ambiance is warm and relaxed.

Art therapy, which had been a part of the healing repertoire at Fann during the time of Collomb and *l'Ecole de Fann*, was abandoned in the 1980s and 1990s, due to a lack of resources and waning interest. In 1999, the Professor scraped together funds to hire an art therapist who could come to Fann for a few hours each week, with the goal of reanimating the workshop. Since that time, the person charged with running the *Atelier*—who was trained as an artist and art educator and had worked for many years at a school for the deaf—has brought the little art studio to life. The *Atelier*, which is open on Monday and Wednesday mornings, has become one of the most successful initiatives of the present-day clinic.

There are two components to the success of the *Atelier*. The first is its welcoming atmosphere, and the second has to do with the national and international visibility that the leader of the *Atelier* has brought to the initiative. To the first point, the *Atelier* is a relaxed space of sociality and exchange that the leader has worked hard to cultivate. Here music, tea, and conversation mix with painting and drawing. Some patient-artists are very serious about their work, while others dabble in a more halfhearted way. Men and women who were once inpatients at Fann but have since been released often stop in to paint alongside current inpatients, and to take part in the conversation. The leader of the *Atelier* does not instruct or critique, though he does offer advice if asked for it, and he does obtrusively foster interaction and reflection. I present here three brief scenes to give a sense of how the *Atelier* works, and to demonstrate the ethos and ambiance of the place.

During my 2017 visit to Fann, I met a patient named Idriss. While I was sitting with a few other patients near the front entrance of the clinic one day, he walked out slowly, saying, "Maybe you all hate me, I can't tell. Do you hate me?" We all said that no, of course we didn't hate him, and we invited him to sit down with us. We introduced ourselves, and I introduced my research project to him. Idriss was from a small village in the Bakel region in northeastern Senegal. This was his third time at the clinic—his first stay was in 2004—and he had been at Fann for a few of weeks already. As he explained it, things go fine for him for long periods. Then all of a sudden, he gets agitated, aggressive. He cannot still himself. He lashes out at the people around him, his family even. Each time it has been like this. Then he gets to Fann, and they give him the drugs (this time, he reported to me, he was prescribed Largactil, Nozinan, and Tegratol) and after about two days, that agitation— that aggression—is gone, but it is replaced, he says, by an exhaustion so profound that when he wakes up from sleeping he not only doesn't want to get up, he just wants to die. "I don't want to be here anymore," he said to us on the steps that day, "I want to go back to the village. My wife is in the village. My kids are there." He repeated these last two lines to us three times, slowly and desperately. We tried to console him and told him that he would surely be going home in a few weeks. One of the other patients suggested that he attend art therapy, to help him relax and think of other things. A few days later, Idriss showed up in the *Atelier*. He was, at first, shy and reluctant to paint. He had never really done it before, he said, and did not have an idea of what he should paint. As he told the group about his family in Bakel and the place to which he desired so much to return, the head of the *Atelier* suggested he draw or paint his house. On the surface it was a simple suggestion, and the way Idriss was best able to visualize and represent the house was by painting its floorplan. As Idriss worked, he used the images he produced to guide his commentary about what his home meant to him, about who was there waiting for him, and about how he wanted it to be upon his return. Idriss's paintings allowed him to articulate ideas about kinship and intimacy, nostalgia and regret, forgiveness and possibility. In so doing, he was able to communicate with and be heard by others who were in the *Atelier* that day.

Another patient who frequented the *Atelier* during those same weeks in 2017 was Aby, a woman in her forties who described herself as being of Wolof ethnicity and devoutly Muslim. Because Aby had worked as a schoolteacher, everyone in the *Atelier* started calling her *la Maîtresse* (in Senegal as in France, elementary school children typically call their teachers *Maître* or *Maîtresse*). Aby did not want to do art. Rather, she wanted to lead dictations of poems and fables that she had memorized, and that she had likely taught in her classrooms. She spoke loudly and with a firm voice as she read. A couple of other patients watched her, curiously. The head of the *Atelier* too listened along, and then chuckled in his easygoing way. "These dictations are

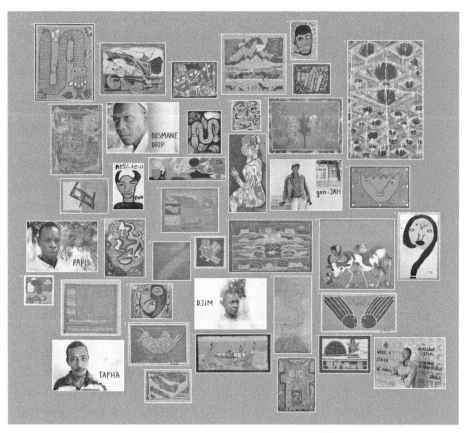

FIGURE 6 AND FIGURE 7. Poster, published on the occasion of the exhibition "Friedl Kubelka: Atelier d'Expression (Dakar)," Camera Austria (Graz), 2016. Copyright: The artists and Camera Austria.

difficult! I bet nobody in here could write them out without any mistakes. In fact, I'll give 5,000 fcfa ($10) from my own pocket to the person who can write out a perfect dictation!" Suddenly more people were involved, and the contest was on. Nobody won in the end (myself included; the dictation was no joke), but the activity led to a lively exchange with much laughter.

The third scene that speaks to the kind of ambiance cultivated within the *Atelier* took place in 2015. A young man in his twenties, Moctar, had been attending the *Atelier* for a couple of weeks. Moctar had not spoken a word in more than two months; instead he relied on gestures to communicate. He appeared to be a very talented artist. An older man, Ibou, was no longer an inpatient at Fann but had been attending art therapy sessions regularly for nearly a year. His skills were more elementary. Citing a paper shortage and

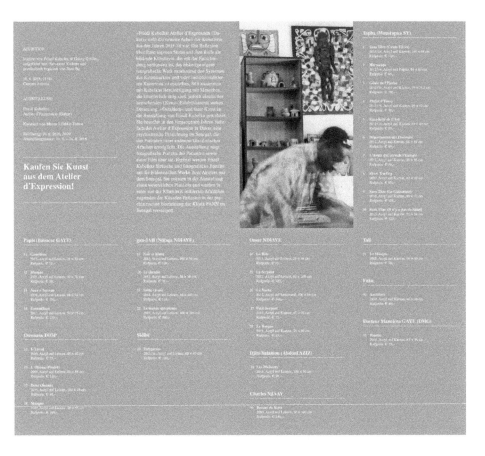

limited supplies, the head of the *Atelier* suggested the two men work on a painting together. As I watched the two of them communicate and try to collaborate I was struck by the subtle kind of magic that the head of the *Atelier* had worked by this suggestion. Here, and at so many other moments in the *Atelier*, art was not treated as a tool of individual self-expression or a key to a hidden unconscious mind, but rather as a medium that could inspire (but not force) exchange, intersubjectivity, connection, and camaraderie.

Along with the welcoming ambiance of the studio, the other important facet of the workshop's enduring success relates to the way the head of the *Atelier* has quietly and skillfully brought national and international visibility to the group, and used this visibility to tap into transnational flows of funding. Since taking up his post at Fann, he has championed art therapy in Dakar and has tirelessly sought funding and support. Since the early 2000s, he has organized art exhibitions of patients' work during the Dak'Art Biennial of Contemporary African Art. These shows, which have been organized with the assistance of l'Atelier Graphoui (Brussels) and Wallonie-Bruxelles International, among other organizations, have been part of the Dak'Art exhibitions, which are shows displayed outside of the main venues and around Dakar. In 2008, the head of the *Atelier* himself created an organization, Rescap'art, which is geared toward finding appropriate local and international partnerships to materially support artists who have been or are patients at the Fann clinic and to help finance the exhibition of their art. In 2016, in collaboration with Camera Austria, 33 paintings created by 11 Fann artists were displayed in a show called "Friedl Kubelka: Atelier d'Expression (Dakar)," all of which were sold. These exhibits have been wildly successful, and have brought great acclaim to the *Atelier* as well as to the larger Fann Psychiatric Clinic.

And so it was that by 2017, a key feature of the *Atelier* was the frequent presence of local and international students, researchers, and potential funders. The *Atelier* has been able to flourish in the neoliberal present precisely because it has been able to tap into transnational networks and insert itself into global flows of capital, interest, and valuation as an important and meaningful node.

Over the past two decades and during the Wade years in particular, uneven investments (both foreign-sourced and domestic, intergovernmental and NGOs) across Dakar have created new opportunities for those who have been lucky enough to channel or to be part of these resource flows. For many others, however, the uneven distribution of these investments has led to new forms of exclusion, erasure, and dispossession. In tandem with these new opportunities and exclusions have come new forms of distinction that, above all, highlight and display global membership and the ability to draw upon resources from abroad. This chapter has considered how such changes have impacted and become perceptible at Fann, in the afterlives of practices and arrangements that were first put into place during Collomb's era. Each of the four examples featured here—infrastructural changes and new forms of distinction at Fann, the normalization of the *accompagnant mercenaire*, the changing form and function of the *pénc*, and the reanimation of art therapy within the clinic—is born out of and describes both the material effects of Senegal's neoliberal turn and the new forms of subjectivity it promotes.

Although their storylines tell a somewhat familiar story of neoliberalism, it is also important to draw attention to places or moments in these stories that might disrupt or push beyond sealed periodization and predictable narratives to suggest new openings and possibilities—presents and futures that are not foreclosed. Perhaps the most obvious of these is the sociality that is cultivated in the *Atelier d'Ex-pressions*, and the way the studio is experienced by Modou and others as a space in which one "can breathe." Within the *accompagnant mercenaire* arrangement, too, which I described above as a form of commodified care, AMs are at times involved with the intimate, quotidian processes of illness and recovery; they do *take care* in a very powerful way (Mol et al. 2010). AMs draw upon and establish new sets of moral codes, obligations, debts, and expectations in their day-to-day interactions at the clinic—with patients, family members, and staff alike—to create new webs of social relations that are often maintained long after the patients are released.[9] These and other moments of sociality and care in the present-day Fann clinic may hold within themselves the possibility for new lines of flight—other futures—that may themselves bear traces of the earlier forms of sociality and care for which Fann has come to be remembered, by Demba and others.

Conclusion

THERE WERE DAYS WHEN I WOULD ARRIVE at Fann in the early morning and find Demba waiting for me, ready to talk regardless of what else I told him I needed to do that day. There were also periods in which many weeks would go by without my seeing him at all. When Demba was around, I spent a lot of time sitting in the courtyard with him and listening to him talk. Like any self-proclaimed artist, he certainly had a lot to say. Our time together oscillated between enjoyable, annoying, and difficult, for both of us I think. There were moments when we laughed and joked with one another. He was intensely interested in my life back in New York, my family, my romantic interests; I shared my own story as he shared his. Twice he pushed me to tears with words that were intentionally hurtful; several times I scribbled in my field journal that I was done talking with him. Demba's frequent use of sexual innuendo was sometimes more than I could take. And then there were the times when, as we sat together, I just could not make sense of what he was talking about—sometimes I couldn't understand his words and sometimes I couldn't understand his ideas. Stories about events in his life changed drastically from one telling to the next, which frustrated me to no end. Several times he accused me of being able to transmogrify: he was certain I turned myself into a cat each night so I could try to enter his room and spy on him.

Our relationship was rocky at best, our understanding of each other partial at most. Still, my own learning about the past and present Fann Psychiatric Clinic has been—and continues to be—entangled with and punctuated by the conversations we had together, just as Demba's own life has been entangled with the history of the Fann clinic. As something of a revenant, Demba thus comes and goes in the pages of this book in much the same way that he came and went during my time at Fann, the same way that he had been haunting the clinic for so many years.

To tell and untell, to unmake while also making. I have endeavored here to write a history of the Fann clinic—one that might also stand as a history of postcolonial psychiatry in Senegal and its relation to the Senegalese state—while at the same time seeking to trouble the very narrative that I write and the making of history more generally. This book, then, has attempted to grapple with ghosts and simultaneously allowed itself to be haunted. Because Fann's past and present are unsettled, dynamic, and in some ways, uncontainable, I have worked in these chapters to expose the seams of my own and others' stories. I have likewise sought to leave openings and create spaces for things to be imagined otherwise. Frantz Fanon's letter to Léopold Senghor requesting employment is a powerful example of this. I have detailed contested pasts and stories that do not match up—such as the claims made by retired nurses about *ndëpp* (possession) rites being performed in the courtyards of Fann—and lingered on bits that usually get left out, as with the use of psychopharmaceuticals and electroshock treatment during the early years of Fann. While the book's chapters appear in more or less chronological order, starting first with colonial psychiatry in Senegal and the establishment of Fann before building toward the present, I have also tried to disrupt its chronologics by remaining attentive to pasts that might have been, and once-imagined futures that never came into being. Perhaps, then, this book both *is* and *is not* a history of the Fann clinic.

Described in these pages are many inheritances that might be called *impossible*, most of which bring into sharp relief the enduring legacy of colonialism and the ways it has remained entangled with the postcolonial and neoliberal eras. While the title of this book refers primarily to Collomb's culturalist project as an *impossible inheritance* in the hands of the generation of Senegalese psychiatrists who took over at Fann after Collomb's departure, it is also meant to invite reflection upon all of the other transfers and transitions that have been preempted, aborted, rejected, or foreclosed before they happen, or that remain unassimilable, partial, violent, or incomplete to the present, both at Fann and beyond. Inheritance may affirm kinship and connection—to inherit is, to a certain extent, to acknowledge one's place in a lineage and to recognize a debt to past generations. But inheritance, like memory, can also be troubled and troubling, messy and contested, intimate and devastating. For instance, take Demba's claim that he was "like a son" to Collomb (which means also that Demba was, in a sense, abandoned by

Collomb when he left). Or consider the untimely death of Moussa Diop, Collomb's protégé, who many say was being groomed to take Collomb's place as director of the clinic. The brutal and dehumanizing colonial psychiatric practices that existed in Senegal before Fann stood as yet another kind of impossible inheritance for the clinic, born as it was in an era of welfare colonialism, on the eve of independence. Likewise, Senghor's Negritude-inspired political philosophy was an impossible inheritance to the period of heavy structural adjustment that followed it, and to the neoliberal policies and *grands travaux* undertaken by Wade.

When memory work draws lines of affinity, inheritance, or distinction between past and present, there is always (and perhaps, necessarily) much that gets cast to the side. The work of these chapters, then, has been to show how pasts, real and imagined, may linger, even and especially when they have been forgotten, disavowed, or disinherited. In seeking out the material and affective afterlives of Fann's early years and of the history of psychiatry in Senegal more generally, I have attended to how these pasts may make claims on, push their way into, or indeed haunt the present. Perhaps it is precisely this haunting—of colonial occupation and dispossession, of violence disguised as care, of aborted hopes and optimism turned sour, of futures foreclosed—that is Fann's inheritance.

I come back around to a provocation I made in the introduction, one that is crucially important and yet infinitely complex. *Why remember, anyway?* A simple answer, perhaps, is that the past stays with us and continues to affect us in complicated ways, whether we remember or not. Remembrance is a necessary component of larger political projects that pave the way for justice, liberation, and an end to oppression; it is a first step toward reconciliation, reparation, and healing. And the remembrance of even deeper pasts—times before violence, war, or colonial subjugation, for example—may lay the groundwork for new futures. From this perspective, we have an ethical obligation to the past, and our ability to live in the present and future depends precisely on this reckoning. To challenge the imperative to remember that is at the heart of these political projects—to even pose the question *why remember?*—seems especially pernicious in these reactionary times. But who is to choose which pasts must be remembered and by whom, which ghosts must be addressed, and how this remembrance must take shape? What if some forms of remembrance actually have the capacity to inflict or prolong violence, stall liberation, or foreclose future possibility? Memory's "truth-claim," as Ricoeur has argued, may be of ultimate ethical importance, but it might nevertheless be necessary to remember selectively and creatively, and to even forget sometimes.

I shall end, then, with Demba, and with two quotes by André Malraux that tangle me up each time I think about him. The first, from *Les voix du silence* [*Voices of Silence*] (1951: 122): *"L'art est un anti-destin"* (Art is a revolt against fate). The second is one that I stumbled upon when I finally got around to reading *L'Espoir*, many years after Demba had first mentioned it to me: *"[L]a tragédie de la mort est en ceci qu'elle transforme la vie en destin, qu'à partir d'elle rien ne peut plus être compensé"* (1937: 225) ([T]he terrible thing about Death is that it transforms Life into Destiny. After death, nothing can be compensated for [translation mine]).

It was upon my return to Fann in March 2013 that I learned that Demba had passed away. During my flight to Dakar, I had rehearsed what I was going to say to him when I saw him again; I had imagined how our conversation would go. He would be angry with me, I was sure of it, for staying away for so long, for not finding him an agent, for wasting his time. He would be deeply disappointed in me and tell me I had let him down. As I sat on the plane thinking about Demba, I thought also of the small, leather-bound journal and set of colored pens I had brought to give him. These seemed painfully, even insultingly, small next to the unfulfilled expectations he had for me, for our relationship. Although I knew he would love these gifts, I knew also that there was a chance he might not accept them, and I felt deeply ashamed. After my too-long absence from Fann, Demba was the person I was most nervous to see.

The circumstances of Demba's death, as they were recounted to me, were profoundly disturbing, and I will not go into the details here. But in a very real sense, Demba's absence now haunts Fann as much as (perhaps more than) his presence as a living revenant ever did. No longer does Demba leave and come back, or yell insults at the doctors, or brag about how he was like Collomb's own son; gone is this troubled and troubling man who refused to allow Fann to relinquish a very specific iteration of its own past. And for my part, although I remain just as conflicted about Demba and the difficulties of our relationship as I ever was, I am nevertheless filled with a great sadness when I think of him. I deeply regret that I was never quite able to be the person he wanted me to be; I was never quite able to get things right or make things right for him. His absence will undoubtedly continue to haunt me, as it does Fann, for many years to come.

When I read the two Malraux quotes in relation to Demba and his art, his life, and his death, then, they propel me in two directions at once. On the one hand, *art revolts against fate, but death transforms life into destiny*—here I run up against futility, finality, unavoidable endings, disappointments, and regrets. The other reading, however, suggests a glimmer of something else: *death transforms life into destiny, but art revolts against fate.* I take this not as a grand gesture toward transcendence or redemption, but rather as a small nod toward the way in which art, much like memory work, may trouble, suspend, and remake both life and death as it opens new avenues for what is to come.

NOTES

INTRODUCTION

1. The three major ethnic groups of Senegal are Wolof (43% of the population), Pulaar (24%), and Serer (15%). People of Lebu ethnicity number about 50,000 and live primarily along the coast near Dakar. The widespread privileging of the Wolof language in postcolonial Senegal has created a Wolof hegemony that has not gone uncontested; it is sometimes referred to as the "Wolofization" of Senegal (Cruise O'Brien 1979, 1998).

2. This despite the fact that upwards of 92 percent of Senegal's population identify as Muslim. While Senegal is a secular state, Islam dominates public life. Islam in Senegal is dominated by four main Sufi brotherhoods: Tijaniyyah, Muridiyyah (Mourides), Qadiriyyah, and Layene.

3. "[A]ll ethnography is history," writes Christopher Griffin (2008: 20).

4. CEMETRA, an experimental center for the research of traditional medicine and healing practices, was created in 1989 under the auspices of the Dakar-based PROMETRA, an international organization dedicated to the promotion of indigenous knowledge throughout Africa.

5. The 2000 election of Abdoulaye Wade was the first time that Senegal had experienced *l'alternance*, the transfer of power from one political party to another (in this case, from the PS [*Parti Socialiste*]—the political party of Léopold Senghor and Abdou Diouf—to the PDS [*Parti Démocratique Sénégalais*]).

6. As Kleinman et al. (1978: 254) suggest, it is "[t]hrough diagnostic activities and labeling [that] health care providers negotiate with patients medical 'realities' that become the object of medical attention and therapeutics."

7. Emiko Ohnuki-Tierney (1990: 4n5) prefers the term "historicity" over "historical consciousness" because it allows her to "avoid the inference that how people think of and experience history is always conscious." Michel-Rolph Trouillot (1995: 2) describes historicity as "the facts of the matter and a narrative of those facts, both 'what happened' and 'that which is said to have happened.'" Put differently, he says,

historicity relates to how "[t]he ways in which what happened and that which is said to have happened are and are not the same may itself be historical" (4).

8. Maurice Halbwachs ([1925] 1992: 38) expounded upon the "ultimate opposition between collective memory and history." Pierre Nora (1989: 14) went much farther to describe history as both the death and destroyer of memory; he repeatedly refers to what he calls the "terrorism of historicized memory." In his view, history threatens to colonize memory; it forecloses the very possibility of memory taking place.

9. Historian Jacques Le Goff (1992: xi), for example, describes memory as "the raw material of history." See also Crane 1997; Klein 2000.

10. Komaromy (2011: 64) asserts: "Memory is aporetic not simply because the general problem of representation pertains to it, but because it simultaneously claims the identity and the difference of the original object of memory and the mnemonic copy."

11. In Spinoza's view, memory relates to the image-making of that which is not present: "The affections of the human body present whose ideas present [*repraesentant*] external bodies as present [*praesentia*] to us, we shall call images of things, though they do not reproduce [*referunt*] the figures of things. And when the mind regards [*contemplatur*] bodies in this way, we shall say that it imagines" (Ethics, Part 2, S17; Curley translation). Later, Spinoza extends this idea even further as he attributes imaginative capacity to nonhumans, and even to things.

12. Already in 1992, anthropologist Nancy Munn (1992: 115–16) raised questions about the expansion of memory studies and the "close attention that was being given to 'the past in the present'" in anthropology, to the exclusion of other temporal considerations. In a similar vein, Jane Guyer (2007: 418) likewise remarks upon "how the anthropology of time settles so quickly into the 'past in the present' and memory."

13. Anthropology's preoccupation with memory is itself a topic worthy of interrogation. As a concept closer to experience, perhaps, than history, memory makes reference to the past as *experience lived* by social actors and agents—it is no wonder that so many ethnographic encounters have been attuned to this line of inquiry. Furthermore, the act of writing post-fieldwork is itself a re-membering—we ourselves are engaged in these powerful acts of remembering.

14. See, for example, Klein 2000; Radstone 2000; Winter and Sivan 1999.

15. Historian James Young (1993: xi), for example, sent out an early warning regarding the dangers of "apply[ing] individual psychoneurotic jargon to the memory of . . . groups."

16. In Freud, the past leaves its mark one way or another; what is forgotten is never truly forgotten. In "Remembering, Repeating, and Working-Through," Freud explains that when instinctual impulses and painful past experiences are repressed they become inaccessible to intellectual memory or recollection. In lieu of remembering, the patient acts out that which is seated at the source of his neuroses. "He reproduces it not as a memory but an action; he repeats it, without, of course, knowing that he is repeating it" ([1914] 1958: 150).

17. George Santayana (1905: 284) famously wrote, for example, that "[t]hose who cannot remember the past are condemned to repeat it." I can't help but also think of Mrs. Berman's response to Slazinger in Kurt Vonnegut's *Bluebeard*, after Slazinger comments upon her disinterest in history. "I've got news for Mr. Santayana," Mrs. Berman says. "We're doomed to repeat the past no matter what. That's what it is to be alive. It's pretty dense kids who haven't figured that out by the time they're ten."

18. In order to create, for example, what Ricoeur (2006: 68) has called a "just memory" [*une mémoire juste*], or "an idea that will take shape . . . through our reflection on the abuses of a memory manipulated by ideology."

19. Also from Nietzsche's *Untimely Meditations*: "We wish to use history only insofar as it serves living. But there is a degree of doing history and a valuing of it through which life atrophies and degenerates" ([1874] 2006: 1).

20. The concept of "entanglement" has gotten much play recently. As a way of thinking not just about time or temporality, but also about the intertwined relationships between particles, people, things, and animals, these various deployments of "entanglement" attempt to move beyond tropes of difference to think instead about cohabitation, togetherness, and co-constitution. Sarah Nuttall (2009), for example, elaborates upon Mbembe's "time of entanglement" to apprehend social transformations and future possibilities in post-apartheid South Africa. She describes entanglement as a "condition of being twisted together or entwined, involved with; it speaks of an intimacy gained, even if it was resisted, or ignored or uninvited" (1). To focus on entanglement, she writes, is to think about how things that were "once thought of as separate—identities, spaces, histories—come together or find points of intersection in unexpected ways" and to explore their "terrains of mutuality" (11). It is also to make space to accommodate a "complex temporality . . . in which the time of potential . . . exists in complex tandem with new kinds of closure and opposition" (11). To be entangled, however, is also *to be caught*. Archeologist Ian Hodder has described the entanglement of humans and things in terms of relations of dependence (2011, 2012) and even entrapment (2014). Noting what he refers to as the "darker side" of entanglements between humans and things, Hodder (2014: 19) suggests that entanglements "are often asymmetrical, leading to entrapments in particular pathways from which it is difficult to escape." Likewise, literary theorist Rey Chow (2012) challenges us to look more critically at the tangle itself. While much of the recent literature on entanglement has stressed the conjoining of that which is entangled, Chow goes against the grain to question whether "entanglement could not also be a figure for meetings that are not necessarily defined by . . . affinity" (1–2).

21. Biehl ([2005] 2013) tells the story of Catarina, a woman left for mad in the Brazilian asylum that he refers to as Vita. Caterina was a prolific writer; unlike Demba, however, she did not call herself an artist or refer to her writing as poetry or art, but said she was composing her own dictionary to make sense of her life, "'writing to not forget the words'" (5). Biehl approaches Catarina's dictionary as not only an expression of her subjectivity but as the key to her survival. He seeks to understand the truth of Caterina's condition, which turns out to be genetic rather than psychiatric, and he reads her writing as a critical commentary on the forces that

led her to this "zone of social abandonment" in the first place. Similarly, Demba's stories and drawings offer him a means of expression and survival, primarily because they allow him to assert himself as an artist and reaffirm the identity that connects him back to Collomb. Demba's art—not just its creation but also its circulation and display—allows him to become *himself.*

RUPTURE: CHASING A GHOST

1. The Wolof *rab*—which translates as "animal" in English—is usually thought to be wild or untamed, compared to the domesticated *tuur. Djinné*, or jinn, are invisible beings or spirits of the Islamic tradition. I discuss this in more detail in chapter 2.

CHAPTER 1

1. *L'Afrique Occidentale Française* (AOF), or French West Africa, refers to the federation of French colonial territories, consolidated in 1895. The first territories to be included were Senegal, French Sudan (Mali), French Guinea (Guinea), and Côte d'Ivoire. These were joined later by Dahomey (Benin), Mauritania, Upper Volta (Burkina Faso), and Niger.

2. The first African to serve as a deputy in the French National Assembly was Blaise Diagne, who took up the post in 1914. Previous deputies had either been of European or *métis* (mixed African and European) ancestry. This sole deputy who represented the Communes in the French National Assembly was the only representative of any African community in a European parliament until 1940.

3. *L'indigénat* was finally abolished in the French Constitutional Assembly laws of December 22, 1945, and February 20, 1946 (Crowder 1976).

4. The French Lunacy Law of 1838, or the *Loi sur les aliénés, 30 juin 1838* (IX Bull. DLXXXI, number 7443), can be accessed in its entirety in a recently digitized version of the *Collection Complete des Lois, Decrets, Ordonnances, Reglements,* by Jean Baptiste Duvergier, which was originally published by Oxford University in 1841: https://play.google.com/books/reader?id = OVUUAAAAYAAJ&printsec = frontcover&output = reader&authuser = 0&hl = en&pg = GBS.PP1 (accessed August 10, 2014).

5. A 1947 copy of the *Bilan Hebdomadaire* in the Senegalese National Archives (ANS) takes a critical look at the strengths and drawbacks of the 1838 law.

6. The Royal Order of 1840, or *l'Ordonnance organique du 7 septembre 1840* (IX Bull. DCCLXX, number 8984) can be accessed in its entirety in Duvergier, *Collection Complete des Lois, Decrets, Ordonnances, Reglements.*

7. ANS, 1 H 74, Rapport sur les aliénés du Senegal par le Dr. Morin (18 Décembre 1910).

8. Roger Cheneveau was a military doctor who held the high rank of *Médecin-commandant des troupes colonials*. It is worth noting that Cheneveau was an early proponent of referring to mentally disturbed persons as *les malades* (patients; the sick) rather than *les aliénés* (lunatics; lit. the alienated).

9. ANS, Série Police et Prisons [*en voie de classement*]; cited also in Reboul and Régis 1912: 82.

10. Within the Cape Colony, the Robben Island Lunatic Asylum opened in 1846 (Deacon 1996), the Grahamstown Mental Hospital opened in 1875 (Burrows 1958), and the Valkenberg Lunatic Asylum opened in 1891 (Swartz 1995a, 1995b; Marks 1999).

11. The British would likewise erect many more asylums throughout Africa by 1910, including the Yaba Lunatic Asylum in Nigeria in 1906 (Sadowsky 1999), the Itgusheni in Southern Rhodesia in 1908 (Jackson 2005), the Mathari Mental Hospital in Kenya in 1910 (McColloch 1995), and the Zomba Lunatic Asylum in Nyasaland in 1910 (Vaughan 1983).

12. It is important here to remember that French Algeria was not administered as a colony or part of the protectorate, but rather as part of France itself. The territory was divided into three veritable French *départements* in the north (Oran, Alger, Constantine) and four territories (Oasis, Touggourt, Aïn-Sefra, Ghardaïa) in the south. *L'Asile de Saint-Pierre* was rather ambitious when it came to procuring—or at the very least, accepting—overseas patient transfers; the asylum also went on to sign a treaty with Tunisia (a protectorate) in 1899 and Guinea in 1905. The treaty with Tunisia reserved ten beds (for an annual fee of 8,000FF) for psychiatric patients who were to be transferred to Marseille (Planchon 2013: 141). Treaties were also made with New Caledonia in 1879 and with French Indochina in 1902, although these were aimed specifically at the repatriation of French patients working in those colonies (Collignon 2002; Edington 2013).

13. The full treaty was reproduced in Borreil (1908); it is from this document that I have drawn the details that follow.

14. ANS, Série Police et Prisons: "L'Assistance des aliénés au SN et en AOF" (1927).

15. ANS 1 H 74 (163), Letter from Dr. Berne to the Services de Psychiatrie en AOF.

16. ANS 1 H 74 (163) 1067, Letter from the Services de Psychiatrie en AOF to Dr. Berne.

17. The Université Cheikh Anta Diop (UCAD), formerly the University of Dakar, was part of the French university system until it established its autonomy in 1969. It evolved out of *l'Ecole des Hautes Etudes*, which had been built in Dakar in 1918.

INTERLUDE: MANY BATTLES

1. I did read *l'Espoir*, but only many years later. Written between 1936–39, the novel chronicles the Spanish Civil War, and in particular, the cooperation of the socialist, communist, and anarchist contingents that fought Francisco Franco's

fascist regime. Malraux, a member of the French Communist Party, was himself present in Spain during this time, fighting for the Republican side. *L'Espoir* is a modernist tale of resistance, hope, and unlikely camaraderie, but perhaps most interesting to me were its brilliant flashes of description that captured the evening light and the stillness, the flocks of pigeons in flight, the blood on the cobblestones. While I did not find a passage referring to a "battle of Titans," I did come across another that I cannot resist including here: *"Le fou copie l'artiste, et l'artiste ressemble au fou"* ("The madman copies the artist, and the artist resembles the madman") (Malraux 1937: 60).

CHAPTER 2

1. *Psychopathologie africaine* was an influential journal launched by Henri Collomb in 1965.

2. From 1951 until 1953, Collomb served as a medical officer for colonial troops in Indochina, based at the Grall Hospital in Saigon (Arnaut 2006). According to an interview with Collomb published by Boussat and Boussat (2002), Collomb later recalled his stint in Saigon as a "horrible memory. In Indochina it was war, and an incredibly incoherent war. There were cultures, civilizations, certainly well superior to ours and I could not understand why we were fighting . . . I asked myself why we were there, what were we doing there, who imposed this war on us?" (419; also cited in Bullard 2005a).

3. *Professeur agrégé* is a title conferring the highest academic rank in the French university system. In order to receive this nomination, one must pass the highly competitive *agrégation* examination. Since Fann serves as a teaching clinic for the University of Dakar, the director is required to hold this title.

4. Not only did Collomb want the clinic to become more "village-like," he also championed the establishment of "psychiatric villages" throughout Senegal. Two of these (Kénia in Casamance and Botu in Tambacounda) were started during the 1970s (Collomb 1978; Collignon 2000; Guèye 1984). Collomb was not the first to promote psychiatric villages in sub-Saharan Africa; Lambo in Nigeria had founded the Aro Village and Hospital near Abeokuta (cf. Ben-Tovim 1987; Boroffka 1975; Lambo 1966, 1974; Margetts 1962; Swift and Asuni 1975). The Kénia village still exists but maintains no ties to Fann.

5. Senghor claimed, for example, that the writer who contributed the most to his elaboration of Negritude was the German ethnologist Leo Frobenius (1873–1938). He once insisted that "no one better than Frobenius revealed Africa to the world and *Africans to themselves*" (Senghor's preface to a Frobenius anthology entitled *Leo Frobenius 1873 / 1973*, ed. Eike Haberland, cited in Miller 1990: 16).

6. Zempléni was born in Hungary and trained in ethnology, psychology, and linguistics at the Sorbonne in Paris, receiving his PhD under Roger Bastide in 1968.

7. The salvage paradigm is animated by what Baker (1996: 82) has described as the "logic of loss and control" that typifies the archival impulse. The paradox, of course,

is that the agents doing the "salvaging" and preserving for posterity's sake are almost always part of the very same apparatus that has made them vulnerable in the first place.

8. Devereux, in his *Mohave Ethnopsychiatry* (1969: 1; original published in French in 1961), described the book as "a kind of 'Mohave textbook' of psychiatry, dictated by Mohave 'psychiatrists' to the anthropologist fieldworker" (also cited in Gaines 1992).

9. In Senegal, *marabout* can refer to a Muslim spiritual leader, a teacher of the Qur'an, or a *cheikh*. It can also mean "diviner" or "healer," or refer to a person who has magical knowledge or means at their disposal to bring harm to—or protect— others. While some *marabouts* work exclusively with the Qur'an (writing verses of the Qur'an, reciting verses and prayers) many use the Qur'an in combination with other objects (some, for example, make talismans containing Qur'anic verses or prepare special water in which their followers are told to bathe), and others do not use the Qur'an at all. Many of my devoutly Muslim friends in Dakar cringe at the use of the word *marabout* in the latter case. *Liggeey* can also be put on someone by a *borom xam-xam* (a Wolof phrase meaning "proprietor of knowledge"), a *jabarkat*, or a *fajkat* (Wolof words meaning "healer"); both *jabarkat* and *fajkat* indicate a healer working outside of Islam, and the latter usually implies a person who works with advanced knowledge of medicinal plants.

10. According to András Zempléni (1966: 302), "The distinction between *tuur* and *rab* is rather fluid. *Tuur* are *rab*, and a ritual held regularly for a *rab* will elevate it to the rank of a *tuur*. The difference is in the degree of notoriety and the amount of time the alliance has endured."

11. Elements of *rab* and *tuur* possession resemble forms of possession that have been well documented in anthropology, such as the *zar* in Ethiopia and Sudan (Leiris [1958] 1980; I. M. Lewis [1971] 2003; Boddy 1989; Kenyon 1995), *voudoun* in Haiti (Hurston 1990; Métraux 1989; Deren 1970), and *condomblé* in Brazil (Bastide 2001; Wafer 1991).

12. In a 1979 review of hospitalization data collected from psychiatric clinics and hospitals across Africa from the 1950s–1970s, Corin and Murphy (1979: 148) likewise note: "the percentage of admissions carrying this diagnosis [schizophrenia] varies from 70 percent in Nigeria (Boroffka 1973) and 57 percent in South Africa (Moffson 1955) to 15 percent for Senegal (Collomb 1965) and 11 percent for Zaire (Vyncke 1957). These percentage differences would be of great interest if they were reliable, but most of the variation probably results from the difficultly in fitting the acute reactive psychoses into the British and international diagnostic classifications. Some psychiatrists include these psychoses among the schizophrenias for want of a better place, and others resist this practice."

13. In the third edition of *Oedipe africain* (1984), the Ortigues distanced them-selves from this Lacanian-inspired inquiry, removing a substantial chapter (Chapter 2) that had been devoted to this analysis. For a more in-depth discussion of these changes, see Bullard 2005b.

14. In the introduction to *Psychiatry Inside Out: Selected Writings of Franco Basaglia*, Scheper-Hughes (1987: 48) writes that Basaglia's reconstruction of

psychiatry and the psychiatric institution "heed[ed] Foucault's call to 'give madness back its voice.' In Basaglia's terms, this mean[t] an empowerment through words, an understanding that even delusional or delirious speech may be a febrile voice of protest, the only possible resistance available to those who are usually silenced, disgraced, or excluded."

15. See Cooper 1967; Laing 1960; Basaglia [Scheper-Hughes and Lovell, eds.] 1987; Szasz 1974.

16. Lise Tripet had also studied ethnology at the University of Neuchâtel prior to her work at Fann. From 1971–79, Tripet returned to Dakar to continue her work as a psychoanalyst. During that period, she worked at Fann while also maintaining her own private practice.

17. Abdou Anta Ka is considered by some to be one of the more original and underappreciated writers of the early post-independence era. Ka was a patient at Fann, treated for alcohol abuse. He later wrote a play based on his experiences at the clinic entitled "Pinthioum-Fann: Farce, comédie, drame ou tragédie?" which won the Arts d'Afrique award in 1969. The play was published in a 1972 collection called *Théâtre: Quatre pièce d'Abdou Anta Ka.*

18. Césaire's "Cahier d'un retour au pays natal," or "Notebook of a Return to the Native Land," was originally published in 1939 in the Parisian journal *Volontés*, no. 20, p. 42.

19. Senghor served in a regiment of French colonial infantry and fought with the French army during World War II. In 1942, Senghor was captured by German forces and imprisoned for eighteen months. After the war, Senghor was appointed to the faculty of *l'École Nationale de la France d''Outre-Mer* as a professor of African languages, and during the next several years he became a well-known writer. In 1947, his collaboration with Senegalese intellectual Alioune Diop produced the cultural and literary journal *Présence africaine*, which explored issues of African identity and elaborated the notion of Negritude through writing, poetry, and the arts. Among those on the advisory board of *Présence africaine* were André Gide, Albert Camus, and Jean-Paul Sartre (Hymans 1971; Spleth 1985).

20. In 1945 and 1946, Senghor was elected to the French parliament to represent Senegal in the French Constituent Assemblies, and until 1958 he continued to be elected to the French National Assembly. When Senegal joined the Sudanese Republic to form the Federation of Mali in 1958, Senghor was named president of the federal assembly, and when Senegal separated from the Federation of Mali in 1960, Senghor was elected the first president of Senegal (Hymans 1971; Spleth 1985).

21. The brand of secularism written into Senegal's constitution referred "neither [to] atheism . . . nor [to] the desire to banish from the public sphere, through intense propaganda, religions" but was instead aimed at "guarantee[ing] the 'autonomy' of the religious communities" (Diagne 2009: 4–5).

22. "Si l'on parle de l'Ecole de Dakar, c'est grâce à la psychiatrie," *Le Soleil*, Jeudi 17 septembre 1998.

23. These words were part of Senghor's opening speech at an exhibition called *Picasso en Nigrité*, which was held at Dakar's *Musée Dynamique* in 1972.

CHAPTER 3

1. Arriving hand in hand with a resurgence of interest in memory both within and outside academia, nostalgia began to emerge as a topic of serious anthropological inquiry during the mid- to late 1980s. Since then, much has been written about the deeply nostalgic origins of contemporary social theory and anthropology (see Berliner 2012; Shaw and Chase 1989; Frow 1997; Robertson 1990; Rosaldo 1989; Strathern 1995; Turner 1987). Recently, Berliner (2014: 19) has argued that this very same "nostalgic proclivity still permeates anthropologists' postures" in the present day, apparent in what Kulick et al. (2006) and Robbins (2013) have termed "masochistic" or "suffering slot" anthropology, respectively. On other fronts, anthropologists have explored nostalgia's relationship with late capitalism and postmodern subjectivity (cf. Ivy 1995; Jameson 1989; Stewart 1988). Van Rijk (1998: 155) has even suggested, after Robertson (1990) and Strathern (1995), the importance of putting forth a "theory of nostalgia." Alongside all of this, numerous studies have grappled with the nostalgia that anthropologists encountered "in the field." Bissell (2005), for example, has considered the theoretical and political implications of the colonial nostalgia he encountered among Zanzibari youth, while van Rijk (1998), in his study of African Pentecostalism in urban Malawi, has addressed the anti-nostalgia that is at the heart of the growing "Born-Again" movement and looks at its effects on both cultural memory and the state. Kathleen Stewart (1996) has written of the nostalgic stories that circulate in disenfranchised communities of rural West Virginia. Ivy (1995: 65) has considered the production and consumption of nostalgia in contemporary Japan, where the object of nostalgia is "a Japan that is kept on the verge of vanishing, stable yet endangered (and thus open for commodifiable desire)." Battaglia (1995) has written of what she has called "practical nostalgia" among urban Trobrianders, and Werbner (1991) has considered the nostalgic narratives that are recounted by Kalanga elders living in Zimbabwe.

2. These categories closely resemble Marilyn Strathern's (1995) "substantive" versus "synthetic" nostalgia.

3. Walter Benjamin expressed a wholly different opinion about both the power of the past in the present and the demise of the French Revolution. Whereas Marx viewed the conjuring of the past as that which necessarily *foils* revolutions, Benjamin (1969: 263, Thesis XVII) considered the "blast[ing of] a specific era out of the homogeneous course of history" and into what he referred to as "the time of the now" or *Jetztzeit,* to be of extraordinary revolutionary power. Although he admits that *Jetztzeit* is always at risk of being used as an instrument of domination by the ruling class, he claims that the downfall of the revolution and the establishment of French bourgeois society were not the result of the conjuring of the past, but of that which came after the dialectic moment had passed. See also Benjamin 1969: 261, Thesis XIV.

4. The establishment of the Senegalese bourgeoisie has a long history, with its origins dating back to the founding of the Four Communes (Clark and Phillips 1994; Diouf 1998; Harney 2004).

1. *S'exhilent* is the third-person-plural conjugation for the transitive verb *s'exhiler*. *S'exhiler,* however, is not a word. I and others who have read the poem have tended to assume it to be a case of mistaken orthography, and we have translated it as the verb *s'exiler* (to exile oneself). However, Demba also could have meant to write *s'exhaler,* to rise, to rise up, or to escape.

CHAPTER 4

1. Moussa Diop began his medical studies in Dakar. He completed his specialization in psychiatry in Bordeaux in 1958 and then returned to Dakar, where he worked at the Fann clinic until his death.

2. Witches are thought to prey on people while they sleep and feed on their vital energy *(fit)*, which is located in the liver. That Moussa Diop had cancer of the liver seemed to confirm that witchcraft was indeed at work.

3. Around Dakar in the late 1990s, I often heard people joke that Senghor must have occult forces at his disposal. How else could he have risen so high and still be alive? (Senghor died in 2001, at the age of 95.) Friends of mine speculated in jest about Senghor being a Freemason, about him sacrificing his own children for political advancement, about his secret relations with a local *marabout,* and so on. Ashforth (2005: 14) too notes that "[t]alk of witches and their craft in Soweto is mostly conducted with the warm convivial malice of good gossip accompanied by plentiful laughter and jokes." He adds: "People rarely feel free to talk of such things when they do not feel free to laugh. Good stories are rewarded with guffaws. The fact of laughter, however, does not detract from the importance of the information."

4. The second, Baaba Ly, worked at the Salpiètre in Paris during the 1960s before returning to Senegal to work at the psychiatric hospital in Thiaroye. Daouda Sow was the most junior of the group. Sow did clinical work at Fann, but left psychiatry to pursue a career in politics.

5. Babakar Diop was not related to Moussa Diop.

6. The original French text: "Rencontrer l'autre (malade) est également lourd de conséquences pour le psychiatre africain formé à l'école française. Il commet une transgression en pénétrant dans le domaine de la maladie mentale réservé traditionnellement au guérisseur investi de la fonction de guérir" (Diop 1968: 169–70). The paper was published in *Bulletins et Mémoires de la Faculté de Médicine et de Pharmacie de Dakar.*

7. This mimetic movement of "becoming other," which was noted numerous times in discussions about both Collomb and Senghor, deserves further attention, especially in light of Levinas [1961] 1969, [1972] 2006; Deleuze and Guattari 2004; Taussig 1993.

8. Itself a product of Enlightenment ideals, it might be said that conventional psychiatry also has as its main objective the "disenchantment of the world; the

dissolution of myths and the substitution of knowledge for fancy" (Adorno and Horkheimer [1944] 1997: 3).

9. None of Collomb's publications from 1959–62 hinted at a political consciousness on his part, nor did they reflect the social transformations taking place as struggles for decolonization erupted across Africa at that time. Instead, as noted in chapter 2, many of his papers focused on the organic causes of mental illness. According to Sarr, Seck, and Ba (1997: 218), it is not incidental that this "organic phase" occurred when it did; i.e., during a time of major political transition in Senegal. "For the psychiatrist from the colonizing country . . . it was easier . . . to make reference to the organic causes of mental illness" than to have taken a more critical approach that would have directly implicated colonial regimes of power and their relationship to mental health.

10. Philippe told me that Collomb remained interested in what was happening in neurology even after it had split off from psychiatry, and spent each Wednesday visiting patients and talking with the doctors in the service. He also continued to participate in weekly brain dissections (*les coupures de cerveau*), and assisted in the training of new staff each Thursday morning.

11. In 1982, Lambo "urged psychiatrists practicing in the developing world to 'decontaminate intellectually from Freudian and neo-Freudian theories'" (Heaton 2013: 73, quoting Lambo 1982).

CHAPTER 5

1. The SICAPs (*Société Immobilière de Cap Vert*) are popular residential neighborhoods in Dakar. The first SICAP neighborhoods, built in the 1950s by the colonial government, were meant to house an emerging middle class. Houses in these neighborhoods are separated into compounds and divided by high cement walls, and the door of each opens onto a small street or laneway.

2. Compelling anthropological accounts of the effects of structural adjustment and neoliberalism on everyday life in Senegal include works by Foley (2008, 2009, 2010), who has drawn connections among the rise of neoliberalism, ecological degradation, newly emerging and precarious migration patterns, increased vulnerability to illness, and new forms of both inequality and structural violence. Likewise, Buggenhagen (2001, 2004) has written on how neoliberal reforms have affected migration, bridewealth, romantic love, and even ideas of personhood, and Melly (2010, 2011) has written of changing migration patterns and infrastructural transformation.

3. For a full account of the troubled modern history of the Université Cheikh Anta Diop, see Max 2009; Tamba 2009. Max (2009: 45) writes that while the "student and faculty activism" surrounding the *année blanche* of 1988–89 "focused on the declining conditions for students and professors, they also began to dovetail with more widespread opposition to the IMF and World Bank and a general recognition of the reemergence of international influence over economic and social policy

in Senegal." While 1988–89 was a canceled year for university students, the *année invalide* of 1993–94 was even more punitive—enrolled students were forced to take zeros on all of their coursework for that year. Students were "evicted . . . from the campus and their dormitories by force" and they "had only a few hours to gather their things and leave" (45). Thousands of students dropped out or were forced from university as a result; Max notes that "[i]n interviews with former students, they estimated as many as 50 percent of their classmates ended their university careers as a result of the invalid year" (50).

4. Goorgoorlou is not just a name but is also a frequently used Wolof word: *goórgoórlu*, as it is written in standardized Wolof orthography, can take the form of a verb or a noun. As a verb, its meaning approximates "to try hard" or "to struggle through" or "to make do" (similar, perhaps, to the French verb se *débrouiller*); it suggests at once difficulty, work, adversity, and making one's way against the odds. With the word *goór* (man) as its root, it also evokes masculinity and the work of "being a man," and there is something about the word that is suggestive of public sphere activities and aspirations. Nevertheless, in its common usage from the 1990s up to the present, the word *goórgoórlu* is used to describe the actions of women and men alike.

5. *Le Cafard Libéré* is a double entendre—the word "cafard" means "cockroach," while the idiomatic expression "avoir le cafard" means "to have the blues" or "to be depressed." *Le Cafard Libéré* thus means both "the liberated cockroach" and "the liberated doldrums / blues." The paper's name (*Le Cafard Libéré*) is also a take-off on a French satirical paper—*Le Canard Enchaîné*, which means both "the chained duck" and "the chained newspaper" (as "canard" is a slang term for "paper").

6. For example, Novartis, the manufacturer of thioridazine (Mellaril), ended up voluntarily discontinuing the drug in 2005 because it was shown to cause cardiac arrhythmia and cardiac arrest.

7. Fann psychiatrists frequently consulted the DSM-IV (Diagnostic and Statistical Manual of Mental Disorders). Less frequently, they also consulted the ICD (International Statistical Classification of Diseases and Related Health Problems) and the French INSERM (*Institut National de la Santé et de la Recherche Médicale*) classification manual.

8. In a context separate from the conference, the chair once told me that he had wanted to start a reading group at the clinic—everyone working at Fann, he said, should read Collomb's work. Regrettably, though, there had been little interest. In other conversations, he seemed to intimate that people (including researchers like me) spent too much time thinking about Collomb and the institution's past. I also remember hearing him mutter while going though papers in Fann's document center that Collomb must have been a government spy.

9. Although participants were in fact taken on a tour of Fann and invited to a delicious lunch at the facility, the conference itself was held at the CESAG (*Centre Africain d'Etudes Superieures en Gestion*, or the African Center for Higher Management Studies) campus a few miles away.

10. Tobie Nathan, "Le thérapeute doit négocier avec l'invisible," interview by Marie-Laure Théodule, *La Recherche*, no. 403 (December 1, 2006), www

.larecherche.fr/tobie-nathan-%C2%AB-le-th%C3%A9rapeute-doit-n%C3%A9gocier-avec-l'invisible-%C2%BB (accessed January 22, 2015).

11. The harshest critiques of Nathan's work came from anthropologists, and I certainly sensed an antagonism toward anthropologists (and anthropology) during our conversation together. Even though I had told him while introducing myself that I was an anthropologist interested in the history of the Fann clinic, Nathan later stopped me abruptly and asked in a half-joking but suspicious tone: "What are you, exactly? What kind of work do you do?" When I reminded him, he nodded and laughed: "*Ah, une anthropophage!*" An *anthropophage* is an anthropophagus, or a devourer of humans.

12. Tobie Nathan, "Freud ressemblait un peu à un guérisseur africain," interview by Dominique Dhombres, *Le Monde*, October 22, 1996.

13. Indeed, critiques related to the field's enduring commitment to relativism (and its overinvestment in ideas of "cultural difference") abounded during the late 1990s and early 2000s. James Ferguson (2006: 19) insisted that anthropologists were too fixated on cultural difference and needed to shift their focus toward political economic analyses that took as their point of departure an interrogation of material inequality, for "the question of cultural difference itself is . . . tightly bound up with questions of inequality." Mahmood Mamdani (2004) criticized "culture talk" from another angle, insisting that it is wrongheaded to view culture as some discrete, timeless essence that in turn generates "politics."

14. Responding to an interview that was provocatively titled "*Freud ressemblait un peu à un guérisseur africain*" ("Freud was a bit like an African healer"), Tunisian psychoanalyst Fethi Benslama criticized Nathan's clinical approach, his showmanship, and his politics (not to mention his take on Freud). "Claiming to wield the tools of psychology, psychoanalysis, shamanism, and ethnology," wrote Benslama, "Mr. Nathan occupies every position of knowledge about the other and his soul. This stance clearly demonstrates the reality of his ethnopsychiatric approach: it is a totalizing practice that hinges upon what Guy Debord has called the nature of the spectacle" (Fethi Benslama, "L'illusion ethnopsychiatrique," *Le Monde*, December 4, 1996).

15. Nathan, "Le thérapeute doit négocier avec l'invisible."

16. The conference's official title was the International Conference on Primary Health Care at Alma-Ata.

CHAPTER 6

1. www.seaplazadakar.com/fr/business-directory/wpbdm-category/divertissement/ (accessed July 17, 2014).

2. Mehdi Ba, "Sénégal: Dakar s'embourgeoise," *Jeune Afrique*, July 25, 2013, http://economie.jeuneafrique.com/regions/afrique-subsaharienne/18554-senegal-dakar-sembourgeoise.html (accessed July 17, 2014).

3. Michael Pauron, "Sea Plaza: Un temple sénégalais à la recherche de ses adeptes," *Jeune Afrique*, March 11, 2011, www.jeuneafrique.com/Article/ARTJAJA2616po70-072.xmlo/ (accessed July 17, 2014).

4. In the intervening years, many of Rico's friends managed to make their way to France, Italy, Spain, or the United States, either legally or *sans papiers*, but Rico had not. Carling (2002) has described the migration experiences of people from Cape Verde and Senegal not only from the perspective of those who leave, but also from the perspective of those who are "involuntarily immobile," unable to leave despite their efforts.

5. The autoroute was a public / private venture. It will be expanded incrementally over the next two decades. An article published on *Africa Nouvelles* listed the total budget for the project as an estimated 380.2 billion fcfa / $785 million, financed by the Senegalese state (193.5 billion fcfa / $400 million), Eiffage Group (61 billion fcfa / $126 million), the World Bank (52.5 billion fcfa / $108 million), the French Development Agency (40 billion fcfa / $82.5 million), and the African Development Bank (33.2 billion fcfa / $66.6 million). Milton Kwami, "SENEGAL: Ouverture de l'autoroute à péage Dakar-Diamniadio," *Africa Nouvelles*, August 1, 2013, www
.africanouvelles.com/varietes/varietes/evenements/senegal-ouverture-de-
lautoroute-a-peage-dakar-diamniadio.html (accessed July 18, 2014).

6. Motorcycles pay 800 fcfa (approx. $1.65), while *cars rapides* and minibuses pay 2,000 fcfa (approx. $4.10), and buses and trucks pay 2,700 fcfa (approx. $5.55).

7. Saliou Diouf, "Sénégal: L'autoroute à péage Dakar-Diamniadio fait débat," *Jeune Afrique*, July 29, 2013, http://economie.jeuneafrique.com/regions/afrique-
subsaharienne/18788-senegal-lautoroute-a-peage-dakar-diamniadio-fait-debat.html (accessed July 18, 2014).

8. James Ferguson (2012: 559) reminds us that social inequalities are "often naturalized, made invisible, or made to seem inevitable, by the walls, pipes, wires, and roads that profoundly shape our urban environments." In the introduction to the same special issue of the journal *Ethnography* in which Ferguson's above-quoted article appears, Rodgers and O'Neill (2012) introduce the term "infrastructural violence" to describe the active and passive ways in which seemingly "neutral" infrastructure may not only render visible, but also create new forms of, exclusion and inequity. Once such projects have been completed, they tend to take their place as "apolitical" and even natural features of the cityscape, around which people must necessarily re-pattern their daily habits and aspirations (as well as reconfigure their dissent).

9. In this way, my observations are in line with recent scholarship that describes the intimacy of relations that are forged and negotiated within the domain of paid domestic care (e.g., Brown 2012; Näre 2011; Glenn 2010; Paerregaard 2010; Stacey 2011) and that insist that such commodified care relations are not necessarily amoral, mechanistic, cold, or void of "true" care.

BIBLIOGRAPHY

NATIONAL ARCHIVES OF SENEGAL (ANS)

Anonymous. 1914. "Rapport Sur L'aliénation Mentale Dans Le Haut-Sénégal-Niger (Rapport Anonyme)." Dossier 1 H 74. National Archives of Senegal (ANS).

———. 1927. "Rapport Sur l'Assistance Des Aliénés Au Sénégal et En A. O. F. (Destiné Au Département)." Dossier 1 H 74. National Archives of Senegal (ANS).

———. 1932. "Plans D'un Asile D'aliénés En A. O. F, T. P. Du Sénégal." Dossier 1 H 74. National Archives of Senegal (ANS).

———. 1947. "Le Problème de l'Assistance Aux Malades Mentaux." Bilans Hebdomadaires, Bulletin du Centre de Documentation sociale, économique et politique. Dossier 1 H 74 (163). National Archives of Senegal (ANS).

Berne, Eric. 1955. "Letter to the Directeur de La Santé Publique de l'A. O. F. (Director of Public Health in French West Africa)," January 29. Dossier 1 H 74 (163). National Archives of Senegal (ANS).

Cazanove, Frank. 1912. "Note Sur l'Assistance Des Aliénés En A. O. F." Dossier 1 H 74. National Archives of Senegal (ANS).

———. 1931. "Rapport Sur Le Projet D'un Asile d'Aliénés." Dossier 1 H 74. National Archives of Senegal (ANS).

Cheneveau, Roger. 1938. "Rapport Sur La Création D'un Service D'assistance Psychiatrique En Afrique Occidentale Française." Gouvernement général de L'A. O. F. (l'Inspection générale des services sanitaires et médicaux). Dossier 1 H 74 (163). National Archives of Senegal (ANS).

Morin, Paul. 1910. "Rapport Sur Les Aliénés Du Sénégal." Dossier 1 H 74. National Archives of Senegal (ANS).

Talec, Désiré-Alain. 1955. "Letter Responding to Dr. Eric Berne," March 5. Dossier 1 H 74 (163). National Archives of Senegal (ANS).

Abraham, Nicolas, and Maria Torok. 1994. *The Shell and the Kernel: Renewals of Psychoanalysis.* Chicago: University of Chicago Press.

Ade Ajayi, Jacob F., and Michael Crowder, eds. 1987. *History of West Africa.* 2nd edition. Vol. II. Harlow, England: Longman.

Adorno, Theodor W., and Max Horkheimer. [1944] 1997. *Dialectic of Enlightenment.* New York: Verso.

Anagnostou, Yiorgos. 2009. *Contours of White Ethnicity: Popular Ethnography and the Making of Usable Pasts in Greek America.* Athens: Ohio University Press.

Andoche, J. 2001. "Culture et santé mentale: Les avatars français de l'ethnopsychiatrie." In *Critique de la santé publique: Une approche anthropologique,* edited by J. P. Dozon and D. Fassin, 281–308. Paris: Balland.

Angé, Olivia, and David Berliner, eds. 2014. *Anthropology and Nostalgia.* New York: Berghahn Books.

Appadurai, Arjun. 1996. *Modernity at Large: Cultural Dimensions of Globalization.* Minneapolis: University of Minnesota Press.

Archer-Shaw, Petrine. 2000. *Negrophilia: Avant Garde Paris and Black Culture in the 1920s.* New York: Thames and Hudson.

Arnaut, Robert. 2006. *La folie apprivoisée: L'Approche unique du professeur Collomb pour traiter la folie.* Paris: De Vecchi.

Arnold, A. James. 1999. *Modernism and Negritude: The Poetry and Poetics of Aimé Césaire.* Lincoln, NE: iUniverse.

Ashforth, Adam. 2005. *Witchcraft, Violence, and Democracy in South Africa.* Chicago: University of Chicago Press.

Attoun, Lucien. 1970. "Aimé Césaire et Le Théâtre Nègre." *Le Théâtre* 1: 111–12.

Aubin, Henri. 1938. "Assistance Psychiatrique Indigène Aux Colonies." In *Rapport Au XLI Le Congrès Des Médecins Aliénistes et Neurologistes de Langue Française,* 147–76. Algiers.

Austen, Ralph A. 2006. "Interpreters Self-Interpreted: The Autobiographies of Two Colonial Clerks." In *Intermediaries, Interpreters, and Clerks: African Employees in the Making of Colonial Africa,* edited by Benjamin N. Lawrance, Emily Lynn Osborn, and Richard L. Roberts, 159–79. Madison: University of Wisconsin Press.

———. 2011. "Colonialism from the Middle: African Clerks as Historical Actors and Discursive Subjects." *History in Africa* 38(1): 21–33.

Back, Irit. 2004. "Communities of Ideas: Blyden, Senghor and the Evolution of the Discourse between Pan-Africanism and Islam." In *Community, Identity and the State: Comparing Africa, Eurasia, Latin America and the Middle East,* edited by Moshe Gammer, 142–56. New York: Routledge.

Baker, George. 1996. "Photography between Narrativity and Stasis: August Sander, Degeneration, and the Decay of the Portrait." *October* 76: 73–113.

Bartoli, Daniel. 1968. "Aménagement de L'environnement Des Malades Mentaux À Dakar." Special edition (Psychiatrie au Sénégal). *Études Médicales,* 18–25.

Basaglia, Franco. 1987. *Psychiatry Inside Out: Selected Writings of Franco Basaglia.* Edited by Nancy Scheper-Hughes and Anne M. Lovell. New York: Columbia University Press.

Bastide, Roger. 2001. *Le Candomblé de Bahia.* Paris: Plon.

Battaglia, Debbora. 1995. "On Practical Nostalgia: Self-Prospecting among Urban Trobianders." In *Rhetorics of Self-Making*, edited by Debbora Battaglia, 77–96. Berkeley: University of California Press.

Bégué, Jean-Michel. 1989. "Un Siècle de Psychiatrie Française en Algérie (1830–1939)." Mémoire de CES de psychiatrie. Paris: Université Pierre et Marie Curie, Faculté de Médecine Saint Antoine.

———. 1997. "Genèse de l'ethnopsychiatrie, un texte fondateur de la psychiatrie coloniale française: Le Rapport de Reboul et Régis au Congrès de Tunis en 1912." *Psychopathologie Africaine* 28(2): 177–220.

Benjamin, Walter. 1969. *Illuminations: Essays and Reflections.* New York: Schocken Press.

———. 1999. *The Arcades Project.* Edited by Rolf Tiedemann. Cambridge, MA: Harvard University Press.

Benoist, Joseph-Roger de, and Hamidou Kane. 1998. *Léopold Sédar Senghor.* Paris: Beauchesne.

Benslama, Fethi. 1996. "L'Illusion Ethnopsychiatrique." *Le Monde*, December 4.

Ben-Tovim, David. 1987. *Development Psychiatry: Mental Health and Primary Health Care in Botswana.* London: Tavistock.

Berliner, David. 2005. "The Abuses of Memory: Reflections on the Memory Boom in Anthropology." *Anthropological Quarterly* 78(1): 197–211.

———. 2012. "Multiple Nostalgias: The Fabric of Heritage in Luang Prabang (Lao PDR)." *Journal of the Royal Anthropological Institute* 18(4): 769–86.

———. 2014. "Are Anthropologists Nostalgist?" In *Anthropology and Nostalgia*, edited by Olivia Angé and David Berliner, 17–34. New York: Berghahn Books.

Bessire, Lucas. 2014. *Behold the Black Caiman: A Chronicle of Ayoreo Life.* Chicago: University of Chicago Press.

Betts, Raymond F. 1961. *Assimilation and Association in French Colonial Theory: 1890–1914.* New York: Columbia University Press.

Bhabha, Homi. 1994. "Remembering Fanon: Self, Psyche and the Colonial Condition." In *Colonial Discourse and Post-Colonial Theory: A Reader*, edited by Patrick Williams and Laura Chrisman, 112–13. New York: Columbia University Press.

Biehl, João. [2005] 2013. *Vita: Life in a Zone of Social Abandonment.* 2nd rev. ed. Berkeley: University of California Press.

Bissell, William C. 2005. "Engaging Colonial Nostalgia." *Cultural Anthropology* 20(2): 215–48.

Blake, Casey Nelson. 1999. "The Usable Past, the Comfortable Past, and the Civic Past: Memory in Contemporary America." *Cultural Anthropology* 14(3): 423–35.

Boddy, Janice. 1989. *Wombs and Alien Spirits: Women, Men, and the Zar Cult in Northern Sudan.* Madison: University of Wisconsin Press.

Boroffka, Alexander. 1975. "The Provision of Psychiatric Services in Developing Countries: Nigeria, an Example." *African Journal of Psychiatry* 2: 117–32.

Borreil, Paul. 1908. "Considérations sur l'Internement des Aliénés Sénégalais en France." Medical thesis. Montpellier, France: University of Montpellier.

Bourdieu, Pierre. 1977. *Outline of a Theory of Practice*. Translated by Richard Nice. Cambridge: Cambridge University Press.

———. 1984. *Distinction: A Social Critique of the Judgement of Taste*. Translated by Richard Nice. Cambridge, MA: Harvard University Press.

Boussat, Stéphane, and Michel Boussat. 2002. "À propos de Henri Collomb (1913–1979): De la psychiatrie coloniale à une psychiatrie sans frontières." *L'Autre* 3(3): 409–24.

Boyarin, Jonathan. 1991. *Polish Jews in Paris: The Ethnography of Memory*. Bloomington: Indiana University Press.

Boym, Svetlana. 2001. *The Future of Nostalgia*. New York: Basic Books.

Brooks, Van Wyck. 1918. "On Creating a Usable Past." *The Dial* 64(11): 337–41.

Brown, Tamara Mose. 2012. "Who's the Boss? The Political Economy of Unpaid Care Work and Food Sharing in Brooklyn, USA." *Feminist Economics* 18(3): 1–24.

Brunschwig, Henri. 1983. *Noirs et Blancs Dans l'Afrique Noire Française, Ou, Comment Le Colonisé Devient Colonisateur, 1870–1914*. Paris: Flammarion.

Buggenhagen, Beth Anne. 2001. "Prophets and Profits: Gendered and Generational Visions of Wealth and Value in Senegalese Murid Households." *Journal of Religion in Africa* 31(4): 373–401.

———. 2004. "Domestic Object(ion)s: The Senegalese Murid Trade Diaspora and the Politics of Marriage Payments, Love, and State Privatization." In *Producing African Futures: Ritual and Reproduction in a Neoliberal Age*, edited by Brad Weiss, 21–53. Leiden: Brill.

Bulhan, Hussein Abdilahi. 1985. *Frantz Fanon and the Psychology of Oppression*. New York: Plenum Press.

Bullard, Alice. 2005a. "The Critical Impact of Frantz Fanon and Henri Collomb: Race, Gender, and Personality Testing of North and West Africans." *Journal of the History of the Behavioral Sciences* 41(3): 225–48.

———. 2005b. "L'Oedipe Africain, A Retrospective." *Transcultural Psychiatry* 42(2): 171–203.

Burke, Peter. 1989. "History as Social Memory." In *Memory: History, Culture and the Mind*, edited by Thomas Butler, 97–113. Oxford: Blackwell.

Burrows, Edmund H. 1958. *A History of Medicine in South Africa Up to the End of the Nineteenth Century*. Cape Town, South Africa: A. A. Balkema.

Buse, Peter, and Andrew Stott, eds. 1999. "Introduction: A Future for Haunting." In *Ghosts: Deconstruction, Psychoanalysis, History*. London: Palgrave Macmillan.

Carling, Jørgen. 2002. "Migration in the Age of Involuntary Immobility: Theoretical Reflections and Cape Verdean Experiences." *Journal of Ethnic and Migration Studies* 28(1): 5–42.

Carothers, John Colin. 1951. "Frontal Lobe Function and the African." *British Journal of Psychiatry* 97 (406): 12–48.

———. 1953. *The African Mind in Health and Disease: A Study in Ethnopsychiatry.* Geneva, Switzerland: World Health Organization.

Castel, Robert. 1976. *L'ordre psychiatrique: L'âge d'or de l'aliénisme.* Paris: Éditions de Minuit.

Cazanove, Frank. 1912. "La Folie Chez les Indigènes de l'Afrique Occidentale Française." *Annales d'Hygiène et de Médecine Coloniales* 15: 894–97.

———. 1927. "Mémento de Psychiatrie Coloniale Africaine." *Bulletin Du Comité Historique et Scientifique de l'Afrique Occidentale Française,* 133–77.

Centre Hospitalier de Fann, Service de Neuropsychiatrie (Dakar). 1968. "Psychopathologie et Environnement Familial En Afrique." *Psychopathologie Africaine* 4(2): 173–226.

Certeau, Michael de. 1988. *The Writing of History.* New York: Columbia University Press.

Césaire, Aimé. 1939. "Le Cahier d'un Retour au Pays Natal." *Volontés* 20: 23–51.

———. 1976. *Œuvres complètes: Poèmes.* Vol. 1. Fort-de-France: Désormeaux.

———. 1979. "Notebook of a Return to the Native Land." *Montemora* 6: 9–37.

Cherki, Alice. 2006. *Frantz Fanon: A Portrait.* Translated by Nadia Benabid. Ithaca, NY: Cornell University Press.

Chow, Rey. 2012. *Entanglements, Or Transmedial Thinking about Capture.* Durham, NC: Duke University Press.

Clark, Andrew F., and Lucie Colvin Phillips. 1994. *Historical Dictionary of Senegal.* Metuchen, NJ: Scarecrow Press.

Clifford, James. 1986. "Introduction: Partial Truths." In *Writing Culture: The Poetics and Politics of Ethnography,* edited by James Clifford and George E. Marcus, 1–26. Berkeley: University of California Press.

———. 1988. *The Predicament of Culture: Twentieth-Century Ethnography, Literature, and Art.* Cambridge, MA: Harvard University Press.

———. 1989. "The Others: Beyond the 'Salvage' Paradigm." *Third Text* 3(6): 73–78.

Cole, Jennifer. 2001. *Forget Colonialism?: Sacrifice and the Art of Memory in Madagascar.* Berkeley: University of California Press.

Collignon, René. 1976. "Quelques Propositions Pour Une Histoire de La Psychiatrie Au Sénégal." *Psychopathologie Africaine* 12(2): 245–73.

———. 1978. "Vingt Ans de Travaux à la Clinique Psychiatrique de Fann-Dakar." *Psychopathologie Africaine* 14(2 / 3): 133–342.

———. 1995. "Some Reflections on the History of Psychiatry in French Speaking West Africa: The Example of Senegal." *Psychopathologie Africaine* 27(1): 37–51.

———. 1999. "La Construction du Sujet Colonial: Le Cas Particulier des Malades Mentaux. Difficultés d'une Psychiatrie en Terre Africaine." In *La Psychologie Des Peuples et Ses Dérives,* edited by Michel Kail and Geneviève Vermès, 165–81. Paris: Centre National de Documentation Pédagogique.

———. 2000. "Santé Mentale entre Psychiatrie Contemporaine et Pratique Traditionnelle: Le Cas du Sénégal." *Psychopathologie Africaine* 30(3): 283–98.

———. 2002. "Pour une histoire de la psychiatrie coloniale française: A partir de l'exemple du Sénégal." *L'Autre* 3(3): 455–80.

———. 2004. "Pour une prise en compte de l'histoire." In *Psychiatrie, Psychanalyse, Culture* (Premier Congrès panafricain de Santé mentale) / *Psychiatry, Psychoanalysis, Culture* (First Panafrican Conference on Mental Health), edited by René Collignon and Momar Guèye, 105–20. Dakar: Société de Psychopathologie et d'Hygiène Mentale de Dakar.

———. 2006. "French Colonial Psychiatry in Algeria and Senegal: Outline of a Historical Comparison." *Revue Tiers Monde* 187(3): 527–46.

Collignon, René and Momar Guèye. 2003. *Psychiatrie, Psychanalyse, Culture (Premier Congrès panafricain de Santé mentale) / Psychiatry, Psychoanalysis, Culture* (First Panafrican Conference on Mental Health). Dakar: Société de Psychopathologie et d'Hygiène Mentale de Dakar.

Collomb, Henri. 1965a. "Assistance Psychiatrique en Afrique (Expérience Sénégalaise)." *Psychopathologie Africaine* 1(1): 11–84.

———. 1965b. "Les Bouffées Délirantes en Psychiatrie Africaine." *Psychopathologie Africaine* 1(2): 167–239.

———. 1967a. "Les Problèmes Psychiatriques en Afrique Noire." *La Gazette Médicale de France* 3(3): 1723–32.

———. 1967b. "Methodological Problems in Cross-Cultural Research." *International Journal of Psychiatry* 3: 17–19.

———. 1967c. "Moussa Diop (1923–1967)." *Psychopathologie Africaine* 3(2): 181–82.

———. 1968. "Psychiatrie 'Africaine.'" *Études Médicales*, 1–9.

———. 1972. "Psychothérapies Non Verbales Traditionnelles en Afrique." *Actualités psychiatriques* 3: 27–34.

———. 1975. "Histoire de La Psychiatrie en Afrique Noire Francophone." *African Journal of Psychiatry* 1(2): 87–115.

———. 1976. "Psychiatrie Africaine." In *Conférence Illustré de Diapositives*. Paris, France.

———. 1978a. "La Sorcellerie-Anthropophagie. Genèse et Fonction." *L'Évolution Psychiatrique* 43(3): 499–520.

———. 1978b. "L'économie des Villages Psychiatriques." *Social Science and Medicine* 12 C (1–2): 113–15.

Collomb, Henri, and Henri Ayats. 1962. "Les migrations au Sénégal: Étude psychopathologique." *Cahiers d'd'Études Africaines* 2(8): 570–97.

Collomb, Henri, Paul Martino, and Moussa Diop. 1964. "Les Difficultés Du Psychiatre À Propos Du Meurtre D'un Sorcier." *Bulletin de La Société Médicale d'Afrique Noire de Langue Française* 9(4): 415–17.

Collomb, Henri, and Jacques Zwingelstein. 1961. "Depressive States in an African Community (Dakar)." In *Conference Report*, edited by T. Adeoye Lambo, 227–34. Ibadan, Nigeria: Government Printer.

Comaroff, Jean, and John L. Comaroff, eds. 1993. "Introduction." In *Modernity and Its Malcontents: Ritual and Power in Postcolonial Africa*, xi–xxxvii. Chicago: University of Chicago Press.

Comaroff, John L., and Jean Comaroff. 1987. "The Madman and the Migrant: Work and Labor in the Historical Consciousness of a South African People." *American Ethnologist* 14(2): 191–209.

Comité du souvenir de la personne et de l'œuvre d'Henri Collomb. 1980. *Henri Collomb: Professeur Agrégé de Médecine, 1913–1979; Son Œuvre, Son Humanité.* Valbonnais, France.

Conklin, Alice L. 1997. *A Mission to Civilize: The Republican Idea of Empire in France and West Africa, 1895–1930.* Stanford, CA: Stanford University Press.

Cooper, David G. 1967. *Psychiatry and Anti-Psychiatry.* London: Tavistock.

Cooper, Frederick. 2002. *Africa Since 1940: The Past of the Present.* Cambridge: Cambridge University Press.

Corin, Ellen. 1997. "Playing with Limits: Tobie Nathan's Evolving Paradigm in Ethnopsychiatry." *Transcultural Psychiatry* 34(3): 345–58.

Corin, Ellen and H. B. M. Murphy. 1979. "Psychiatric Perspectives in Africa, Part I: The Western Viewpoint." *Transcultural Psychiatric Research Review* 16(2): 147–78.

Couloubaly, Pascal B. F. 1997. "Réflexions Critiques sur l'Ethnopsychiatrie." In *La Folie au Sénégal,* edited by Ludovic d'Almeida, 85–113. Dakar: Association des Chercheurs Sénégalais (ACS).

Coulthard, Glen S. 2007. "Subjects of Empire: Indigenous Peoples and the 'Politics of Recognition' in Canada." *Contemporary Political Theory* 6(4): 437–60.

———. 2014. *Red Skin, White Masks: Rejecting the Colonial Politics of Recognition.* Minneapolis: University of Minnesota Press.

Crane, Susan A. 1997. "Writing the Individual Back into Collective Memory." *American Historical Review* 102(5): 1372–85.

Crapanzano, Vincent. 1980. *Tuhami: Portrait of a Moroccan.* Chicago: University of Chicago Press.

———. 2003. "Reflections on Hope as a Category of Social and Psychological Analysis." *Cultural Anthropology* 18(1): 3–32.

Crapanzano, Vincent and Vivian Garrison, eds. 1977. *Case Studies in Spirit Possession.* New York: Wiley.

Crowder, Michael. [1968] 1976. *West Africa under Colonial Rule.* Evanston, IL: Northwestern University Press.

Cruise O'Brien, Donal B. 1979. "Langue et nationalité au Sénégal: L'enjeu politique de la wolo sation." *Année Africaine* 319–35.

———. 1998. "The Shadow-Politics of Wolo Sation." *Journal of Modern African Studies* 36(1): 25–46.

Daniel, E. Valentine. 1997. "Suffering Nation and Alienation." In *Social Suffering,* edited by Arthur Kleinman, Veena Das, and Margaret M. Lock, 309–38. Berkeley: University of California Press.

Deacon, Harriet Jane. 1996. "Madness, Race and Moral Treatment: Robben Island Lunatic Asylum, Cape Colony, 1846–1890." *History of Psychiatry* 7(26): 287–97.

de Bures, Idelette. 2006. "À propos de la loi sur les aliénés du 30 juin 1838." *Histoire des Sciences Médicales* 40(3): 301–4.

Deleuze, Gilles, and Félix Guattari. 2004. *A Thousand Plateaus: Capitalism and Schizophrenia*. London and New York: Continuum.

Deliss, Clémentine. 2011. "Some Thoughts on the Transformational Psyche of Objects." In *Antje Majewski—The World of Gimel: How to Make Objects* Talk, edited by Adam Budak. Berlin: Sternberg Press.

Dembele, Demba Moussa. 2005. "The International Monetary Fund and World Bank in Africa: A 'Disastrous' Record." *International Journal of Health Services* 35(2): 389–98.

Deren, Maya. 1970. *Divine Horsemen: Voodoo Gods of Haiti*. New York: Chelsea House.

Derrida, Jacques. 1976. *Of Grammatology*. Translated by Gayatri Chakravorty Spivak. Baltimore, MD: Johns Hopkins University Press.

———. 1978. *Writing and Difference*. Chicago: University of Chicago Press.

———. 1994. *Specters of Marx: The State of the Debt, the Work of Mourning, and the New International*. New York: Routledge.

Desclaux, Alice. 2004. "Equity in Access to AIDS Treatment in Africa: Pitfalls among Achievements." In *Unhealthy Health Policy: A Critical Anthropological Examination*, edited by Arachu Castro and Merrill Singer, 115–32. Walnut Creek, CA: AltaMira Press.

Devereux, George. [1961] 1969. *Mohave Ethnopsychiatry and Suicide: The Psychiatric Knowledge and the Psychic Disturbances of an Indian Tribe*. Washington, DC: U.S. Government Printing Office.

Dia, Alhousseynou. 1976. "Une Communauté Thérapeutique: Le Pinth de Fann." *African Journal of Psychiatry* 2(1): 147–51.

———. 1977. "Du Pénc de Fann aux Réunions Institutionnelles à l'hôpital de Jour du 17e Arrondissement de Paris." *Psychopathologie Africaine* 8(3): 371–96.

Dia, Alhousseynou, Chantal de Préneuf, and Jean-Paul Salaün. 1976. "Psychodrame en Afrique. Expérience Sénégalaise." *African Journal of Psychiatry*, Actes de 3e Congrès Pan-Africain de Psychiatrie, Khartoum, 1972, 2(1): 247–52.

Diagne, Souleymane Bachir. 2009. "Religion and the Public Sphere in Senegal: The Evolution of a Project of Modernity." *Institute for the Study of Islamic Thought in Africa (ISITA) Working Paper Series* 09–008.

Dijk, Rijk van. 1998. "Pentecostalism, Cultural Memory, and the State: Contested Representations of Time in Postcolonial Malawi." In *Memory and the Postcolony: African Anthropology and the Critique of Power*, edited by Richard P. Werbner, 155–81. London: Zed Books.

Diop, Babakar. 1967. "Docteur Moussa Diop (1923–1967)." *Bulletin de la Société Médicale d'Afrique Noire de Langue Française* 12(2): 177–78.

———. 1968. "Sur la Formation des Psychiatres Négro-Africains en France." In *IIe Colloque Africain de Psychiatrie*, 16: 169–70. Dakar: Bulletins et Mémoires de la Faculté Mixte de Médecine et de Pharmacie de Dakar.

Diop, Babakar and Maurice Dorès. 1976. "L'Admission d'un Accompagnant du Malade à l'hôpital Psychiatrique." *Perspectives Psychiatriques* 59(5): 359–68.

Diop, Momar-Coumba, ed. 2002. *Le Sénégal contemporain*. Paris: Karthala.

Diop, Moussa, and Henri Collomb. 1965. "Pratiques Mystiques et Psychopathologie: À Propos d'un Cas." *Psychopathologie Africaine* 1(3): 304–22.

Diop, Moussa, András Zempléni, and Paul Martino. 1966. "Les Techniques Thérapeutiques Traditionnelles des Maladies Mentales au Sénégal." *Médecine d'Afrique Noir* 4: 115–16.

Diouf, Mamadou. 1998. "The French Colonial Policy of Assimilation and the Civility of the Originaires of the Four Communes (Senegal): A Nineteenth-Century Globalization Project." *Development and Change* 29(4): 671–96.

Diouf, Mamadou Lamine, Marième Ndiaye, René Collignon, and Amadou Makhtar Seck. 2008. "Entre Événements de Vie et Croyances Culturelles: Un Délire à la Croisée des Chemins." *L'Évolution Psychiatrique* 73(1): 135–44.

Diouf, Mamadou, and Mohamed Mbodj. 1997. "L'administration coloniale du Sénégal et la question de l'aliénation mentale: 1840–1956." In *La Folie au Sénégal*, edited by Ludovic d'Almeida, 13–55. Dakar: Association des Chercheurs Sénégalais (ACS).

Dorès, Maurice. 1996. "Comment Soigner Les Troubles Psychologiques Des Immigrants? Le Psy, le Chaman et le Charlatan." *Libération*, December 4.

Dorès, Maurice and Gérard Tourame. 1975. "Vie Quotidienne dans une Institution Psychiatrique au Sénégal." *Bulletin de l'Association Mondiale de Psychiatrie* 1: 22–26.

Duvergier, Jean Baptiste. 1841. *Collection Complète Des Lois, Décrets, Ordonnances, Réglements, et Avis Du Conseil d'Etat*. Paris.

Easterly, William. 2005. "What Did Structural Adjustment Adjust?: The Association of Policies and Growth with Repeated IMF and World Bank Adjustment Loans." *Journal of Development Economics* 76(1): 1–22.

Ebong, Ima. 1991. "Negritude: Between Flag and Mask: Senegalese Cultural Ideology and the 'École de Dakar.'" In *Africa Explores: African Art in the 20th Century*, edited by Susan Vogel, 198–209. New York: Center for African Art.

Edington, Claire Ellen. 2013. "Beyond the Asylum: Colonial Psychiatry in French Indochina, 1880–1940." PhD diss., Columbia University, New York. http://gradworks.umi.com/35/68/3568704.html.

Englund, Harri. 1996. "Witchcraft, Modernity and the Person: The Morality of Accumulation in Central Malawi." *Critique of Anthropology* 16(3): 257–79.

Estroff, Sue E., William S. Lachicotte, Linda C. Illingworth, and Anna Johnston. 1991. "Everybody's Got a Little Mental Illness: Accounts of Illness and Self among People with Severe, Persistent Mental Illnesses." *Medical Anthropology Quarterly* 5(4): 331–69.

Fabian, Johannes. 1999. "Remembering the Other: Knowledge and Recognition in the Exploration of Central Africa." *Critical Inquiry* 26(1): 49–69.

———. 2007. *Memory against Culture: Arguments and Reminders*. Durham, NC: Duke University Press.

Fanon, Frantz. [1961] 1963. *The Wretched of the Earth*. Translated by Constance Farrington. New York: Grove Press.

———. [1952] 1967. *Black Skin, White Masks*. Translated by Charles Lam Markmann. New York: Grove Press.

Farmer, Paul. 1992. "The Birth of the Klinik: A Cultural History of Haitian Professional Psychiatry." In *Ethnopsychiatry: The Cultural Construction of Professional and Folk Psychiatries*, edited by Atwood D. Gaines, 251–72. Albany: SUNY Press.

Fassin, Didier. 1999. "L'Ethnopsychiatrie et ses Réseaux. L'Influence qui Grandit." *Genèses* 35(1): 146–71.

———. 2000. "Les Politiques de L'ethnopsychiatrie: La Psyché Africaine, des Colonies Africaines Aux Banlieues Parisiennes." *L'Homme* 153: 231–50.

Fassin, Didier and Richard Rechtman. 2005. "An Anthropological Hybrid: The Pragmatic Arrangement of Universalism and Culturalism in French Mental Health." *Transcultural Psychiatry* 42(3): 347–66.

Ferguson, James. 1999. *Expectations of Modernity: Myths and Meanings of Urban Life on the Zambian Copperbelt*. Berkeley: University of California Press.

———. 2006. *Global Shadows: Africa in the Neoliberal World Order*. Durham, NC: Duke University Press.

———. 2012. "Structures of Responsibility." *Ethnography* 13(4): 558–62.

Fichte, Hubert. 1980. *Psyche*. Frankfurt am Main: Verlag.

Foley, Ellen. 2008 "Neoliberal Reform and Health Dilemmas: Illness, Social Hierarchy, and Therapeutic Decision-Making in Senegal." *Medical Anthropology Quarterly* 22(3): 257–73.

———. 2009. "The Anti-politics of Health Reform: Household Power Relations and Child Health in Rural Senegal." *Anthropology and Medicine* 16(1): 61–71.

———. 2010. *Your Pocket Is What Cures You: The Politics of Health in Senegal*. New Brunswick, NJ: Rutgers University Press.

Fons, T. T. (Alphonse Mendy). 1999. *Goorgoorlou et la dévaluation*. Dakar: Editions Clair Afrique.

Foster, Stephen William. 1988. *The Past Is Another Country: Representation, Historical Consciousness and Resistance in the Blue Ridge*. Berkeley: University of California Press.

Foucault, Michel. 1965. *Madness and Civilization: A History of Insanity in the Age of Reason*. New York: Vintage Books.

———. 1973. *The Birth of the Clinic: An Archaeology of Medical Perception*. New York: Vintage Books.

———. 1978. *History of Sexuality: An Introduction, Vol. 1*. New York: Vintage Books.

———. 1988a. "Confinement, Psychiatry, Prison." In *Politics, Philosophy, Culture: Interviews and Other Writings, 1977–1984*, edited by Lawrence Kritzman, 178–210. New York: Routledge.

———. 1988b. *Politics, Philosophy, Culture: Interviews and Other Writings, 1977–1984*. Edited by Lawrence Kritzman. New York: Routledge.

Freud, Sigmund. [1917] 1957. "Mourning and Melancholia." In *The Standard Edition of the Complete Psychological Works of Sigmund Freud*, edited by James Strachey, Vol. XIV: *On the History of the Psycho-Analytic Movement, Papers on Metapsychology and Other Works*, 243–58. London: Hogarth Press.

———. [1914] 1958. "Remembering, Repeating and Working-Through: (Further Recommendations on the Technique of Psycho-Analysis II)." In *The Standard Edition of the Complete Psychological Works of Sigmund Freud*, edited by James Strachey, Vol. XII, *The Case of Schreber, Papers on Technique and Other Works*, 146–56. London: Hogarth Press.

Frobenius, Leo. 1973. *Leo Frobenius, 1873–1973: An Anthology*. Edited by Eike Haberland. Wiesbaden, Germany: Franz Steiner.

Frow, John. 1997. *Time and Commodity Culture: Essays on Cultural Theory and Postmodernity*. Oxford: Oxford University Press.

Gagnon, Marilou, Jean Daniel Jacob, and Dave Holmes. 2010. "Governing through (In)security: A Critical Analysis of a Fear-Based Public Health Campaign." *Critical Public Health* 20(2): 245–56.

Gaines, Atwood D., ed. 1992. *Ethnopsychiatry: The Cultural Construction of Professional and Folk Psychiatries*. Albany: SUNY Press.

Gates, Henry Louis, Jr. 1991. "Critical Fanonism." *Critical Inquiry* 17(3): 457–70.

Gautron, Jean Claude. 1964. "L'évolution des rapports franco-sénégalais." *Annuaire français de droit international* 10(1): 837–50.

Gbikpi, Paul, and Roselyne Auguin. 1978. "Evaluation d'une pratique institutionnelle à Fann: l'admission d'un accompagnant de malade à l'hôpital." *Psychopathologie Africaine* 14(1): 5–68.

Gellar, Sheldon. 1982. *Senegal: An African Nation between Islam and the West*. Boulder, CO: Westview Press.

Geschiere, Peter. 1997. *The Modernity of Witchcraft: Politics and the Occult in Postcolonial Africa*. Charlottesville: University of Virginia Press.

Giordano, Cristiana. 2011. "Translating Fanon in the Italian Context: Rethinking the Ethics of Treatment in Psychiatry." *Transcultural Psychiatry* 48(3): 228–56.

———. 2014. *Migrants in Translation: Caring and the Logics of Difference in Contemporary Italy*. Berkeley: University of California Press.

———. 2015. "Lying the Truth." *Current Anthropology* 56(S12): S211–21.

Glenn, Evelyn N. 2010. *Forced to Care: Coercion and Caregiving in America*. Cambridge, MA: Harvard University Press.

Goldstein, Jan E. [1990] 2002. *Console and Classify: The French Psychiatric Profession in the Nineteenth Century*. Chicago: University of Chicago Press.

Good, Byron. 1994. *Medicine, Rationality, and Experience: An Anthropological Perspective*. Cambridge: Cambridge University Press.

Gordon, Avery F. 1997. *Ghostly Matters: Haunting and the Sociological Imagination*. Minneapolis: University of Minnesota Press.

Griffin, Christopher. 2008. *Nomads under the Westway: Irish Travellers, Gypsies and Other Traders in West London*. Hertfordshire, UK: University of Hertfordshire Press.

Guèye, Momar. 1984. "Situation Actuelle de La Santé Mentale Au Sénégal." In *Congrès Internationale Psychiatrique et Social de Langue Français*, 17–22. Paris, France.

———. 1998. "Serigne Mbaye Babakar Diop (1933–1998) Ou L'art D'accomplir Sa Destinée." *Psychopathologie Africaine* 29(1): 3–6.

Guyer, Jane I. 2007. "Prophecy and the Near Future: Thoughts on Macroeconomic, Evangelical, and Punctuated Time." *American Ethnologist* 34(3): 409–21.

Halbwachs, Maurice. 1992. *On Collective Memory*. Translated by Lewis A. Coser. Chicago: University of Chicago Press.

Hanna, William John. 1975. *University Students and African Politics*. New York: Holmes & Meier.

Harney, Elizabeth. 2004. *In Senghor's Shadow: Art, Politics, and the Avant-Garde in Senegal, 1960–1995*. Durham, NC: Duke University Press.

Harrison, Christopher, Tukur Bello Ingawa, and Susan M. Martin. 1987. "The Establishment of Colonial Rule in West Africa, c. 1900–1914." In *History of West Africa*, edited by Jacob F. Ade Ajayi and Michael Crowder, 2nd edition, II: 485–545. Harlow, England: Longman.

Hart, Keith. 1973. "Informal Income Opportunities and Urban Employment in Ghana." *Journal of Modern African Studies* 11(1): 61–89.

Harvey, David. 2005. *A Brief History of Neoliberalism*. New York, Oxford: Oxford University Press.

Headrick, Rita. 1994. *Colonialism, Health and Illness in French Equatorial Africa, 1885–1935*. Edited by Daniel R. Headrick. Atlanta: African Studies Association Press.

Heaton, Matthew M. 2013. *Black Skin, White Coats: Nigerian Psychiatrists, Decolonization, and the Globalization of Psychiatry*. Athens: Ohio University Press.

Hecht, David, and Abdumaliq Simone. 1994. *Invisible Governance: The Art of African Micropolitics*. New York: Autonomedia.

Hesseling, Gerti. 1985. *Histoire Politique du Sénégal: Institutions, Droit et Société*. Paris: Karthala.

Hodder, Ian. 2011. "Human-Thing Entanglement: Towards an Integrated Archaeological Perspective." *Journal of the Royal Anthropological Institute* 17(1): 154–77.

———. 2012. *Entangled: An Archaeology of the Relationships between Humans and Things*. Malden, MA: John Wiley & Sons.

———. 2014. "The Entanglements of Humans and Things: A Long-Term View." *New Literary History* 45(1): 19–36.

Höller, Christian. 2002. "Africa in Motion: An Interview with the Post-Colonialism Theoretician Achille Mbembe." *Springerin* 3(2). www.springerin.at/dyn/heft_text.php?textid = 1195&lang = en#fussnoten.

Humbert, Agnes, and Barbara Mellor. 2009. *Résistance: A Woman's Journal of Struggle and Defiance in Occupied France*. New York: Bloomsbury.

Hunt, Nancy Rose. 1999. *A Colonial Lexicon of Birth Ritual, Medicalization, and Mobility in the Congo*. Durham, NC: Duke University Press.

Hurston, Zora Neale. 1990. *Tell My Horse: Voodoo and Life in Haiti and Jamaica*. New York: Harper Perennial.

Huyssen, Andreas. 2003. *Present Pasts: Urban Palimpsests and the Politics of Memory*. Stanford, CA: Stanford University Press.

Hymans, Jacques Louis. 1971. *Léopold Sédar Senghor: An Intellectual Biography*. Edinburgh: Edinburgh University Press.

Idowu, H. Oludare. 1969. "Assimilation in 19th Century Senegal." *Cahiers d'Études Africaines* 9 (34): 194–218.

Irele, Abiola. 1990. *The African Experience in Literature and Ideology.* Bloomington: Indiana University Press.

Ivy, Marilyn. 1995. *Discourses of the Vanishing: Modernity, Phantasm, Japan.* Chicago: University of Chicago Press.

Jackson, Lynette. 2005. *Surfacing Up: Psychiatry and Social Order in Colonial Zimbabwe, 1908–1968.* Ithaca, NY: Cornell University Press.

Jameson, Fredric. 1989. "Nostalgia for the Present." *South Atlantic Quarterly* 88(2): 517–37.

———. 1995. "Marx's Purloined Letter." *New Left Review* 209: 75–109.

Johnson, G. Wesley Jr. 1971. *The Emergence of Black Politics in Senegal: The Struggle for Power in the Four Communes, 1900–1920.* Stanford, CA: Stanford University Press.

Kâ, Abdou Anta. 1972. " 'Pinthioum Fann': Farce, Comédie, Drame Ou Tragédie? Théâtre, Quatre Pièces d'Abdou Anta Kâ." *Présence Africaine.*

Keller, Richard. 2001. "Madness and Colonization: Psychiatry in the British and French Empires, 1800–1962." *Journal of Social History* 35(2): 295–326.

Kelly, Valerie, Thomas Reardon, Bocar Diagana, and Amadou Abdoulaye Fall. 1995. "Impacts of Devaluation on Senegalese Households: Policy Implications." *Food Policy* 20(4): 299–313.

Kenyon, Susan M. 1995. "Zar as Modernization in Contemporary Sudan." *Anthropological Quarterly* 68(2): 107–20.

Klein, Kerwin Lee. 2000. "On the Emergence of Memory in Historical Discourse." *Representations* 69: 127–50.

Kleinman, Arthur. 1988. *The Illness Narratives: Suffering, Healing, and the Human Condition.* New York: Basic Books.

Kleinman, Arthur, Leon Eisenberg, and Byron Good. 1978. "Culture, Illness, and Care: Clinical Lessons from Anthropologic and Cross-Cultural Research." *Annals of Internal Medicine* 88(2): 251–58.

Komaromy, Zsolt. 2011. *Figures of Memory: From the Muses to Eighteenth-Century British Aesthetics.* Lewisburg, PA: Bucknell University Press.

Koselleck, Reinhart. 1985. *Futures Past: On the Semantics of Historical Time.* Cambridge, MA: MIT Press.

Kulick, Don, Michael Billig, Virginia Dominguez, P. Steven Sangren, Mary Weismantel, Unni Wikan, and Don Kulick. 2006. "Theory in Furs: Masochist Anthropology." *Current Anthropology* 47(6): 933–52.

Kwon, Heonik. 2008. *Ghosts of War in Vietnam.* Cambridge: Cambridge University Press.

Laing, Ronald David. 1960. *The Divided Self: An Existential Study in Sanity and Madness.* London: Tavistock.

Lakoff, Andrew. 2005. *Pharmaceutical Reason: Knowledge and Value in Global Psychiatry.* Cambridge: Cambridge University Press.

Lambek, Michael. 1996. "The Past Imperfect: Remembering as Moral Practice." In *Tense Past: Cultural Essays in Trauma and Memory*, edited by Paul Antze, 235–54. New York: Routledge.

Lambert, Michael C. 1993. "From Citizenship to Négritude: 'Making a Difference' in Elite Ideologies of Colonized Francophone West Africa." *Comparative Studies in Society and History* 35(2): 239–62.

Lambo, T. Adeoye. 1966. "Patterns of Psychiatric Care in Developing African Countries: The Nigerian Village Program." In *International Trends in Mental Health*, edited by Henry Philip David, 147–53. New York: McGraw-Hill.

———. 1974. "Psychotherapy in Africa." *Psychotherapy and Psychosomatics*, What Is Psychotherapy? *Proceedings of the 9th International Congress on Psychotherapy* 24: 311–26.

Larchanché, Stephanie. 2010. *"Anxiétés culturelles et régulation institutionnelle: Santé mentale 'spécialisée' et 'souffrance immigrée' à Paris."* PhD diss., École des hautes études en sciences sociales (Paris) and Washington University (Saint Louis, MO).

Last, Murray, and G. L. Chavunduka. 1986. The *Professionalization of African Medicine*. Manchester: Manchester University Press.

Lawrance, Benjamin N., Emily Lynn Osborn, and Richard Roberts, eds. 2006. "Introduction: African Intermediaries and the 'Bargain' of Collaboration." In *Intermediaries, Interpreters, and Clerks: African Employees in the Making of Colonial Africa*, 3–34. Madison: University of Wisconsin Press.

Le Goff, Jacques. 1992. *History and Memory*. Translated by Steven Rendall and Elizabeth Claman. New York: Columbia University Press.

Le Soleil. 1978. "Après 18 Ans Au Sénégal, Le Professeur Collomb Nous Quitte," July 19.

———. 1998. "Si L'on Parle de l'École de Dakar, C'est Grâce À La Psychiatrie," September 17.

Le Vine, Victor T. 2004. *Politics in Francophone Africa*. Boulder, CO: Lynne Rienner.

Lebeau, Yann, and Mobolaji Ogunsanya, eds. 2015. "Index Des Textes En Francais." In *The Dilemma of Post-Colonial Universities: Elite Formation and the Restructuring of Higher Education in Sub-Saharian Africa*, 325–34. Dynamiques Africaines. Ibadan: Institut Français de Recherche en Afrique.

Leiris, Michel. [1958] 1980. *La possession et ses aspects théâtraux chez les Éthiopiens de Gondar, précédé de La croyance aux génies zâr en Éthiopie du Nord*. Paris: Le Sycomore.

Levinas, Emmanuel. [1961] 1969. *Totality and Infinity: An Essay on Exteriority*. Translated by Alphonso Lingis. Pittsburgh: Duquesne University Press.

———. [1972] 2006. *Humanism of the Other*. Translated by Nidra Poller. Champaign: University of Illinois Press.

Lévi-Strauss, Claude. 1963. "The Effectiveness of Symbols." In *Structural Anthropology*, 186–205. New York: Basic Books.

Lévy-Bruhl, Lucien. 1922. *La Mentalité Primitive*. Paris: Librairie Félix Alcan.

Lewis, I. M. [1971] 2003. *Ecstatic Religion: A Study of Shamanism and Spirit Posses-sion.* New York: Routledge.

Lewis, Martin Deming. 1962. "One Hundred Million Frenchmen: The 'Assimila-tion' Theory in French Colonial Policy." *Comparative Studies in Society and History* 4(2): 129–53.

Lock, Margaret, and Vinh-Kim Nguyen. 2010. *An Anthropology of Biomedicine.* Chichester, UK: Wiley-Blackwell.

Luhrmann, Tanya M. 2000. *Of Two Minds: An Anthropologist Looks at American Psychiatry.* New York: Vintage Books.

Mahone, Sloan, and Megan Vaughan. 2007. *Psychiatry and Empire.* London: Pal-grave Macmillan.

Malraux, André. 1937. *L'Espoir.* Paris: Gallimard.

———. 1992. *Les Vois du Silence.* Paris: Gallimard.

Mamdani, Mahmood. 2004. *Good Muslim, Bad Muslim: America, the Cold War, and the Roots of Terror.* New York: Doubleday.

Margetts, Edward Lambert. 1962. "Psychiatry and Mental Health in Africa: Pros-pects for the Future." In *Conference Report,* 186–95. Ibadan, Nigeria: Govern-ment Printer.

Markovitz, Irving Leonard. 1969. *Léopold Sédar Senghor and the Politics of Negri-tude.* New York: Atheneum.

Marks, Shula. 1999. "Every Facility That Modern Science and Enlightened Human-ity Have Devised: Race and Progress in a Colonial Hospital, Valkenberg Mental Asylum, Cape Colony, 1894–1910." In *Insanity, Institutions and Society, 1800–1914: A Social History of Madness in Comparative Perspective,* edited by Joseph Melling and Bill Forsythe, 268–92. London: Routledge.

Mars, Louis. 1947. *La Lutte Contre la Folie.* Port-Au-Prince, Haiti: Imprimerie de l'Etat.

Martino, Paul. 1968. "Les Représentations Culturelles des Maladies Mentales: L'Étape Nécessaire de Leur Reconnaissance—Leur Intégration Aux Techniques Occidentales de Diagnostic et D'assistance." *Études Médicales,* 10–17.

———. 1989. "Henri Collomb 1913–1979." *Psychiatrie Française* 2: 41–47.

Martino, Paul, Michel Simon, and Henri Collomb. 1968. "Bouffées Délirantes et Schizophrénie: Réflexions Méthodologiques pour une Étude Nosologique." In *Deuxième Colloque Africain de Psychiatrie.* Dakar, Senegal.

Martino, Paul, András Zempléni, and Henri Collomb. 1965. "Délire et Représenta-tions Culturelles: À Propos du Meurtre d'un Sorcier." *Psychopathologie Africaine* 1(1): 151–57.

Marx, Karl. 1972. "The Eighteenth Brumaire of Louis Bonaparte." In *The Marx-Engels Reader,* edited by Robert C. Tucker, 436–525. New York: Norton.

Max, Rosemary. 2009. "The Décalage and Bricolage of Higher Education Policy-making in an Inter / National System." In *Critical Approaches to Comparative Education: Vertical Case Studies from Africa, Europe, the Middle East, and the Americas,* edited by Frances Vavrus and Lesley Bartlett, 39–55. New York: Pal-grave Macmillan.

Mbembe, Achille. 1992. "Provisional Notes on the Postcolony." *Africa: Journal of the International African Institute* 62(1): 3–37.

———. 2001. *On the Postcolony.* Berkeley: University of California Press.

McCann, Lisa I., and Laurie Anne Pearlman. 1990. "Vicarious Traumatization: A Framework for Understanding the Psychological Effects of Working with Victims." *Journal of Traumatic Stress* 3(1): 131–49.

McClintock, Anne. 1992. "The Angel of Progress: Pitfalls of the Term 'Post-Colonialism.'" *Social Text* 31(32): 84–98.

McCulloch, Jock. 1995. *Colonial Psychiatry and the African Mind.* Cambridge: Cambridge University Press.

Melly, Caroline. 2010. "Inside-Out Houses: Urban Belonging and Imagined Futures in Dakar, Senegal." *Comparative Studies in Society and History* 52(1): 37–65.

———. 2011. "Titanic Tales of Missing Men: Reconfigurations of National Identity and Gendered Presence in Dakar, Senegal." *American Ethnologist* 38(2): 361–76.

———. 2013. "Ethnography on the Road: Infrastructural Vision and the Unruly Present in Contemporary Dakar." *Africa* 83(3): 385 – 402.

Métraux, Alfred. 1989. *Voodoo in Haiti.* Translated by Hugo Charteris. New York: Pantheon.

Miller, Christopher L. 1990. *Theories of Africans: Francophone Literature and Anthropology in Africa.* Chicago: University of Chicago Press.

Moncrieff, Joanna. 2008. "Neoliberalism and Biopsychiatry: A Marriage of Convenience." In *Liberatory Psychiatry: Philosophy, Politics and Mental Health,* edited by Carl I. Cohen and Sami Timimi, 235–55. Cambridge: Cambridge University Press.

Moore, Henrietta L., and Todd Sanders, eds. 2001. *Magical Interpretations, Material Realities: Modernity, Witchcraft and the Occult in Postcolonial Africa.* New York: Routledge.

Moro, Marie Rose, Quitterie de la Noé, and Yaram Mouchenik. 2006. Manuel de psychiatrie transculturelle: Travail clinique, travail social. Grenoble: La Pensée Sauvage.

Morrison, Toni. 1987. *Beloved.* New York: Alfred A. Knopf.

Mphahlele, Ezekial. 1962. *The African Image.* London: Faber and Faber.

Mueggler, Erik. 2001. *The Age of Wild Ghosts: Memory, Violence, and Place in Southwest China.* Berkeley: University of California Press.

Munn, Nancy D. 1992. "The Cultural Anthropology of Time: A Critical Essay." *Annual Review of Anthropology* 21: 93–123.

Näre, Lena. 2011. "The Moral Economy of Domestic and Care Labour: Migrant Workers in Naples, Italy." *Sociology* 45(3): 396–412.

Nathan, Tobie. 1986. "L'utérus, le chaman et le psychanalyste: Ethnopsychanalyse du cadre thérapeutique." *Psychothérapie sans frontières, NRE* 5.

Nathan, Tobie. 1988. *Le sperme du diable: Éléments d'ethnopsychothérapie.* Paris: Presses universitaires de France, 1988.

———. 1994. *L'influence qui guérit.* Paris: Odile Jacob.

————. 1996. "Freud ressemblait un peu à un guérisseur africain." Interview by Dominique Dhombres. *Le Monde.*

————. 1997. "Spécificité de L'ethnopsychiatrie." *Nouvelle Revue d'Ethnopsychiatrie* 34: 7–24.

————. 2006. "Le thérapeute doit négocier avec l'invisible." Interview by Marie-Laure Théodule. *La Recherche* (304).

Ndoye, Omar, Anne Devos, and Momar Guèye. 2000. "L'ethnopsychiatrie À Fann Aujourd'hui." *Psychopathologie Africaine* 30(3): 265–82.

Nerone, John. 1989. "Professional History and Social Memory." *Communication* 11(2): 89–104.

Niermann, Inge. 2005. "Capturing Psyche: Leonore Mau." *032c* 9: 112–16.

Nietzsche, Friedrich. [1874] 2006. *The Use and Abuse of History.* Reprint, New York: Cosimo.

Nora, Pierre. 1989. "Between Memory and History: Les Lieux de Mémoire." *Representations* 26: 7–24.

Nuttall, Sarah. 2009. *Entanglement: Literary and Cultural Reflections on Post Apartheid.* Johannesburg: Wits University Press.

O'Brien, Donal Brian Cruise, Momar Coumba Diop, and Mamadou Diouf. 2002. *La construction de l'Etat au Sénégal.* Paris: Karthala.

O'Hara, Vincent. 2013. *Struggle for the Middle Sea.* Annapolis, MD: Naval Institute Press.

Ohnuki-Tierney, Emiko, ed. 1990. *Culture through Time: Anthropological Approaches.* Stanford, CA: Stanford University Press.

Olick, Jeffrey K., and Joyce Robbins. 1998. "Social Memory Studies: From 'Collective Memory' to the Historical Sociology of Mnemonic Practices." *Annual Review of Sociology* 24(1): 105–40.

Ortigues, Marie-Cécile, and Paul Martino. 1965. "Psychologie Clinique et Psychiatrie en Milieu Africain." *Psychopathologie Africaine* 1(2): 121–47.

Ortigues, Marie-Cécile, Paul Martino, and Henri Collomb. 1967. "L'Utilisation des Données Culturelles dans un Cas de Bouffée Délirante." *Psychopathologie Africaine* 3(1): 121–47.

Ortigues, Marie-Cécile, and Edmond Ortigues. 1966. *Oedipe Africain.* Paris: Librarie Plon.

————. 1984. *Oedipe Africain.* Paris: L'Harmattan.

Ortigues, Marie-Cécile, András Zempléni, and Jacqueline Rabain. 1968. "Psychologie Clinique et Ethnologie (Sénégal)." *Bulletin de Psychologie de La Sorbonne* 21(15–19): 950–58.

Paerregaard, Karsten. 2012. "Commodifying Intimacy: Women, Work, and Care in Peruvian Migration." *Journal of Latin American and Caribbean Anthropology* 17(3): 493–511.

Pandolfo, Stefania. 2000. "The Thin Line of Modernity: Some Moroccan Debates on Subjectivity." In *Questions of Modernity*, edited by Timothy Mitchell, 115–47. Minneapolis: University of Minnesota Press.

Parin, Paul, Fritz Morgenthaler, and Goldy Parin-Matthey. 1967. "Considérations Psychanalytiques Sur Le Moi de Groupe." *Psychopathologie Africaine* 3(2): 195–206.

Petryna, Adriana, and Arthur Kleinman. 2006. "The Pharmaceutical Nexus." In *Global Pharmaceuticals: Ethics, Markets, Practices*, edited by Adriana Petryna, Andrew Lakoff, and Arthur Kleinman, 1–32. Durham, NC: Duke University Press.

Petryna, Adriana, Andrew Lakoff, and Arthur Kleinman, eds. 2006. *Global Pharmaceuticals: Ethics, Markets, Practices*. Durham, NC: Duke University Press.

Pinthioum Fann. 1970 (November). Centre Hospitalier Universitaire de Fann (CHU de Fann), Service de Psychiatrie.

Piot, Charles. 2010. *Nostalgia for the Future: West Africa after the Cold War.* Chicago: University of Chicago Press.

Planchon, Michel. 2013. "Psychiatrie Coloniale et Hospitalière En Métropole, Notamment À Marseille (1840–1940)." In *XXIIe Congrès National de Généalogie À Marseille: Retour Aux Sources, Marseille Carrefour Des Cultures.* Marseilles, France.

Plato. 1975. *Philebus.* Oxford: Clarendon Press.

———. 1987. *Theaetetus.* London: Penguin Books.

Policar, Alain. 1997. "La Dérive de L'ethnopsychiatrie." *Libération*, June 20.

Povinelli, Elizabeth A. 2002. *The Cunning of Recognition: Indigenous Alterities and the Making of Australian Multiculturalism.* Durham, NC: Duke University Press.

Rabinow, Paul, and Nikolas Rose. 2006. "Biopower Today." *BioSocieties* 1(2): 195–217.

Radstone, Susannah, ed. 2000. "Working with Memory: An Introduction." In *Memory and Methodology*, 1–22. New York: Berg.

Rainaut, Jean. 1981. "Historique de La Création Du Service de Neuropsychiatrie de Fann." *Psychopathologie Africaine* 17(1–2–3): 431–35.

Rappaport, Joanne. 1990. *The Politics of Memory: Native Historical Interpretation in the Colombian Andes.* Cambridge: Cambridge University Press.

Reboul, Henry, and Emmanuel Régis. 1912. "L'assistance des aliénés aux colonies." In *XXIIe Congrès des médecins aliénistes et neurologistes de France et des pays de langue française (Tunis, 1–7 avril 1912).* Paris: Masson.

Repetti, Massimo. 2007. "African Wave: Specificity and Cosmopolitanism in African Comics." *African Arts* 40(2): 16–35.

Ricœur, Paul. 1974. "A Philosophical Interpretation of Freud." In *The Conflict of Interpretations: Essays in Hermeneutics*, edited by Don Ihde, 160–76. Evanston, IL: Northwestern University Press.

———. 1991. "Life in Quest of Narrative." In *On Paul Ricœur: Narrative and Interpretation*, edited by David Wood, 20–33. London: Routledge.

———. 1999a. "Imagination, Testimony and Trust: A Dialogue with Paul Ricœur." In *Questioning Ethics: Contemporary Debates in Philosophy*, edited by Richard Kearney and Mark Dooley, 12–17. London: Routledge.

———. 1999b. "Memory and Forgetting." In *Questioning Ethics: Contemporary Debates in Philosophy*, edited by Richard Kearney and Mark Dooley, 5–11. London: Routledge.

_____. 2006. *Memory, History, Forgetting*. Translated by Kathleen Blamey and David Pellauer. Chicago: University of Chicago Press.

Robbins, Joel. "Beyond the Suffering Subject: Toward an Anthropology of the Good." *Journal of the Royal Anthropological Institute* 19: 447–62.

Roberts, Richard L., Emily Lynn Osborn, and Benjamin N. Lawrance, eds. 2006. *Intermediaries, Interpreters, and Clerks: African Employees in the Making of Colonial Africa*. Madison: University of Wisconsin Press.

Robertson, Roland. 1990. "After Nostalgia?: Wilful Nostalgia and the Phases of Globalization." In *Theories of Modernity and Postmodernity*, edited by Bryan S. Turner, 45–61. London: Sage.

Rodgers, Dennis, and Bruce O'Neill. 2012. "Infrastructural Violence: Introduction to the Special Issue." *Ethnography* 13(4): 401–12.

Rosaldo, Renato. 1980. *Ilongot Headhunting, 1883–1974: A Study in Society and History*. Stanford, CA: Stanford University Press.

_____. 1989. *Culture and Truth: The Remaking of Social Analysis*. Boston: Beacon Press.

Russell, Catherine. 1999. *Experimental Ethnography: The Work of Film in the Age of Video*. Durham, NC: Duke University Press.

Sadowsky, Jonathan. 1999. *Imperial Bedlam: Institutions of Madness in Colonial Southwest Nigeria*. Berkeley: University of California Press.

Samuel, Raphael. 1994. *Theatres of Memory: Past and Present in Contemporary Culture*. London: Verso.

Santayana, George. 1905. *The Life of Reason, Vol. 1: Reason in Common Sense*. Mineola, NY: Dover.

Saris, A. Jamie. 1995. "Telling Stories: Life Histories, Illness Narratives, and Institutional Landscapes." *Culture, Medicine and Psychiatry* 19(1): 39–72.

Sarr, Doudou, Amadou Makhtar Seck, and Moussa Ba. 1997. "Quarante Ans de Psychiatrie au Sénégal (1938–1978)." In *La Folie au Sénégal*, edited by Ludovic d'Almeida, 201–27. Dakar: Association des Chercheurs Sénégalais (ACS).

Sartre, Jean-Paul. 1976. *Black Orpheus*. Paris: Présence Africaine.

Sembéne, Ousmane. 1975. *Xala*. New Yorker Films (USA).

Senghor, Léopold Sédar. 1963. "Négritude et Civilisation de l'Universel." *Présence Africaine* 46: 8–13.

_____. 1964. *Liberté: Négritude et humanisme*. Vol. 1. Paris: Seuil.

_____. 1966. "Négritude: A Humanism of the 20th Century." *Optima* 16(1): 1–8.

_____. 1977. *Liberté: Négritude et civilisation de l'universel*. Vol. 3. Paris: Seuil.

_____. 1979. "Henri Collomb (1913–1979) Ou L'art de Mourir Aux Préjugés." *Psychopathologie Africaine* 15(2): 137–39.

_____. 1980. *La Poésie de l'action: Conversations avec Mohamed Aziza*. Paris: Stock.

Sharp, Lesley A. 2000. "The Commodification of the Body and Its Parts." *Annual Review of Anthropology* 29(1): 287–328.

_____. 2002. *The Sacrificed Generation: Youth, History, and the Colonized Mind in Madagascar*. Berkeley: University of California Press.

Shaw, Christopher, and Malcolm Chase, eds. 1989. *The Imagined Past: History and Nostalgia*. Manchester, UK: Manchester University Press.

Shobe, Katharine Krause, and John F. Kihlstrom. 2002. "Interrogative Suggestibility and 'Memory Work.'" In *Memory and Suggestibility in the Forensic Interview*, edited by Mitchell L. Eisen, Jodi A. Quas, and Gail S. Goodman, 309–27. Mahwah, NJ: Lawrence Erlbaum Associates.

Simone, AbdouMaliq. 2004. *For the City Yet to Come: Changing African Life in Four Cities*. Durham, NC: Duke University Press.

———. 2010. *City Life from Jakarta to Dakar: Movements at the Crossroads*. New York: Routledge.

Soyinka, Wole. 1976. *Myth, Literature, and the African World*. Cambridge: Cambridge University Press.

Spinoza, Benedictus de. 1996. *Ethics*. Translated by Edwin M. Curley. Penguin Books.

Spleth, Janice. 1985. *Léopold Sédar Senghor*. Boston: Twayne.

Stacey, Clare L. 2011. *The Caring Self: The Work Experiences of Home Care Aides*. Ithaca, NY: Cornell University Press.

Stewart, Kathleen. 1988. "Nostalgia—A Polemic." *Cultural Anthropology* 3(3): 227–41.

———. 1996. *A Space on the Side of the Road: Cultural Poetics in an "Other" America*. Princeton, NJ: Princeton University Press.

Stewart, Susan. 1984. *On Longing: Narratives of the Miniature, the Gigantic, the Souvenir, the Collection*. Baltimore: John Hopkins University Press.

Stoler, Ann Laura, and Karen Strassler. 2000. "Castings for the Colonial: Memory Work in 'New Order' Java." *Comparative Studies in Society and History* 42(1): 4–48.

Storper-Perez, Danielle. 1974. *La Folie Colonisée*. Paris: François Maspero.

Strathern, Marilyn. 1995. "Nostalgia and the New Genetics." In *Rhetorics of Self-Making*, edited by Debbora Battaglia, 97–120. Berkeley: University of California Press.

Streit, Ursula. 1997. "Nathan's Ethnopsychoanalytic Therapy: Characteristics, Discoveries and Challenges to Western Psychotherapy." *Transcultural Psychiatry* 34(3): 321–43.

Swartz, Sally. 1995a. "The Black Insane in the Cape, 1891–1920." *Journal of Southern African Studies* 21(3): 399–415.

———. 1995b. "Changing Diagnoses in Valkenberg Asylum, Cape Colony, 1891–1920: A Longitudinal View." *History of Psychiatry* 6(24): 431–51.

Swift, Charles R., and Tolani Asuni. 1975. *Mental Health and Disease in Africa: With Special Reference to Africa South of the Sahara*. Edinburgh: Churchill Livingstone.

Sylla, Aïda, Aby Seydi, Florence Senghor, and Momar Guèye. 2002. "Les Activités Artistiques et Occupationnelles à Visée Thérapeutique au Service de Psychiatrie du CHU de Fann." *Revue Française de Psychiatrie et de Psychologie Médicale* 6(52): 23–26.

Szasz, Thomas S. 1974. *The Myth of Mental Illness: Foundations of a Theory of Personal Conduct*. Revised. New York: Harper & Row.

Tamba, Moustapha. 2009. "La Recherche À La Faculté Des Lettres et Sciences Humaines de l'Université Cheikh Anta Diop de Dakar: Bilan de 50 Ans D'activités." *Journal of Higher Education in Africa / Revue de L'Enseignement Supérieur en Afrique* 7(3): 105–23.

Taussig, Michael. 1993. *Mimesis and Alterity: A Particular History of the Senses*. New York: Routledge.

Taylor, Charles. 1994. "The Politics of Recognition." In *Multiculturalism: Examining the Politics of Recognition*, edited by Amy Guttman, 25–73. Princeton, NJ: Princeton University Press.

Taylor, Diana. 2003. *The Archive and the Repertoire: Performing Cultural Memory in the Americas*. Durham, NC: Duke University Press.

Tedlock, Dennis, and Bruce Mannheim, eds. 1995. *The Dialogic Emergence of Culture*. Urbana: University of Illinois Press.

Thelen, David. 1989. "Memory and American History." *Journal of American History* 75(4): 1117–29.

Tooth, Geoffrey C. 1950. *Studies in Mental Illness in the Gold Coast*. London: His Majesty's Stationery Office.

Tripet, Lise. 1968. "Quelques Exemples d'Expression Picturale chez les Malades Mentaux du Centre Hospitalier de Fann-Dakar." *Psychopathologie Africaine* 4(3): 419–49.

Trouillot, Michel-Rolph. 1995. *Silencing the Past: Power and the Production of History*. Boston: Beacon Press.

Turner, Bryan S. 1987. "A Note on Nostalgia." *Theory, Culture & Society* 4(1): 147–56.

Valdiya, Shailaja. 2010. "Neoliberal Reform and Biomedical Research in India: Globalization, Industrial Change, and Science." PhD diss., Science and Technology Studies Department, Rensselaer Polytechnic Institute.

Vaughan, Megan. 1983. "Idioms of Madness: Zomba Lunatic Asylum, Nyasaland, in the Colonial Period." *Journal of Southern African Studies* 9(2): 218–38.

———. 1991. *Curing Their Ills: Colonial Power and African Illness*. Stanford, CA: Stanford University Press.

Vaughan, Michalina. 1985. "Assimilation versus Association: Separate Recipes for Failure." *Modern and Contemporary France* 21: 3–8.

Wafer, Jim. 1991. *The Taste of Blood: Spirit Possession in Brazilian Candomblé*. Philadelphia: University of Pennsylvania Press.

Wendland, Claire. 2012. "Animating Biomedicine's Moral Order: The Crisis of Practice in Malawian Medical Training." *Current Anthropology* 53(6): 755–88.

Werbner, Richard P. 1991. *Tears of the Dead: The Social Biography of an African Family*. London: Edinburgh University Press for the International African Institute.

———. ed. 1998. *Memory and the Postcolony: African Anthropology and the Critique of Power*. London: Zed Books.

————— and Terence Ranger, eds. 1996. "Introduction: Multiple Identities, Plural Arenas." In *Postcolonial Identities in Africa*, 1–25. London: Zed Books.

White, Luise. 2000. *Speaking with Vampires: Rumor and History in Colonial Africa*. Berkeley: University of California Press.

Winter, Jay. 2006. *Remembering War: The Great War between Memory and History in the 20th Century*. New Haven, CT: Yale University Press.

Werbner, Richard P. and Emmanuel Sivan, eds. 1999. *War and Remembrance in the Twentieth Century*. Cambridge: Cambridge University Press.

World Health Organization. 1978a. "Alma-Ata Declaration."

Winter, Jay. 1978b. "The Promotion and Development of Traditional Medicine," 622. World Health Organization Technical Report Series. Geneva, Switzerland: World Health Organization.

Young, Allan. 2007. "America's Transient Mental Illness: A Brief History of the Self-Traumatized Perpetrator." In *Subjectivity: Ethnographic Investigations*, edited by João Biehl, Byron Good, and Arthur Kleinman, 155–78. Berkeley: University of California Press.

Young, James Edward. 1993. *The Texture of Memory: Holocaust Memorials and Meaning*. New Haven, CT: Yale University Press.

Young, Robert. 1995. *Colonial Desire: Hybridity in Theory, Culture, and Race*. London: Routledge.

Zahar, Renate. 1974. *Frantz Fanon: Colonialism and Alienation, Concerning Frantz Fanon's Political Theory*. Translated by Willfried F. Feuser. New York: Monthly Review Press.

Zeldine, Georges. 1981. "Un Témoignage Sur Fann." *L'Évolution Psychiatrique* 46(1): 131–53.

Zempléni, András. 1966. "La Dimension Thérapeutique du Culte des Rab, Ndöp, Tuuru, et Samp: Rites de Possession chez les Lebou et les Wolof." *Psychopathologie Africaine* 2(3): 295–439.

—————. 1967. "Sur L'Alliance entre la Personne et Le Rab dans le N'döp." *Psychopathologie Africaine* 3(3): 441–50.

—————. 1968. "L'interprétation et la thérapie traditionnelles du désordre mental chez les Wolof et les Lebou (Sénégal)." PhD diss., Université de Paris, Faculté des Lettres et des Sciences Humaines, Paris, France.

—————. 1977. "From Symptom to Sacrifice: The Story of Khady Fall." In *Case Studies in Spirit Possession*, edited by Vincent Crapanzano and Vivian Garrison, 87–140. New York: Wiley.

INDEX

accompagnant(s), 10, 85; accompagnant mercenaire (paid attendant), 192, 201–5, 217; accompagnant policy at Fann, 86–90, 170–71; at pénc meetings, 207, 208–9; sex of, 87; VIP rooms and, 193

Africa, 25, 139; African culture, 6–7; colonial, 40; postcolonial, 24, 81–82; "traditional," 29

"African mind," the, 42, 43, 55, 56, 76

L'Afrique Occidentale Française (AOF). See French West Africa

agency, 21

Aissatou (nurse at Fann), 104, 123; on Collomb and Moussa Diop, 135; on Collomb's vision for Fann, 117–18, 124; on early days of Fann, 72–73; on illness and death of Moussa Diop, 134; on invisible spirit forces protecting Fann, 141, 150

Algeria/Algerian War, 42, 106, 107, 147, 227n12

aliénés, les ("lunatics"), 29, 40, 46; colonial officials' uncertainty about dealing with, 41–42; forced transportation to France, 28, 41; French "lunacy law" (1838) and, 45, 226nn4–5; perceived as threat to others, 61; traditional therapists and, 42; "use" of, 58

Alma Ata Conference (Soviet Kazakhstan, 1978), 179–80, 235n16

Ambohidatrimo asylum (Madagascar), 55

l'Ambulance du Cap Manuel (Dakar). See Cap Manuel

ancestors, 33, 83

anciens, les (the elders, old-timers), 2, 27

Anjanamasina asylum (Madagascar), 57, 58

anthropology, 6, 7, 28, 122; anthropologists' critiques of Nathan, 177, 235n11; difficulty of engagements with nostalgia, 110–13, 231n1; ethnopsychiatry and, 76; studies on memory, 20–21, 224nn12–13

anti-psychiatry movement, 86

archive(s), 18–19, 25, 28–29, 39–66, 228n7; Archives Nationales du Sénégal (ANS), 46, 54, 62

Aro psychiatric hospital (Abeokuta, Nigeria), 82, 146, 148

art therapy, 13, 85, 90, 154; Atelier d'Expression, 193, 211–16, 218; exhibitions of patients' work, 214–15, 216

Ashforth, Adam, 136

l'Asile de St-Pierre (Marseille, France), 28, 41, 47, 48–54, 227n12

l'Association l'AMI (Accompagnement Psychologique et Médiation interculturelle), 172

Auguin, Rosalyne, 87, 89–90, 202, 204

Avicenne Hospital (Paris), 176, 178

Ayats, Henri, 81

Ba, Medhi, 195

Ba, Moussa, 42, 71–72, 233n9

Baker, George, 228n7

Barry, Boubacar, 120

Bartoli, Daniel, 73

Basaglia, Franco, 86, 229–30n14

"baseline mental health," 2
Bastide, Roger, 100, 228n6
Battaglia, Debbora, 231n1
Behold the Black Caiman (Bessire, 2014), 9
Benjamin, Walter, 35–36, 231n3
Benslama, Fethi, 235n14
Berne, Eric, 62–63
Bessire, Lucas, 9
Biehl, João, 225n21
Bien-Hoa asylum (French Indochina), 57, 58
bilejo (expeller of witches), 78
Bintou (nurse at Fann), 116, 118, 123, 124
biomedicine/biomedical psychiatry, 9, 80, 81, 148, 149, 166, 175, 202, 205
Bissell, William C., 113, 118, 231n1; on multiple strands of remembrance, 8, 104, 109, 122; on nostalgia and the object world, 120
Bluebeard (Vonnegut), 225n17
Boas, Franz, 111
border zones, 8, 139, 141
Borreil, Paul, 49–50, 51
bouffées délirantes (temporary delusional states), 27, 80, 94, 95
Boym, Svetlana, 111, 112–13, 122
bricolage, 10, 22, 158, 184
British African colonies, asylums in, 47, 61, 227nn10–11, 227n11
Buggenhagen, Beth Anne, 233n2
Bulhan, Hussein Abdilahi, 106
Bullard, Alice, 84, 97
Burkina Faso, 161, 169, 178

Cafard Libéré, Le (satirical newspaper), 157, 234n5
Cape Colony, British colonial asylums in, 47, 227n10
Cap Manuel (*l'Ambulance du Cap Manuel*), 39–41, 71, 107; as annex of *l'Hôpital Le Dantec,* 60; as carceral horror, 72; closure of, 62; colonial violence and, 60–64
care/caretaking, 87, 95; carceral model of, 61; changes in practices of, 31; commodified, 192, 202, 217, 236n9; family, 86; Foucauldian transition from incarceration to, 43; humane model of, 65;

violence disguised as, 220; welfare colonialism and, 41
Carothers, J. C., 56, 61–62, 76
Cazanove, Frank, 56–58, 61
Centre de Prise en Charge Intégrée de l'Addiction de Dakar (CEPIAD), 199, 200
Centre Expérimental de Médecine Traditionnelle (CEMETRA), 9, 223n4
Centre Georges Devereux (CDG), 175, 176, 177
Centre Hospitalier National Universitaire (CHNU) de Fann, 3, 4, 81, 151, 159, 181, 203
Césaire, Aimé, 25, 98–99; "Cahier d'un retour au pays natal" (1939), 98, 230n18
Cheikh Anta Diop University. *See l'Université Cheikh Anta Diop*
Cheneveau, Roger, 54–56, 59, 61, 63, 227n8
Cherki, Alice, 106
Chow, Rey, 225n20
Civil Code, French, 43, 45
civilization, 56–57, 65
"Civilization of the Universal" (Senghor's vision), 29, 101, 103, 104; cultural exchange and, 143; Negritude philosophy and, 30, 126; replaced by neoliberal vision of consumption, 201; Senegalese modernity and, 131
Clifford, James, 100
Clinique des Mamelles (Dakar), 164, 194
Collignon, René, xi, 60, 75
Collomb, Henri, 2, 5–6, 12, 13, 127; *accompagnant* policy and, 86, 90, 202; Babakar-led group in opposition to, 145–49; career as military doctor in colonies, 71, 228n2; collaboration with local healers, 124, 125, 141, 168, 181; cultural psychiatry promoted by, 130–31; death of (1979), 29, 70; Demba's first meeting with, 13–16; departure from Fann, 123, 132–33, 220; as director of Fann post-independence, 131, 144–45; *l'Ecole de Fann* and, 70–74, 80, 81; Fanon contrasted with, 31, 146–47; as father figure, 147–48; ghost of, 28, 33, 34–35, 37, 38; "Histoire de la Psychiatrie en

Dijk, Rijk van, 110, 231n1

Diop, Alioune, 230n19

Diop, Babakar, 87, 88, 90, 151, 152; death of, 149–50; as first Senegalese director of Fann, 130, 149; opposition to Collomb's extended presence at Fann, 145, 148; on potential dangers of psychiatry in Senegal, 138–39, 140

Diop, Habib, 157

Diop, Moussa: expectation of succeeding Collomb as Fann director, 131, 133, 134, 220; medical studies of, 134, 232n1; *professeur agrégé* title of, 133, 134; relationship with Collomb, 133, 134–35

Diop, Moussa, death of (1967), 30, 138, 141, 144, 220, 232n2; Collomb's project thrown into doubt by, 142, 151; as end of an era at Fann, 132–35, 145, 151; obituary written by Collomb, 134; parallels with Babakar Diop's death, 150; witchcraft blamed for, 131, 136–37, 232n2

Diouf, Abdou, 10, 144, 151

Diouf, Mamadou, 65

djinné (jinn), 15, 34, 69, 77, 226n1; as cause of mental disturbances, 140; relation to *rab,* 79

doctors, 16, 174; *accompagnant* policies and, 88, 89, 171, 203; at *l'Asile de St-Pierre,* 51; demoralization of, 10, 164; departure from Senegal, 164–65; at *pénc* meetings, 207; personnel shortages and, 159, 163–64. *See also* psychiatrists, Senegalese/African

dof (crazy person), 2, 153

dogmatism of equivalence (*le dogmatisme égalitaire*), 96

Dorès, Maurice, 87, 88, 90

Durkheim, Émile, 111

Ebong, Ima, 101, 142

l'Ecole de Dakar (The Dakar School), 70, 84, 102–4, 142–43

l'Ecole de Fann (Fann School), 6, 7, 12, 70–74, 133, 170; Collomb's legacy and, 94; emphasis on culture, 149; local exegeses of mental disturbance and, 80; multidisciplinary team at origin of, 75; psychodynamic approach and, 82;

Senegalese psychiatrists distanced from, 145, 147; studies of spirit beings at, 141

l'Ecole Nationale des Beaux Arts (Dakar), 102, 103

electroshock therapy, 93, 94, 95

El Hadj (Collomb's principal translator), 114–15, 116, 117; on changes in *pénc* sessions, 206; on Collomb's departure from Senegal, 132–33; on death of Moussa Diop, 133

ENDA Santé tiers-monde (Dakar), 9

entanglement, 24–25, 225n20

epilepsy, 72

l'Espoir (Malraux), 68, 221, 227–28n1

ethnography, 75, 100; history and, 8–17; limits of fieldwork and writing, 31, 185

ethnopsychiatry, 76, 77, 174–78, 235n14

Fabian, Johannes, 21

fajkat (healer), 77, 168, 169, 229n9

families/family members, 26, 82, 95, 126, 154, 161–62; *accompagnants* and, 10, 85, 87–90, 192, 202, 204, 205; caretaking and, 87; ethnopsychiatry and, 176, 177; family secrets, 15; Fann community as family, 115; of immigrants in France, 175; institutionalization at request of, 45, 168; *Joola* ferry disaster and, 186, 187; patients rejected by, 96; *pénc* meetings and, 85, 86, 208, 210; rehabilitated patients and, 41; spirit beings and, 33, 78, 79; supernatural powers and, 153; traditional healers and, 167, 169, 183; treatment strategies and, 163; VIP rooms and, 193, 199. *See also* kinship

Fann Psychiatric Clinic, 1, 2, 3–9, 24, 107; *accompagnant* policy, 86–90, 170–71; Atelier d'Ex-pression, 193, 211–16, 218; break from violent colonial past, 65–66; *Cap Manuel* patients transferred to, 39, 40, 64, 65; entrance, 4, 6; establishment of, 62; *L'Étage Droit,* 5; genealogy of, 28; hardships under neoliberalism, 159–65; history of, 16, 20; humane model of care at, 65; Moussa Diop's death as end of an era, 132–35; new therapeutic community at, 84–85; nostalgia for early days of, 109; as product of late colonial regime,

96; *Rez-de-Chaussée Gauche,* 5, 212; "Senegalization" (*sénégalisation*) of, 7, 130–31, 138, 143, 149, 151; Senghor's vision and, 103, 125; spirit of Goorgoorlou at, 159–60, 166; "strategic ambivalence" toward early years of, 165–66, 171–74, 184; VIP rooms, 191–94, 199, 200; wealth and status distinctions within, 11. See also *Pavillon des Dames*

Fann Psychiatric Clinic, "golden age" of, 109, 110, 113, 117, 119; death of Moussa Diop and, 131; modernity as object of nostalgia, 120, 121, 122; nostalgia as view of the present, 123; refusal of "golden age" notion, 165

Fanon, Frantz, 25, 29; Collomb contrasted with, 31, 97, 146–47; letter to Senghor, 106–7, 219; *The Wretched of the Earth* (*Les damnés de la Terre*), 62, 146

Fassin, Didier, 177

Faye, Demba Boudy, 184

Ferguson, James, 110, 121–22, 200, 235n13, 236n8

Fichte, Hubert, 94–95

FIDES (*Fonds d'Investissements pour le Developpement Économique et Social des territoires d'outre-mer*), 62, 64

First Pan-African Conference on Mental Health (Dakar, 2002). *See Premier Congrès Panafricain de Santé Mentale*

Foley, Ellen, 233n2

Fons, T. T. (Alphonse Mendy), 157

forgetting, 24, 165, 221

Foucault, Michel, 40, 50, 65, 230n14

Four Communes (*Quatres Communes*), 43–46, 48, 231n4

France (the Metropole), 28, 35, 42, 62, 91, 139, 172; *aliénés* forcibly transported to, 28, 41, 50; emigration of Senegalese doctors to, 165; independent Senegal and, 107, 126, 143, 144; psychiatric hospitals of, 55, 106; reception of Nathan's ethnopsychiatry in, 176–77

French Indochina, 57, 71, 227n12, 228n2

French language, 1, 2, 27; announcements for Pan-African conference in, 182; black African intellectuals and, 99, 100

French West Africa (L'Afrique Occidentale Française [AOF]), 46, 53, 61; federal asylum plan for, 53–56, 59, 60; reform of psychiatry in, 54; territories of, 226n1(chap. 1); under Vichy control in World War II, 67–68

Freud, Sigmund, 22, 23, 224n16, 235n14; concept of the ego, 74; on melancholia, 112; Oedipus complex and, 82

Frobenius, Leo, 228n5

Gbikpi, Paul, 87, 89–90, 202, 204

ghosts, 8, 16, 17, 112, 184, 219, 220; of Collomb, 28, 33, 34–35, 37, 38; concern for justice and, 37; *Jetztzeit* ("now-time") and, 36; justice and, 36–37; as mediators between past and present, 36; return of, 28, 36. *See also* haunting

Giordano, Cristiana, 176

globalization, 111

Gold Coast (Ghana), 47, 61

Goldstein, Jan E., 45

Goorgoorlou (comic strip character), 157–60, 166, 184, 234n4

Gordon, Avery, 28, 35, 36, 37

Gorée Island, 43, 67–68

Great War (World War I), 28, 41, 54; culture in aftermath of, 100; Senegalese soldiers returned from, 54; transfer of patients to French Metropole suspended, 53

Griaule, Marcel, 100

group ego (*le moi de groupe*), 74, 82

Guèye, Eric, 195

Guèye, Momar, 84, 166, 169–70

Guyer, Jane, 224n12

Halbwachs, Maurice, 224n8

hallucinations, 80, 84

haunting, 7, 28, 32, 35, 37, 185, 221; entanglement and, 24; historical nature of, 28; *Jetztzeit* ("now-time") and, 36. *See also* ghosts

"hauntology," 35

"Health for All in the 21st Century" slogan, 179–80

historicism, 17

historicity, 16, 223–24n7

history, 35, 102; forgetting of, 165; hypertrophy of, 20; memory, 17–20, 224nn8–9; nostalgia and, 112
Hodder, Ian, 225n20
Höller, Christian, 25
hope, nostalgia in relation to, 119–20, 122
l'Hôpital Aristide Le Dantec (Dakar), 3
l'Hôpital Principal (Dakar), 3
l'Hôpital Bicêtre (Paris), 40
l'Hôpital Civil de St-Louis, 46–47, 54; construction of (1853), 28, 41; patients transferred to French Metropole, 48, 52
l'Hôpital Colonial de Dakar, 46
l'Hôpital de Gorée, 46
l'Hôpital Le Dantec (formerly *l'Hôpital des Indigenes*), 3, 54, 60
l'Hôpital Militaire de St-Louis, 46
l'Hôpital Principal (Dakar), 54
"horizon of expectation," 120, 121
Huyssen, Andreas, 20

identity, 21, 139, 225n20; nostalgia and, 113, 121; Senegalese national, 98; social and ethnic, 65; writing and, 132
IGSSM (*Inspection Général des Services Sanitaires et Médicaux*), 59
imagination, 8, 16, 17, 19–20, 102
IMF (International Monetary Fund), 151, 156, 233n3
l'indigénat laws, 44, 226n3
informal economy, 12, 159, 201
infrastructure, 8, 45, 53–54, 190; inadequate and deteriorated, 10, 159; inequality and, 197–98; "infrastructural violence," 236n8; new forms of dispossession and, 192; as priority of Wade government, 11, 194; strategic ambivalence and, 184
inheritance, impossible, 32, 219–20; brutality of early colonial treatment as, 29, 41, 220; disavowed colonial legacy as, 66
ink (*encre*), flow of, 132, 151
l'Institut de Recherche et d'Enseignement de Psychopathologie (IREP), 172
l'Institut national de la santé et de la recherche médicale (INSERM), 9
Islam, 7, 72, 74, 229n9; Eid al-Adha ["Festival of Sacrifice"] (Tabaski, Korité), 116, 156, 208; role in West African tradition

and culture, 101; Sufi brotherhoods, 223n2
Isseu, Dr., 164, 169, 170, 171
Ivy, Marilyn, 231n1

jabarkat (healer working outside Islam), 229n9
Jackson, Lynette, 61
jaraaf (Wolof: "village leader/chief"), 208, 209, 210
Jetztzeit ("now-time"), 36, 231n3
Joola ethnic group and language, 51, 52
Joola ferry disaster (2002), 31, 186–90
justice: ghosts and, 36–37; injustice, 26, 35, 39, 143, 181; remembrance and, 23, 220; restorative nostalgia and, 111

Ka, Abdou Anta, 91, 230n17
Keller, Richard, 42
Ker Xaleyi ("Children's House"), 3
kinship, 87, 193, 219. *See also* families/ family members
Kleinman, Arthur, 163, 207
Komaromy, Zsolt, 224n10
Koselleck, Reinhart, 120

Lacan, Jacques, 83, 148
Lacanian theory, 82–83, 86
Lambek, Michael, 21
Lambo, T. Adeoye, 82, 146, 148, 173, 174, 233n11
Lebovici, Serge, 175
Lebu ethnic group, 6, 223n1, 65; healers of Senegambia region, 140; interpretations of mental illness, 76
Le Guérinel, Norbert, 75
Leiris, Michel, 100
Lévi-Strauss, Claude, 111
liggeey [French: *maraboutage*] (sorcery, spell-casting), 77, 140, 229n9
Lô, Moustapha, 144
Ly, Baaba, 232n4

Madagascar, 55, 57
madness, 6, 8; Foucauldian transition to mental illness, 29; from inability to assimilate to colonial modernity, 62; managed under colonial regime, 41, 42,

memory and, 23–24; roles of doctor and healer distinguished by, 142; transgression of boundaries and, 139–40, 141. See also doctors

psychiatry: demedicalization of, 74, 81, 93, 95; demystification of, 88; *l'Ecole de Dakar* and, 102; Enlightenment ideals and, 232n8; illusions of, 93–96; postcolonial transformation and, 7; psychiatric nosology, 80, 81; transcultural, 7, 29, 30, 82, 114, 117, 178; "universal" language of, 178; Western, 8, 97, 124, 140, 147, 167

psychiatry, colonial, 6, 28, 40, 41, 96; discourse of difference and, 145; Foucauldian transition in, 29; racism/racial theories and, 42, 76; reform of, 54–60, 64; violence and, 60–64

psychoanalysis, 22, 23, 74, 75; cross-cultural, 84; cultural difference overlooked by, 177; ethnopsychiatry and, 176; Fann's turn away from, 148; Lacanian, 86; reformulated theory of, 82

psychodynamic methods, 74, 81–84, 88, 160; downplaying or weakening of, 13, 82, 130, 148, 193, 202, 204, 205; transcultural, 6

Psychopathologie africaine (journal), 70, 150, 228n1

psychosis, 81, 229n12

psychotherapy, 145, 183, 204–5, 206. See also *pénc*

Pulaar ethnic group, 223n1, 194

PWIDs (Persons Who Inject Drugs), 199, 200

Qur'an, 79, 183, 229n9

rab (wild spirits), 15, 34, 77, 84, 226n1; as cause of mental disturbances, 140; Collomb and Fann protected by, 141, 150; relation to *djinné*, 79; relation to *tuur*, 78, 229n10

Rabain, Jacqueline, 75

racism, 62, 76, 99, 146

Rainaut, Jean, 39–40, 64, 71, 97, 107

Reboul, Henri, 53, 55, 56, 60

Régis, Emmanuel, 53, 55, 56, 60

"Remembering, Repeating, and Working-Through" (Freud), 22, 224n16

repertoire, 18–19, 84, 90, 94, 206, 212

Repetti, Massimo, 158

responsibilization, 193, 206, 211

revenants, 35, 218, 221

Ricoeur, Paul, 1, 18, 19–20, 225n18

Robbins, Joyce, 17

Rodgers, Dennis, 198, 236n8

Royal Order (*Ordonnance organique*), 46, 48

Rufisque, city of, 27, 43, 68

Sall, Khalifa, 11

Sall, Macky, 11, 192

salvage paradigm, 76, 228n7

Santayana, George, 225n17

Saris, Jamie A., 209

Sarr, Doudou, 42, 71–72, 233n9

Sartre, Jean-Paul, 19–20, 99

schizophrenia, 80, 81, 229n12

Seck, Amadou Makhtar, 42, 71–72, 233n9

Seck, Daouda, 181

secret societies, 78

Sembene, Ousmane, 77

Sène, Seune, 157

Senegal, 45, 229n12; Casamance region, 51, 52, 72; dominance of Islam/Muslim majority, 223n2, 74; elections, 10–11, 223n5; ethnic groups in, 6, 223n1; in Federation of Mali, 230n19; government corruption in, 10; independence (1960), 5, 25, 29, 41, 105, 145; *Joola* tragedy compared to the *Titanic* and 9/11 attack, 188; Ministry of Culture, 98; neoliberal turn, 119, 156, 192–93, 202, 216; secular governance in, 101, 230n21; sense of "decline" in, 122

"Senegalization" (*sénégalisation*), 7, 130–31, 138, 143, 149, 151

Senegambian region, 77, 140

Senghor, Léopold Sédar, 7, 29, 230nn19–20; assassination attempt on, 144; Collomb and, 103, 104, 117; departure from office (1980), 119, 123, 144; *l'Ecole de Dakar* and, 98–104; Fanon's unanswered letter to, 106–7, 219; *La poésie de l'action* (1980), 102; on positive side of colonialism, 143;

Milton Keynes UK
Ingram Content Group UK Ltd.
UKHW040153270124
436770UK00004B/406

9 780520 300200